KW-252-274

Management Options in Breast Cancer

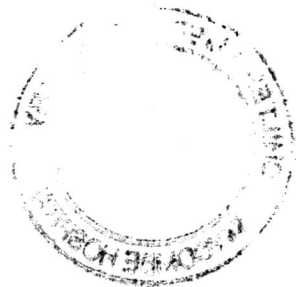

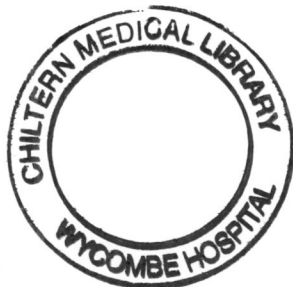

CHILTERN MEDICAL LIBRARY
WYCOMBE HOSPITAL

Management Options in Breast Cancer

Case Histories, Best Practice, and Clinical Decision-Making

John Benson
Cambridge University Hospitals NHS Foundation Trust
Addenbrooke's Hospital
Cambridge, UK

Ismail Jatoi
Uniformed Services University of the Health Sciences
Bethesda, Maryland, USA

informa
healthcare

New York   London

Informa Healthcare USA, Inc.
52 Vanderbilt Avenue
New York, NY 10017

© 2009 by Informa Healthcare USA, Inc.
Informa Healthcare is an Informa business

No claim to original U.S. Government works
Printed and bound in India by Replika Press Pvt. Ltd. on acid-free paper
10 9 8 7 6 5 4 3 2 1

International Standard Book Number-10: 0-415-42310-4 (hardcover : alk. paper)
International Standard Book Number-13: 978-0-415-42310-6 (hardcover : alk. paper)

This book contains information obtained from authentic and highly regarded sources. Reprinted material is quoted with permission, and sources are indicated. A wide variety of references are listed. Reasonable efforts have been made to publish reliable data and information, but the author and the publisher cannot assume responsibility for the validity of all materials or for the consequence of their use.

No part of this book may be reprinted, reproduced, transmitted, or utilized in any form by any electronic, mechanical, or other means, now known or hereafter invented, including photocopying, microfilming, and recording, or in any information storage or retrieval system, without written permission from the publishers.

For permission to photocopy or use material electronically from this work, please access www.copyright.com (http://www.copyright.com/) or contact the Copyright Clearance Center, Inc. (CCC) 222 Rosewood Drive, Danvers, MA 01923, 978-750-8400. CCC is a not-for-profit organization that provides licenses and registration for a variety of users. For organizations that have been granted a photocopy license by the CCC, a separate system of payment has been arranged.

Trademark Notice: Product or corporate names may be trademarks or registered trademarks, and are used only for identification and explanation without intent to infringe.

Library of Congress Cataloging-in-Publication Data

Management options in breast cancer : case histories, best practice, and clinical decision-making / edited by John R. Benson, Ismail Jatoi.
        p. ; cm.
   Includes bibliographical references and index.
   ISBN-13: 978-0-415-42310-6 (hardcover : alk. paper)
   ISBN-10: 0-415-42310-4 (hardcover : alk. paper)
   1. Breast–Cancer. I. Benson, John R., 1959- II. Jatoi, Ismail, 1955-
   [DNLM: 1. Breast Neoplasms–therapy. 2. Patient Care Team. WP 870 M267 2009]
     RC280.B8M352 2009
     616.99'449—dc22
                                                                    2008045962

For Corporate Sales and Reprint Permissions call 212-520-2700 or write to: Sales Department, 52 Vanderbilt Avenue, 16th floor, New York, NY 10017.

Visit the Informa Web site at
www.informa.com

and the Informa Healthcare Web site at
www.informahealthcare.com

This book is dedicated to our friend, colleague and mentor, Uccio

Preface

The incidence of breast cancer continues to increase, and the heterogeneous nature of this disease presents unique management challenges. Treatments are increasingly being tailored to meet the needs of individual patients, although cost issues may influence the decision-making process in some circumstances. Notwithstanding these comments, there are standards of best practice, which are accepted by breast cancer experts in communities around the world, and much consensus now exists in several key areas. This is evident at international meetings, where leading opinion formers share the same principles and philosophies. It is now recognized that diagnostic accuracy, management, and survival rates for breast cancer are superior when practiced within specialized breast teams. Multidisciplinary team (MDT) meetings have helped ensure that as many patients as possible receive optimum standards of care, which can be audited prospectively. These MDT meetings are underpinned by shared protocols and guidelines, though some flexibility and clinical discretion is permissible. There are situations where there is no "right treatment" based on published evidence, and a degree of clinical judgment and personal experience (and even bias) will prevail.

This book exemplifies how guidelines should be followed and the role of clinical judgment in determining management plans for breast cancer patients within the context of the MDT. It is based on a selection of actual clinical cases that have passed through the MDT or "tumor board" meetings. These represent a spectrum of clinical scenarios frequently encountered in routine practice, together with some more unusual and atypical cases. These cases have been grouped under headings with a dominant theme, and each one will be presented in a standard format with (1) clinical history, (2) examination, (3) investigations (mammogram, ultrasound, core biopsy, fine needle aspiration cytology, and tests as appropriate, such as MRI, bone scan, CT scan chest/abdomen/pelvis), (4) treatment, and (5) discussion. Illustrative material includes schematic diagrams, breast imaging results, pathological slides, and clinical photographs (pre-/postoperative). Each case will be followed by a list of summary points, which is intended as a learning tool. Most cases involve multimodality therapies, and cross-referencing has been included to allow the reader *to* compare and contrast similar aspects of treatment between different cases.

This book is aimed for surgeons and oncologists trained in breast disease together with established specialists and clinical nurse practitioners. In addition, physicians in various other disciplines such as radiology and gynecology may find the book a useful guide that highlights problematic and controversial areas within this field.

John R. Benson
Ismail Jatoi

Acknowledgments

The authors are grateful to several individuals for their assistance in the preparation of this manuscript which contains many images and illustrations. Dr Catherine Hubbard and Mr Mohammed Absar helped collate the radiological images whilst Dr Elena Provenzano, Dr Brian Rous and Mr James Neale provided relevant pathological slides for each case. Particular thanks are owed to Catherine Lamoon and Mark Moughton in the departments of medical photography at Addenbrooke's and Hinchingbrooke Hospitals respectively, for producing high quality photographs in sensitive clinical circumstances. Mrs Yvonne Glendenning meticulously uploaded all images onto the publisher's website which greatly facilitated preparation of this book. Finally, we are indebted to all the patients who have kindly agreed to inclusion of their clinical details and images in this book.

Contents

Early Symptomatic Breast Cancer

Part I: Mastectomy

CASE STUDY 1

History

A 65-year-old woman presented with a four-week history of a lump in the superior aspect of the right breast that was slightly tender to palpation but not associated with any nipple discharge. The patient had no previous breast problems and had undergone regular screening mammography until the age of 64 years (never recalled). Several family members had been affected with breast cancer including the patient's sister who developed the disease at the age of 47 years. In addition, both maternal and paternal grandmothers had developed pre- and postmenopausal breast cancer, respectively together with a maternal aunt (postmenopausal disease). The patient had two children both of whom were breast-fed (age at birth of eldest child 22 years). She previously had a hysterectomy with ovarian preservation and had used hormone replacement therapy for a duration of two years in total.

Clinical Findings

On clinical examination, there was an ill-defined irregular mass lying superior to the right nipple-areolar complex measuring 2.5 cm in maximum diameter. This was associated with subtle indrawing of the skin and was suspicious for malignancy (E4). There was no axillary lymphadenopathy (Fig. 1).

Clinical Assessment

The clinical findings were suggestive of a right-sided breast cancer, and the index of suspicion was heightened by a moderately strong family history of breast cancer. This patient was informed of the likely diagnosis and the possible need for mastectomy prior to imaging and biopsy.

Investigations

Mammography

An extra density with an irregular outline was visible in the superior/central aspect of the right breast, which was not present on the previous screening mammogram carried out 12 months previously (R5) (Fig. 2A, B).

Breast Ultrasound

The opacity seen on mammography corresponded to a 1.8-cm hypoechoic mass lesion that appeared lobulated and well defined (U5) (Fig. 2C).

Core Biopsy

Image-guided core biopsy (14-gauge needle) of the right breast mass confirmed an

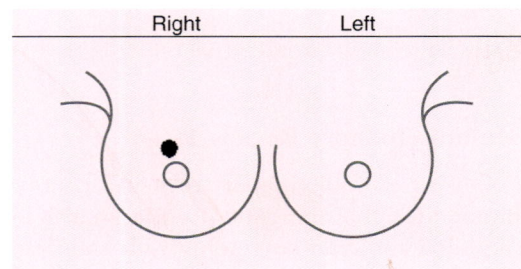

Figure 1

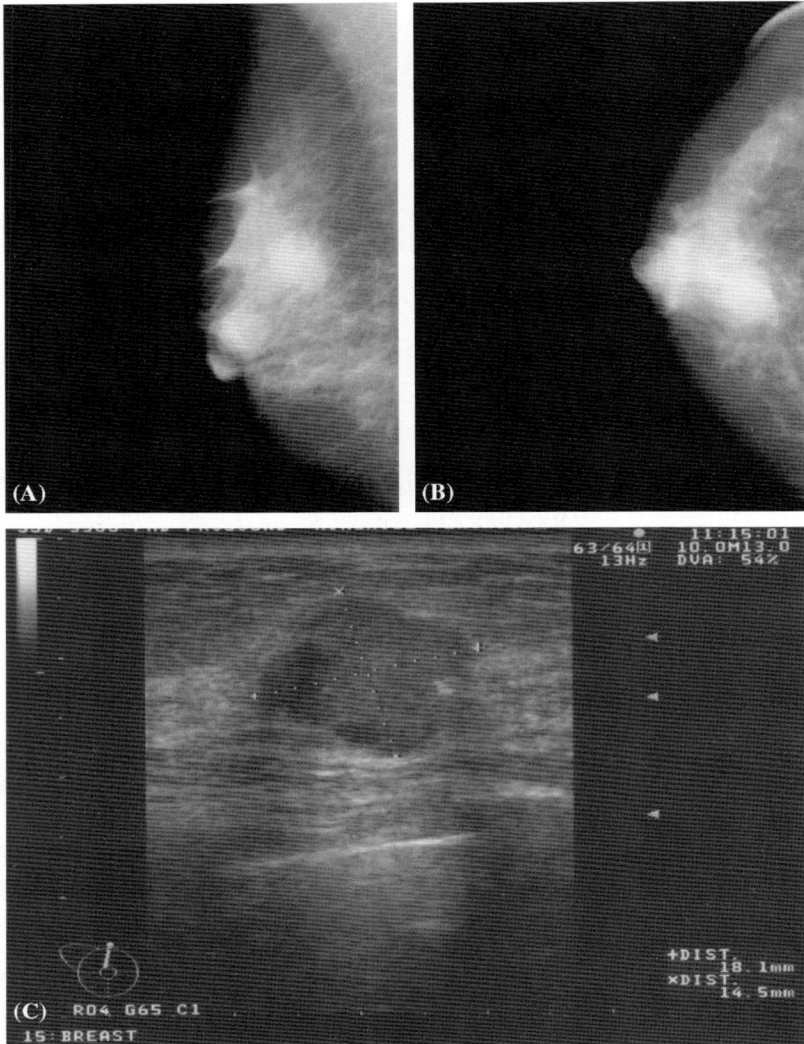

Figure 2

invasive carcinoma (grade II, ER positive) without any in situ component [Fig. 3A (low power), B (high power)].

Diagnosis

Early-stage right breast cancer (T2[a]N0)

Multidisciplinary Review 1

Following multidisciplinary review it was recommended that the patient undergo a right modified radical mastectomy with standard level II axillary lymph node dissection (sentinel node biopsy not routinely offered at the time). The tumor lay close to the nipple and was not amenable to breast-conservation surgery, despite its relatively small size on ultrasound (<2 cm). The tumor appeared larger clinically than the sonographic estimate.

Treatment and Progress

The patient initially expressed some interest in immediate breast reconstruction, and a consultation was arranged with the plastic

---

[a] Clinical assessment T2 but ultrasound measurement <2 cm (T1)

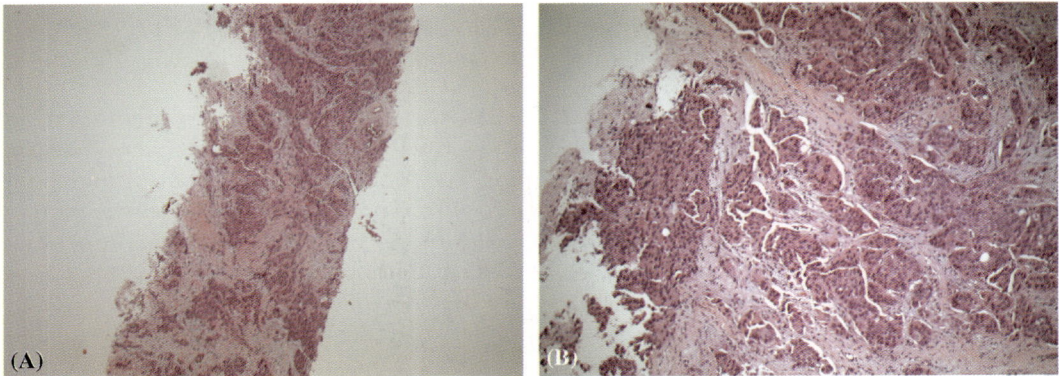

Figure 3

surgeons. However, upon further discussion of reconstructive techniques the patient opted for a right mastectomy only. She made an excellent postoperative recovery without seroma formation, and the mastectomy flaps were healthy. There was a good range of motion of the right shoulder and no "postmastectomy" pain in the region of the axilla and upper inner arm, which is the territory of the intercostobrachial nerve (sacrificed at operation).

Definitive Histology

This showed an invasive ductal carcinoma measuring 20 mm in maximum diameter and was well clear of all radial margins (>40 mm) [Fig. 4A (magnification 20×)].

There was associated ductal carcinoma in situ and lymphovascular invasion [Fig. 4B (low power), C (high power)]. However, none of the 17 nodes retrieved contained metastatic tumor.

Multidisciplinary Review 2

It was recommended that the patient commence the oral aromatase inhibitor Arimidex as adjuvant systemic therapy for a five-year period.

Treatment and Progress

Arimidex was poorly tolerated with troublesome side effects and after three months of treatment was changed to the antiestrogen

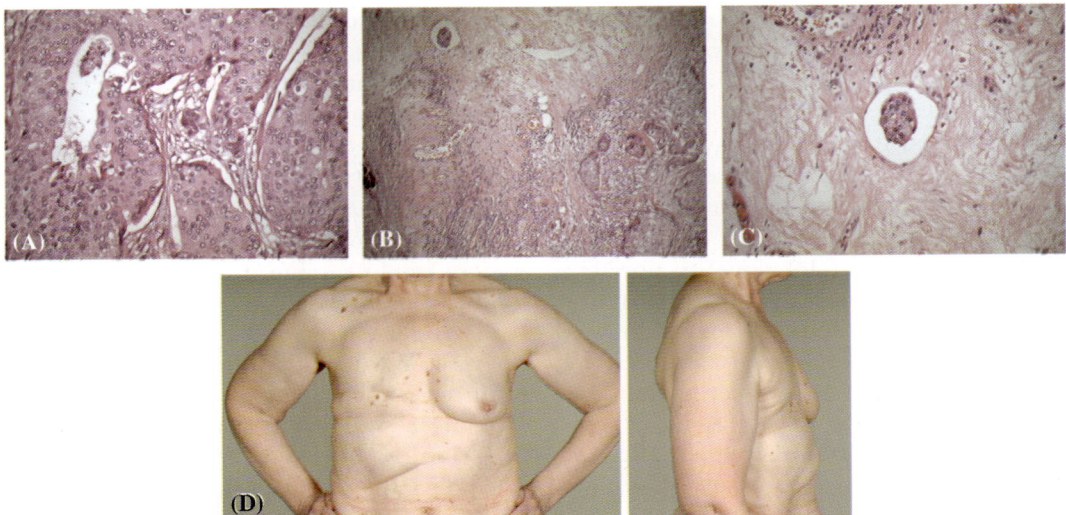

Figure 4

tamoxifen (previously standard adjuvant hormonal treatment for postmenopausal hormone receptor–positive women). Following treatment with tamoxifen for one month, the patient developed bilateral calf pains and pleuritic chest pain. Despite investigations excluding either deep vein thrombosis or pulmonary embolus, tamoxifen was discontinued and another oral aromatase inhibitor commenced (letrozole 2.5 mg daily). Unfortunately, the patient reported persistent aching pains in the wrist and elbows, which were attributed to letrozole. In view of these sequential side effects on different hormonal agents, it was decided (after discussion with the patient) to withhold any further endocrine therapy. Her risk of relapse was low and the estimated survival benefit from an aromatase inhibitor was 2% to 3% at 10 years. The patient remains well and disease-free at three years following surgery and does not desire any form of delayed breast reconstruction (Fig. 4D).

Discussion

This 65-year-old patient presented with a symptomatic cancer of the right breast having undergone a routine screening mammogram 12 months earlier. Review of these screening films revealed no mammographic evidence of any suspicious lesion at that time. Within the context of a screening program, cancers appearing symptomatically in the interval between routine screens can be visualized retrospectively in up to 20% of cases. Interestingly, the upper age limit for the NHS Breast Screening Programme has been increased from 64 to 70 years of age. Randomized controlled trials of breast cancer screening have now confirmed the efficacy of screening in women aged 50 to 70 years for whom reductions in mortality between 25% and 30% are attainable (1–4). When the screening program was implemented in the United Kingdom in the late 1980s, it was considered that the age group 50 to 64 years was most cost-effective, with poor levels of compliance among older women (≥65 years). It is now acknowledged that women within this age group are very keen to continue with screening, and public demand has prompted an expansion of the screening age group within the NHS program.

Breast cancer diagnosis is predicated on the principle of "triple assessment," involving a combination of clinical examination, imaging, and some form of tissue biopsy (core biopsy or fine-needle aspiration). The clinical findings in this case were suspicious for but not diagnostic of malignancy (E4). However, the mass had the typical appearance of a cancer radiologically (R5, U5) and core biopsy confirmed the diagnosis.

Primary surgical therapy is the standard treatment for a 2 cm grade II clinically node-negative breast cancer in a 65-year-old woman. The tumor lay in the central portion of the breast, less than 2 cm from the nipple-areolar complex. Its proximity to the nipple precluded satisfactory breast-conservation surgery. Though it might have been possible to obtain satisfactory margin clearance (2–3 mm microscopic resection margins) by wide local excision, this would have yielded a poor cosmetic result with a "squinting" nipple. Patients with very large pendulous breasts may be suitable for a central segmental resection in which the tumor together with the nipple-areolar complex is incorporated into a horizontally placed wide local excision. Despite loss of the nipple, much of the breast volume is retained and an otherwise good cosmetic outcome is achieved.

At the time this patient underwent surgery, formal axillary lymph node dissection was the standard method for management of the axilla. Patients with a clinically node-negative tumor measuring ≤3 cm would now be offered sentinel lymph node biopsy as an axillary staging procedure. This particular patient had only a 25% to 30% chance of nodal involvement, and sentinel node biopsy would minimize any potential morbidity from a full axillary dissection.

There is currently lack of consensus on the use of aromatase inhibitors in the adjuvant setting. This patient had a Nottingham Prognostic Index (NPI) of 3.4 and would therefore be in a lower category for risk of relapse. Some clinicians would routinely prescribe tamoxifen only for five years in the absence of any contraindication such as a past history of thromboembolism. Others would recommend tamoxifen only for two to three years with an early switch to an aromatase inhibitor. Individual trial data combined with meta-analysis of selected trials suggest that switching from tamoxifen to either exemestane or anastrozole is associated with statistically significant improvements in both disease-free and overall survival compared with tamoxifen alone (5 years duration) (5–11). Results of the BIG 1-98 study have failed to demonstrate a clear advantage from an early switch policy in terms of recurrence rates compared with 5 years of an aromatase inhibitor. At a median follow up of 72 months, there were no significant difference in terms of disease-free survival for 5 years of letrozole compared with either of the switch arms (tamoxifen—letrozole; letrozole—tamoxifen). However, pair wise comparisons suggested a slight advantage for letrozole (5 years) compared with tamoxifen for 2 years followed by letrozole for 3 years. The inverse sequence was equivalent to monotherapy (5). As a consequence of this and other data, some authorities advocate an upfront aromatase inhibitor for patients deemed to be at higher risk of local relapse (larger tumors, node positive, HER2 positive). The amplitude of the initial hazard peak is more effectively suppressed by an aromatase inhibitor administered in the first two to three years than tamoxifen (12).

Though aromatase inhibitors are associated with a lower risk of thromboembolism compared with tamoxifen, patients consistently report a higher incidence of musculoskeletal symptoms that can be troublesome for older women (13). All patients placed on aromatase inhibitors should have a baseline bone density scan. Within the Cambridge Breast Unit, all patients with an NPI <4.4 receive five years of tamoxifen only as adjuvant systemic hormonal therapy. Those patients with an NPI ≥4.4 and ≤5.4 receive tamoxifen for two to three years followed by an early switch to the aromatase inhibitor exemestane. Patients at higher risk of relapse with an NPI >5.4 receive an aromatase inhibitor from the outset with the choice of agent determined by physician discretion. This policy is based on analysis of survival data according to NPI, which shows a highly favorable survival for the excellent, good, and moderate I prognostic groups. It was, therefore, considered that incorporation of an aromatase inhibitor either upfront or after –two to three years of tamoxifen (early switch) was cost-effective for the moderate 2 and poor prognostic groups only within the local healthcare system (14).

Related Cases

Mastectomy without breast reconstruction— *Case Studies 2, 22, and 40*

Axillary lymph node dissection—*Case Studies 2, 3, 9, 22, 28, 32, 40, and 41*

Aromatase inhibitors—*Case Studies 4, 9, 10, 22, and 29*

Learning Points

1. The diagnosis of breast cancer is often established following a "triple assessment": clinical exam, imaging (diagnostic mammogram/ultrasound), and tissue biopsy (core biopsy or FNA).
2. There are two options available for the local therapy of breast cancer: breast-conserving therapy (BCT) or mastectomy.
3. BCT involves removal of only that part of the breast containing the cancer (wide local excision). In BCT, management of the axilla is identical to that of patients opting for mastectomy (sentinel node biopsy/axillary clearance). Radiotherapy to the breast is generally recommended after BCT.
4. Patients who opt for mastectomy generally do not require radiotherapy unless the tumor is large (>5 cm) or there is involvement of the axillary lymph nodes (generally more than 3 nodes containing metastatic disease).
5. For patients with ER-positive tumors, endocrine therapy is usually administered postoperatively. Endocrine therapy generally consists of either tamoxifen (in pre- or postmenopausal women) or an aromatase inhibitor (for postmenopausal women).

References

1. Shapiro S, Venet W, Strax P, et al. Ten- to fourteen-year effect of screening on breast cancer mortality. J Natl Cancer Inst 1982; 69:349–355.
2. Tabar L, Fagerberg CJG, Gad A, et al. Reduction in mortality from breast cancer after mass screening with mammography. Lancet 1985; i:829–832.
3. Fletcher SW, Black W, Harris R, et al. Report of the International Workshop on Screening for Breast Cancer. J Natl Cancer Inst 1993; 85:1644–1656.
4. Nystrom L, Rutqvist LE, Walls S, et al. Breast screening with mammography: overview of Swedish randomised trials. Lancet 1993; 341:973–978.
5. Mouridsen H, Giobbie-Hurder A, Mauriac L, et al. BIG 1-98: a randomized double-blind phase III study evaluating letrozole and tamoxifen in sequence as adjuvant endocrine therapy for postmenopausal women with receptor-positive breast cancer. 31st San Antonio Breast Cancer Symposium, Texas, USA, December 2008.
6. Baum M, Buzdar A, Cuzik J, et al. Anastrozole alone or in combination with tamoxifen versus tamoxifen alone for adjuvant treatment of postmenopausal women with early breast cancer: first results of the ATAC randomized trial. Lancet 2002; 359:2131–2139.
7. ATAC Trialists Group. Results of the ATAC (Arimidex, Tamoxifen, Alone or in Combination) trial after completion of 5 years adjuvant treatment for breast cancer. Lancet 2005; 365:60–66.
8. The Arimidex, Tamoxifen, Alone or in Combination Trialists' Group. Comprehensive side effect profile of anastrozole and tamoxifen as adjuvant treatment for early-stage breast cancer: long-term safety analysis of the ATAC trial. Lancet Oncol 2006; 7:633–643.
9. Coombes RC, Hall E, Gibson LJ, et al. A randomized trial of exemestane after two to three years of tamoxifen therapy in postmenopausal women with primary breast cancer. N Engl J Med 2004; 350:1081–1092.
10. Jonat W, Gnant M, Boccardo F, et al. Switching from adjuvant tamoxifen to anastrozole in postmenopausal women with hormone-responsive early breast cancer: a meta-analysis of the ARNO 95 Trial, ABCSG Trial 8 and the ITA Trial. Breast Cancer Res Treat 2005; 94:S11 (abstr 18).
11. Coombes RC, Kilburn LS, Snowdon CF, et al. Survival and safety of exemestane versus tamoxifen after 2–3 years' tamoxifen treatment (Intergroup Exemestane Study): a randomized controlled trial. Lancet 2007; 369:559–570.
12. Howell A. ATAC trial update. Lancet 2005; 365:1225–1226 (letter).
13. ATAC Trialists Group. Effect of anastrozole and tamoxifen as adjuvant treatment for early stage breast cancer: 100 month analysis of the ATAC trial. Lancet Oncol 2008; 9:45–53.
14. Wishart GW, Greenberg DC, Britton PD, et al. Screen-detected versus symptomatic breast cancer—is improved survival due to stage migration alone? Br J Cancer 2008; 98:1741–1741.

CASE STUDY 2

History

A 44-year-old woman presented to the breast clinic with a three-week history of a tender lump in the right breast. The lump had not changed in size over this time period, and there was no associated nipple discharge. There were no previous breast problems and no family history of breast or ovarian cancer. The patient remained nulliparous (premenopausal) and had never used the oral contraceptive pill. She smoked 20 cigarettes per day.

Clinical Findings

Clinical examination revealed a rather ill-defined area of thickening in the central and superolateral aspects of the right breast with no obviously dominant mass. There was no axillary lymphadenopathy (E2/3) (Fig. 5).

Clinical Assessment

An equivocal lesion in the right breast with an element of clinical suspicion

Investigations

Mammography–

This showed a spiculate mass in the superior and central aspect of the right breast with the appearances of a carcinoma (Fig. 6A, B).

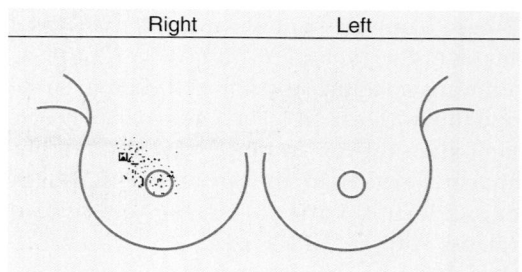

Figure 5

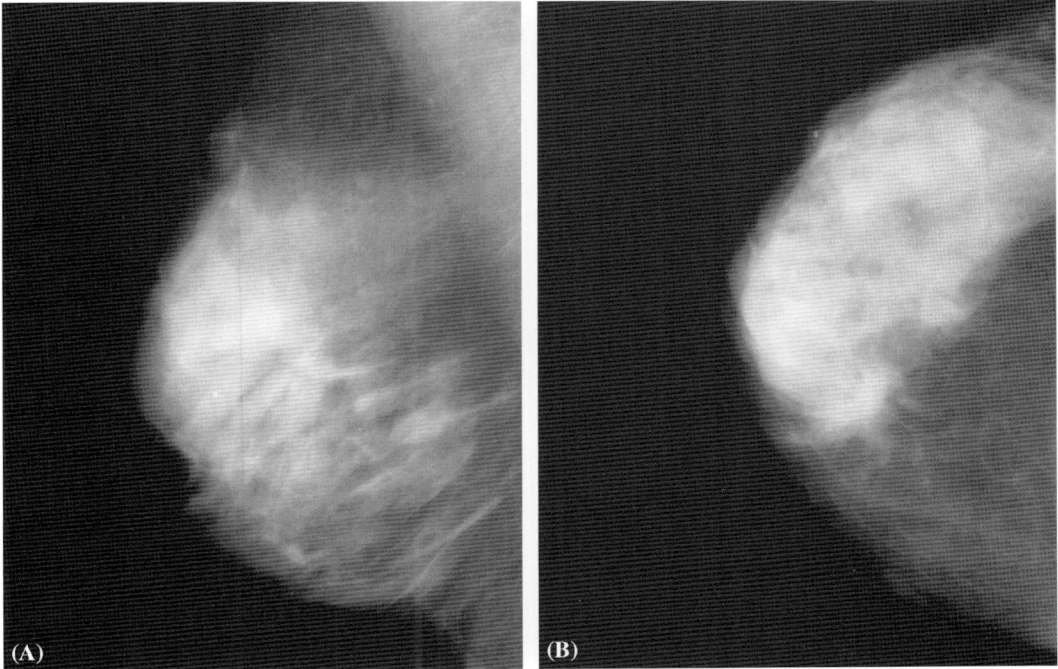

Figure 6

Breast Ultrasound

The sonographic correlate of this lesion was a 24-mm hypoechoic mass lesion with posterior acoustic attenuation (lying between 12 and 1 o'clock) (Fig. 7).

Core Biopsy

Ultrasound-guided core biopsy of the breast mass confirmed an invasive carcinoma (grade II) [Fig. 8A (low power), B (high power)].

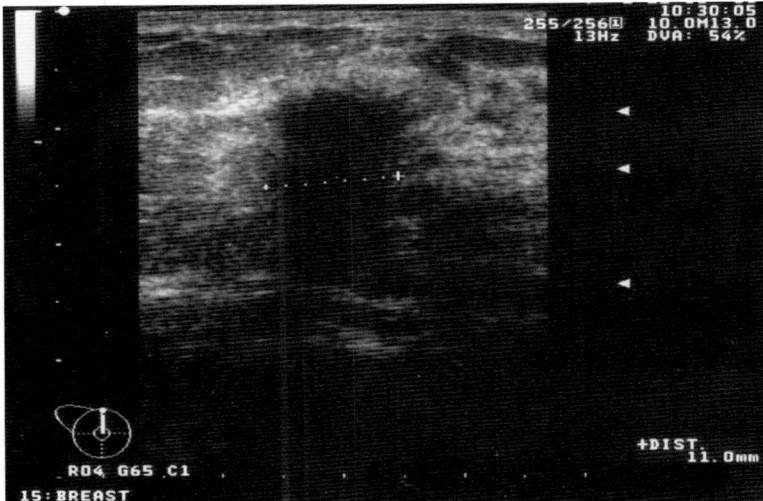

Figure 7

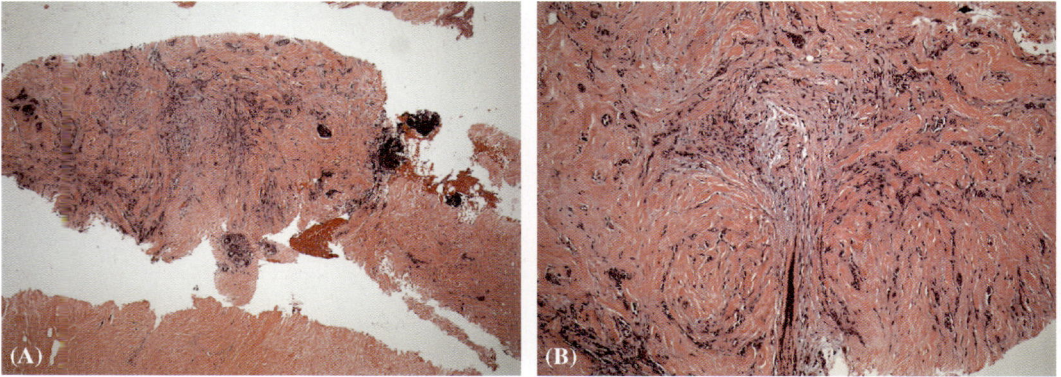

Figure 8

Diagnosis

Early-stage right breast cancer (T2N0)

Multidisciplinary Review 1

Though the radiological extent of the lesion was less than 3 cm, it lay relatively close to the nipple-areolar complex in the central zone of the breast. The lesion was not considered amenable to breast-conservation surgery, and a right modified radical mastectomy was recommended. Sentinel lymph node biopsy was not routinely offered at the time and primary surgery would therefore incorporate a level II axillary lymph node dissection. Immediate breast reconstruction would be offered (relatively young patient).

Treatment and Progress

Though this patient was not suitable for breast-conserving surgery, she adamantly requested a mastectomy whatever the characteristics and location of the primary tumor. Moreover, she declined immediate breast reconstruction with a similar force of conviction and proceeded to a right modified radical mastectomy two weeks later (Fig. 9). She made an uneventful recovery and was discharged on the sixth postoperative day after removal of the second redivac drain. On review in the clinic two weeks after

discharge, there was no evidence of any seroma formation, and the wound was healing nicely. The patient remained well and disease-free after five years of follow-up when she was discharged back to the care of her general practitioner (Fig. 10).

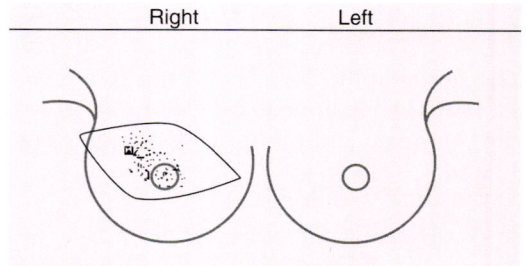

Figure 9

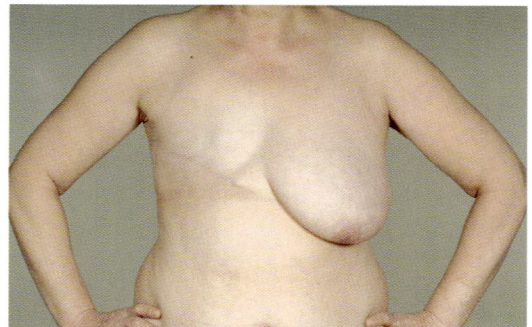

Figure 10

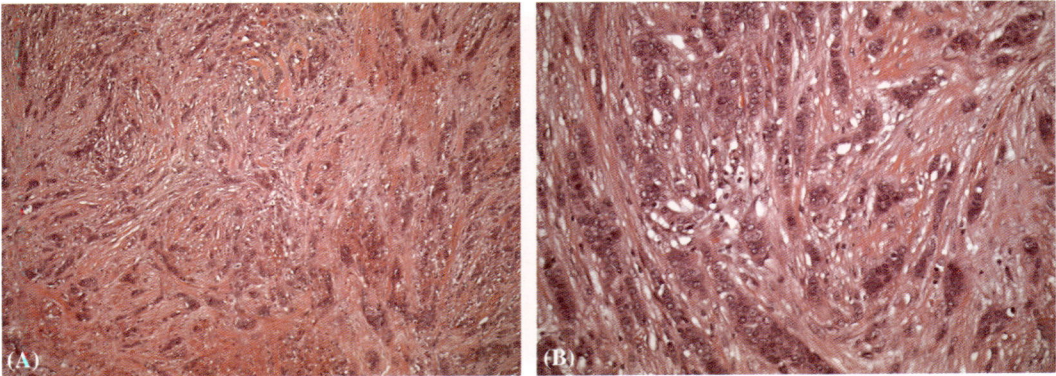

Figure 11

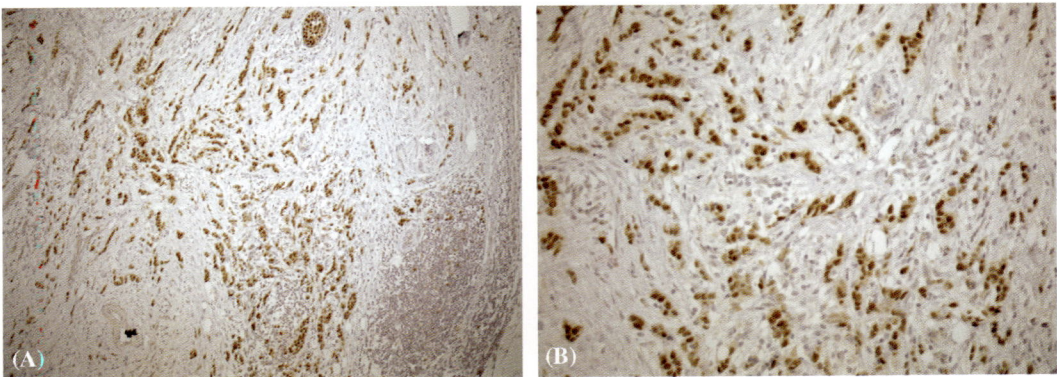

Figure 12

Definitive Histology

This confirmed an invasive carcinoma (grade II) measuring 22 mm in maximum diameter [Fig. 11A (magnification 10×), B (magnification 20×)]. There was associated ductal carcinoma in situ (DCIS) yielding an overall tumor size of 34 mm. Three out of 14 nodes contained metastatic carcinoma, and the tumor was ER positive (90% staining for ER) [Fig. 12A (low power), B (high power)].

Multidisciplinary Review 2

This premenopausal patient had an NPI of [$(0.2 \times 2.2) + 2 + 2 = 4.44$] and fell into the one to three nodes positive category. Adjuvant chemotherapy was recommended (AC × 4 cycles, see Appendix III) together with radiotherapy to the chest wall (not supraclavicular fossa). The patient had an estrogen-sensitive tumor and would be eligible for hormonal manipulation with ovarian suppression and tamoxifen if she remained premenopausal after chemotherapy.

Treatment and Progress

The patient commenced the first cycle of chemotherapy within three weeks of surgery. She was keen to complete chemotherapy as soon as possible in order to go on a previously arranged holiday. She tolerated chemotherapy well, though developed mild nausea, dyspepsia, and hyperactivity (difficulty sleeping). Following the third cycle of adriamycin/cyclophosphamide (AC) chemotherapy, the patient suffered a left-sided pulmonary embolism (confirmed on V/Q scan). She was anticoagulated and the final cycle of chemotherapy delayed by four days. The patient had also become increasingly troubled by daytime hot flushes and night sweats. These were very incapacitating and venlafaxine (37.5 mg twice daily) was prescribed.

Radiotherapy to the chest wall was given immediately upon completion of the final cycle of chemotherapy (the radiotherapy-planning session took place three days after the fourth cycle of AC). The patient received 40 Gy in 15 fractions over three weeks, using megavoltage photons. There was slight erythema of the chest wall, but this responded well to Aqueous Cream.

The patient commenced tamoxifen as adjuvant hormonal therapy after completion of chemotherapy. Despite a history of thromboembolism (a relative contraindication to tamoxifen), the patient remained premenopausal after chemotherapy and was not eligible for an aromatase inhibitor. At 24-month follow-up, the patient reported intermittent bloodstained vaginal discharge. She was referred for gynecological assessment and a transvaginal ultrasound revealed some endometrial thickening (8.1 mm) but no ovarian lesion. A subsequent hysteroscopy and biopsy showed an atrophic endometrium with no polyp formation. Indeed, the endometrial lining was insufficient for adequate biopsy.

In view of the vaginal bleeding and history of pulmonary embolism, there were concerns about continuation of tamoxifen (patient warfarinized indefinitely). Though menstrual activity had resumed immediately postchemotherapy, the patient had not experienced a "normal" period for almost 12 months. Measurement of FSH and LH levels confirmed these to be in the postmenopausal range and, therefore, tamoxifen was switched to the aromatase inhibitor Arimidex (1 mg per day) almost two and a half years after surgery. However, after three months of therapy with Arimidex, the patient experienced a very heavy menstrual bleeding prompting admission to hospital. Interestingly, repeat gonadotrophin levels showed a postmenopausal FSH (27.4) but an LH in the normal range (6.2). It was anticipated that further menstrual activity would occur and management options for ovarian suppression included either a luteinizing hormone–releasing hormone (LHRH) analogue

(Zoladex) injections or laparoscopic bilateral oophorectomy. The patient opted for a total abdominal hysterectomy and bilateral salpingo-oophorectomy after careful discussion with the gynecologists and oncologists. Surgery was expedited on the basis that ovarian suppression constitutes part of the patient's breast cancer treatment.

Discussion

The patient had a clinically indeterminate lesion in the right breast for which the initial index of suspicion was low. At the time of presentation, one-stop style breast clinics with some day imaging had not yet been established. In consequence, there was a significant time lapse between initial clinical assessment and subsequent review with results of radiological investigation and biopsy (25 days). The majority of patients (irrespective of clinical urgency) are now seen within 14 days and basic investigations undertaken in a "one-stop" clinic. Recent evidence suggests that attempts to stratify patients into urgent (14 days) and nonurgent can lead to a significant number of women with cancer being diagnosed through the routine pathway with concomitant delays in treatment. General practitioners do not have access to imaging and cannot undertake triple assessment. Clinical determination of whether a patient has a discrete lump as opposed to a focal area of nodularity can be difficult. It is, therefore, preferable to refer all patients under the two-week rule rather than just those deemed to have a discrete lump (or some other key symptom).

When provided with fully informed consent, some patients will demand mastectomy even when breast-conservation therapy is feasible. For borderline cases, patients may be concerned about risks of local recurrence and choose mastectomy to minimize the chance of any future problems. It is more difficult for surgeons to agree to mastectomy for smaller tumors (<2 cm) situated well away from the nipple-areolar complex in a moderate- to large-breasted woman. Some women wish to avoid radiotherapy, though should be warned that this may be indicated postmastectomy for larger, higher-grade lesions that are node positive. Ultimately, it is the patient's choice if she chooses mastectomy in preference to breast-conservation therapy. Similar considerations apply to a contralateral prophylactic mastectomy in the absence of any strong family history. It should not be assumed that all younger women having mastectomy will seek immediate breast reconstruction. This particular patient had no wish for any form of reconstruction—immediate or delayed.

This premenopausal node-positive patient received chemotherapy with an anthracycline-based regimen. These younger women with nodal involvement are at higher risk of relapse and were the first group to be targeted with adjuvant chemotherapy. Early regimens involved comparison of placebo with either single agents such as melphalan or combination chemotherapy with cyclophosphamide, methotrexate, and 5-fluorouracil (CMF) (1). These early trials of adjuvant chemotherapy for breast cancer were the first to show advantages for both disease-free and overall survival. They spawned a generation of randomized trials investigating CMF alone (shorter vs. longer courses) (2) or CMF with additional agents and other combinations of chemotherapy (namely the anthracycline-containing regimens). Adjuvant chemotherapy was investigated in younger node-negative women with adverse prognosticators relating to primary tumor characteristics (3). The higher risk of relapse for this group justified the potential treatment morbidity from chemotherapy administered to symptomatically well women for whom individual benefits from chemotherapy were unclear.

A series of meta-analyses by the Early Breast Cancer Trialists Collaborative Group (EBCTCG) have assimilated individual patient data from more than 50 trials of chemotherapy involving over 20,000 women. These overviews included 11 trials comparing CMF with anthracycline-containing regimens. The benefits of adjuvant chemotherapy in both younger and older women were confirmed irrespective of nodal status and baseline relapse level. The proportional reductions in mortality and recurrence were higher among younger women under the age of 50 years but similar for node-positive and node-negative women. For women under the age of 50 years, the proportional reductions in risk of relapse and mortality were 35% and 27%, respectively. This translates into absolute mortality reductions at 10 years of 11% for node-positive and 7% for node-negative tumors. For women over 50 years of age, the proportional reductions in risk of relapse and mortality were 20% and 11%, respectively. The corresponding absolute reductions in mortality at 10 years was 3% for node-positive and 2% for node-negative tumors (4).

Initial results from the EBCTCG overview suggested that regimens containing an anthracycline might be more active than CMF. However, the larger NSABP-B15 trial comparing four cycles of AC with CMF failed to demonstrate any superior efficacy for anthracycline regimens but great toxicity for the latter (5). Cardiotoxicity was of particular concern, but nausea, vomiting, and alopecia were also troublesome side effects. An updated analysis by the EBCTCG involving 15,000 (mainly premenopausal) women in 14 trials of anthracycline-containing regimens has confirmed sustained benefits from the latter compared with CMF with a hazard ratio of 0.88 (6). At 10 years, there is an absolute benefit of approximately 4% for recurrence and survival among node-positive women. For node-negative patients, the absolute survival gain at five years is 1.7%. In recent years, regimens incorporating an anthracycline such as AC and FAC have become the standard of adjuvant chemotherapy for early-stage breast cancer. The shorter duration of treatment, shorter hospital stay, and perceived effectiveness have appealed to oncologists around the world. Interestingly, the value of anthracyclines in node-positive disease has recently been called into question; data presented at the 30th San Antonio Breast Cancer Symposium in 2007 suggest that any superior efficacy of anthracyclines is attributable to a minority (8–9%) of HER2-positive patients who co-overexpress topoisomerase II. By implication, there is little evidence for any clear benefit from an anthracycline regimen among the group of HER2-negative patients (75%) (7).

Though all patients undergoing breast-conserving surgery receive some form of breast irradiation, radiotherapy is applied more selectively to the chest wall following mastectomy. All trials have consistently shown that postmastectomy radiotherapy reduces the proportional risk of local failure by two-thirds to three-quarters. However, there remain unresolved issues about the effects of local control on longer-term survival from breast cancer. Indeed, an early meta-analysis of postmastectomy radiotherapy trials showed a poorer overall survival among irradiated patients (8). The EBCTCG published a comprehensive meta-analysis of 40 unconfounded randomized trials involving 20,000 women in 2000. More than half the patients had node-positive disease and radiotherapy fields included not only the chest wall but also the axillary, supraclavicular, and internal mammary nodes. This meta-analysis revealed a reduction in rates of local recurrence from 27.2% to 8.8% at 10 years (9). Though breast cancer–specific mortality was significantly reduced, other causes of death were increased. Many of these data related to outdated modes of radiotherapy and adverse effects (especially cardiotoxicity) are minimized by newer techniques employing tangential fields. A reanalysis of the EBCTCG data with exclusion of pre-1970 trials and small ones with suboptimal protocols supports an overall survival benefit for postmastectomy radiotherapy in selected subgroups. It is important that modern techniques of radiotherapy are used and treatment is with standardized fractionation (10).

Two randomized studies of postmastectomy radiotherapy have shown a survival benefit (approximately 10%) in a subgroup of premenopausal node-positive patients receiving chemotherapy, suggesting that persistence of local or regional disease can lead to distant metastases and impaired survival (11,12). In the smaller Canadian study, 318 node-positive women were randomized to mastectomy and chemotherapy, with or without irradiation. At 15-year follow-up, the overall survival rates were 54% and 46%, respectively for these two groups. In the larger Danish trial, 1708 node-positive or stage III breast cancer patients were similarly randomized, and overall survival rates at 10 years were 54% for the irradiated group compared with 48% for the nonirradiated group ($p < 0.001$). The results of these trials have generated some controversy due to the low number of nodes harvested at axillary dissection and potential understaging of patients due to suboptimal management of the axilla.

In a further landmark publication in 2005, the EBCTCG showed an overall survival benefit at 15 years from local radiation treatment to either the breast following BCT or the chest wall after mastectomy. For those treatment comparisons where the difference in local recurrence rates at five years was less than 10%, survival was unaffected. Among the 25,000 women where differences in local relapse were substantial (>10%), there were moderate reductions in breast cancer–specific and overall mortality. The absolute reduction in local recurrence at five years was 19%, and the absolute reduction in breast cancer mortality at 15 years was 5.0%. This represents one life saved for every four locoregional recurrences prevented by radiotherapy at five years (13).

Postmastectomy radiotherapy does not benefit all subgroups, and the absolute gains in terms of local control and overall survival must be balanced against toxicities and inconvenience to patients together with costs. Patients can be stratified into three risk groups as follows (14):

High risk (>20% chance of locoregional relapse at 10 years)
  – Tumors ≥ 5 cm in maximum diameter
  – ≥4 nodes positive (pathological confirmation)

Moderate risk (10–20% chance of locoregional relapse at 10 years)
  – Tumors <5 cm in maximum diameter
  – 1 to 3 nodes positive (pathological confirmation)

Low risk (<10% chance of locoregional relapse at 10 years)
  – Tumors <5 cm in maximum diameter
  – No pathologically involved nodes

For the high-risk group, there is international consensus for the routine use of chest wall radiotherapy following mastectomy. These patients are also at risk for supraclavicular failure, and irradiation of the supraclavicular nodes is usually undertaken for this group of patients with ≥4 nodes positive. Conversely, patients in the low-risk group should not receive radiotherapy. Those patients who fall into the moderate-risk group with one to three nodes positive have less clear benefits from postmastectomy radiotherapy. The Canadian and Danish trials showed similar proportional benefits in patients with 1 to 3 and ≥4 nodes positive, but with more prolonged follow-up the benefits of radiotherapy are statistically more robust for the higher-risk groups compared with moderate-risk groups. The UK/European SUPREMO study is presently investigating the role of postmastectomy radiotherapy in patients at moderate risk of relapse with smaller tumors (<5 cm) and/or one to three nodes positive (15).

The Cambridge Breast Unit have derived a postmastectomy radiotherapy index to use as a clinical tool for selection of patients for chest wall radiotherapy (16). This ranks patients by a scoring system that is related to known risk factors for locoregional failure (Table 1). Patients receive postmastectomy radiotherapy if the score is ≥3.

Many women over the age of 45 years will experience chemotherapy-induced amenorrhea with permanent cessation of ovarian function (17). The proportional improvement in overall survival from ovarian ablation is 24% in the absence of chemotherapy and only 8% to 10% in those who have received chemotherapy—though the absolute benefits are greatest in those women who continue to menstruate (18). Formal ovarian ablation is often not undertaken for women in their mid to late 40s in expectation of postmenopausal change. Unlike younger women (<35 years), chemotherapy alone is considered adequate treatment within this age group for hormone-sensitive tumors.

This patient underwent delayed ovarian suppression following resumption of menstrual activity after initiation of aromatase inhibitor therapy. This was an unusual situation and bilateral oophorectomy was combined with hysterectomy due to heavy menstrual bleeding. It is unclear beyond what time interval ovarian ablation ceases to be effective in terms of the primary tumor.

Related Cases

Postmastectomy radiotherapy—*Case Studies 3, 18, 22, 25, 26, 27, 28, and 37*

Adjuvant chemotherapy—*Case Studies 3, 6, 8, 11, 36, and 37*

Ovarian suppression—*Case Studies 6, 8, 23, 27, and 37*

Learning Points

1. There is considerable geographic variability in the use of BCT. BCT is more commonly utilized in Europe than in the United States. Furthermore, there is considerable variability in the use of BCT within the United States itself (more commonly utilized in the northeast than in the south).
2. A tumor adjacent to the nipple-areolar complex is not necessarily a contraindication for BCT. Excison of the tumor and nipple-areolar complex is feasible. This is generally followed by radiotherapy.
3. Adjuvant chemotherapy generally begins within six weeks of surgery, and radiotherapy, when indicated, usually follows chemotherapy. Endocrine therapy is commenced after completion of radiotherapy.

Table 1 Postmastectomy Radiotherapy Index

Score	3	2	1
	≥4 nodes	1–3 nodes	Vascular invasion
	tumor size >50 mm/T4	tumor size 30–50 mm	tumor size 20–29 mm
	deep margin <1 mm		grade III or pectoral muscle involvement

4. Adjuvant chemotherapy is usually administered as a combination of drugs, which is more effective than a single anticancer agent. Anthracycline-based regimens have been shown to be more efficacious than classical CMF (cyclophosphamide, methotrexate, 5-fluorouracil), and addition of taxanes may confer additional benefit over and above that of anthracyclines alone.

5. Tamoxifen is associated with about a twofold increased risk of endometrial cancers and thromboembolic events.

6. Postmastectomy radiotherapy is beneficial to both pre- and postmenopausal women who are at high risk for locoregional relapse.

References

1. Bonadonna G, Valagussa P, Moliterni A, et al. Adjuvant cyclophosphamide, methotrexate and fluorouracil in node positive breast cancer. The results of 20 years follow up. N Engl J Med 1995; 332:901–926.

2. Tancini G, Bonadonna G, Valagussi P, et al. Adjuvant MF in breast cancer: comparative 5 year results of 12 versus 6 cycles. J Clin Oncol 1983; 1:2–10.

3. Fisher B, Redmond C, Dimitrov NV, et al. A randomized clinical trial evaluating sequential methotrexate and fluorouracil in the treatment of patients with node negative breast cancer who have estrogen receptor negative tumours. N Engl J Med 1989; 320:473–478.

4. Early Breast Cancer Trialists Collaborative Group. Polychemotherapy for early breast cancer: an overview of the randomized trial. Lancet 1998; 352:930–942.

5. Fisher B, Brown AM, Dimitrov NV, et al. Two months of doxorubicin-cyclophosphamide with and without interval reinduction therapy compared with 6 months of cyclophosphamide, methotrexate and 5-fluorouracil in node positive breast cancer patients with tamoxifen non-responsive tumours: results from the National Surgical Adjuvant Breast and Bowel Project B-15. J Clin Oncol 1990; 8:1483–1496.

6. 5th Meeting of the Early Breast Cancer Trialists Collaborative Group, Oxford, UK, September 21–23, 2000.

7. Slamon D. Another genetic approach to predicting response to anthracyclines: the importance of HER2 and topoisomerase IIa. 30th San Antonio Breast Cancer Symposium, San Antonio, Texas, USA, December 2007.

8. Early Breast Cancer Trialists' Collaborative Group. Effects of radiotherapy and surgery in early breast cancer: an overview of the randomized trials. N Engl J Med 1995; 333:1444–1455.

9. Early Breast Cancer Trialists' Collaborative Group. Favourable and unfavourable effects on long term survival of radiotherapy for early breast cancer. An overview of the randomized trials. Lancet 2000; 355:1757–1770.

10. Van de Steene J, Soete G, Storme G. Adjuvant radiotherapy for breast cancer significantly improves overall survival. Radiol Oncol 2000; 55:263–272.

11. Ragaz J, Jackson SM, Le M, et al. Adjuvant radiotherapy and chemotherapy in node positive premenopausal women with breast cancer. N Engl J Med 1997; 337:956–962.

12. Overgaard M, Hansen PS, Overgaard J, et al. Postoperative radiotherapy in high risk pre-menopausal women with breast cancer who receive adjuvant chemotherapy. Danish Breast Cancer Cooperative Group 82b trial. N Engl J Med 1997; 337:949–955.

13. Early Breast Cancer Trialists Collaborative Group. Effects of radiotherapy and of differences in the extent of surgery for early breast cancer on local recurrence and 15 year survival: an overview of the randomized trials. Lancet 2005; 366:2087–2106.

14. Recht A, Edge SB, Solin SJ, et al. Post-mastectomy radiotherapy: clinical practice guidelines of the American Society of Clinical Oncology. J Clin Oncol 2001; 19:1539–1569.

15. SUPREMO breast cancer trial. Selective Use of Postoperative Radiotherapy after Mastectomy. Available at: www.supremo-trial.com. Accessed November 17, 2008.

16. Wilson CB, Haba Y, Wishart GC. The identification of patients for postmastectomy radiotherapy using the Cambridge index: audit of a prospective series. Breast Cancer Res Treat 2007; 106:S198 (abstr 4093).

17. Del Mastro L, Venturini M, Sertoli MR, et al. Amenorrhoea induced by adjuvant chemotherapy in early breast cancer patients: prognostic role and clinical implications. Breast Cancer Res Treat 1997; 43:183–190.

18. Early Breast Cancer Trialists Collaborative Group. Ovarian ablation in early breast cancer: overview of the randomized trials. Lancet 1996; 348:1189–1196.

CASE STUDY 3

History

A 51-year-old woman presented with a two-week history of an area of fullness and tenderness of the left breast. There was no associated nipple discharge and no previous breast problems or family history of breast cancer. The patient was nulliparous and had used the oral contraceptive pill for a continuous period of almost 20 years.

Clinical Findings

There was a large, firm, irregular mass in the upper outer quadrant of the left breast measuring between 4 and 5 cm. The mass was mobile on the chest wall with no evidence of any skin tethering or infiltration. A hard node was palpable in the left axilla measuring at least 2 cm in diameter (E5) (Fig. 13).

Clinical Assessment

Clinical carcinoma of the left breast with involved axillary lymph nodes

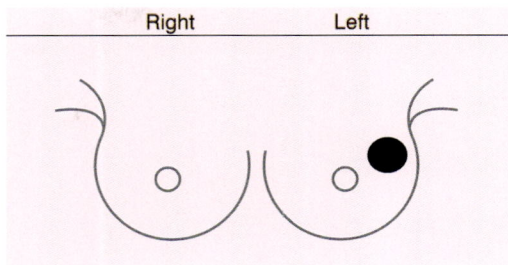

Figure 13

Investigations

Mammography

An asymmetric density was apparent in the upper outer quadrant of the left breast, which contained fine microcalcification (Fig. 14A). Subtle spiculation was seen on the craniocaudal view (Fig. 14B).

Breast Ultrasound

The sonographic correlate of this density was a 42-mm hypoechoic lesion with the radiological features of a carcinoma (U5) (Fig. 15).

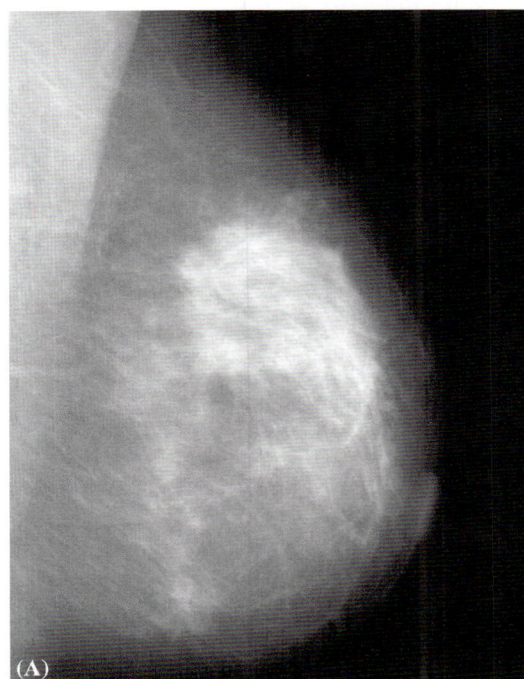

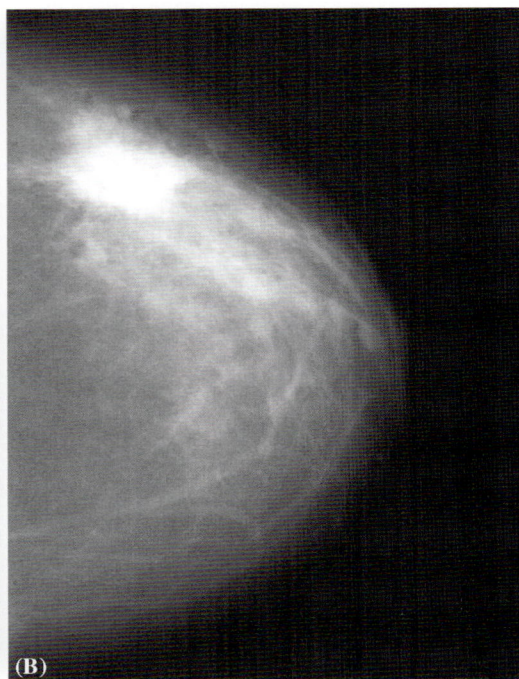

(A)

(B)

Figure 14

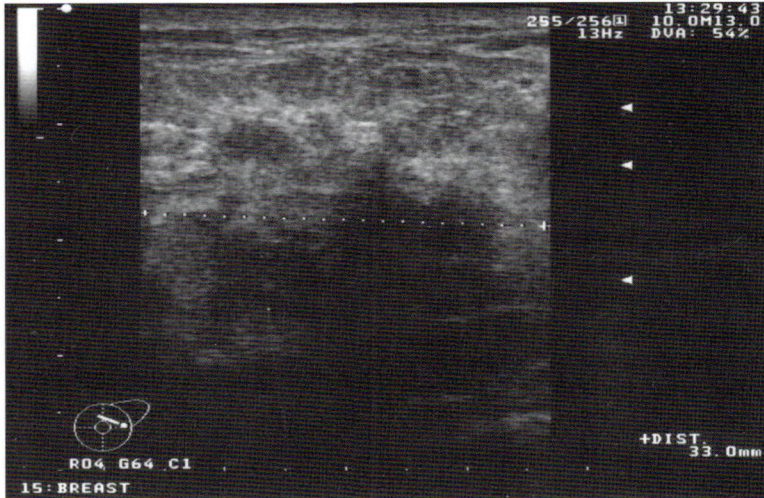

Figure 15

Core Biopsy

Ultrasound-guided core biopsy of the breast mass confirmed an invasive carcinoma (grade II) with associated intermediate nuclear grade DCIS of solid type. Routine ER measurements were not done on core biopsies at the time, and the axilla was not interrogated sonographically [Fig. 16A (low power), B (high power)].

Diagnosis

Early-stage left breast cancer (T2N1).

Multidisciplinary Review 1

It was recommended that the patient undergo a left modified radical mastectomy and be offered immediate breast reconstruc-

tion. The location of the tumor in relation to the nipple made it unlikely that breast-conserving surgery would be feasible after induction chemotherapy. This together with the grade (II) and size of the lesion (<5 cm) prompted the recommendation for primary surgery rather than chemotherapy. The patient was not eligible for sentinel lymph node biopsy on account of the clinically suspicious node in the left axilla (and to some extent tumor size at the time). Radiotherapy to the chest wall would likely be required (large size and clinically node positive).

Treatment and Progress

The patient expressed an interest in immediate breast reconstruction and was reviewed by the plastic surgeon. It was noted that the

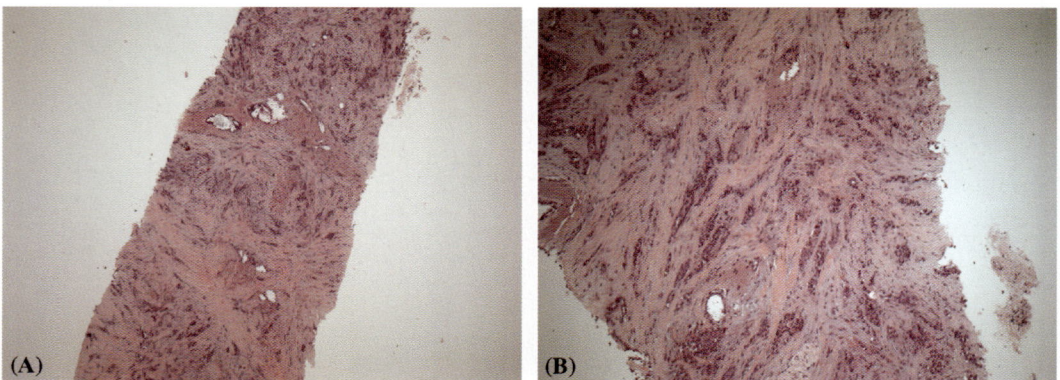

(A)

(B)

Figure 16

patient had a 34D cup and was likely to require both chemotherapy and radiotherapy postoperatively. An implant-only procedure was excluded by the expectation of radiotherapy, and the patient had an inadequate volume of infraumbilical abdominal tissue for a transverse rectus abdominus myocutaneous (TRAM) flap reconstruction.

The patient proceeded to a left modified radical mastectomy and immediate breast reconstruction with a latissimus dorsi flap and implant within four weeks of initial tissue diagnosis. A modified skin-sparing technique was employed to incorporate the nipple-areolar complex and the skin directly over the tumor. She made an excellent recovery and was discharged home on the seventh postoperative day. A seroma was aspirated on two occasions from the donor site on the back.

Definitive Histology

This revealed a grade II invasive ductal carcinoma measuring 35 mm microscopically but approximately 45 mm macroscopically (which was more consistent with the clinical/radio-logical estimate) [Fig. 17A (magnification 10×), B (magnification 20×)]. The invasive tumor was associated with both intermediate and high nuclear grade DCIS with focal comedo necrosis. DCIS did not extend significantly beyond the invasive tumor that was well clear (≥5 mm) of all margins, including the anterior (skin) margin (10 mm). There was extensive lymphovascular invasion and five nodes contained metastatic carcinoma [Fig. 17C (low power), D (high power)]. Immunohistochemical staining for ER was positive, but PgR negative. The Hercep Test for HER2 was borderline 2+ and HER2 FISH was amplified (i.e., HER2 overexpression).

Multidisciplinary Review 2

This patient had a relatively large tumor with extensive regional disease. The calculated NPI was $[(0.2 \times 3.5) + 2 + 3 = 5.7]$, and it was recommended she receive chemotherapy with a taxane-based schedule together with radiotherapy to the chest wall and supraclavicular fossa. Tamoxifen would be given as adjuvant systemic hormonal therapy

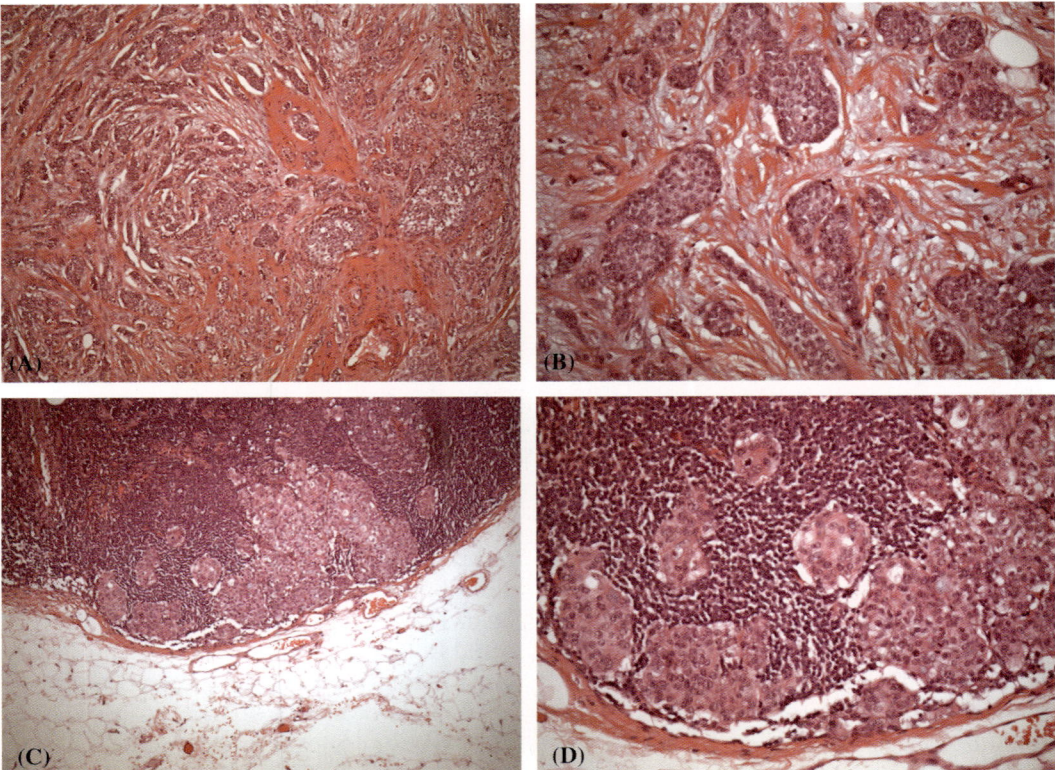

Figure 17

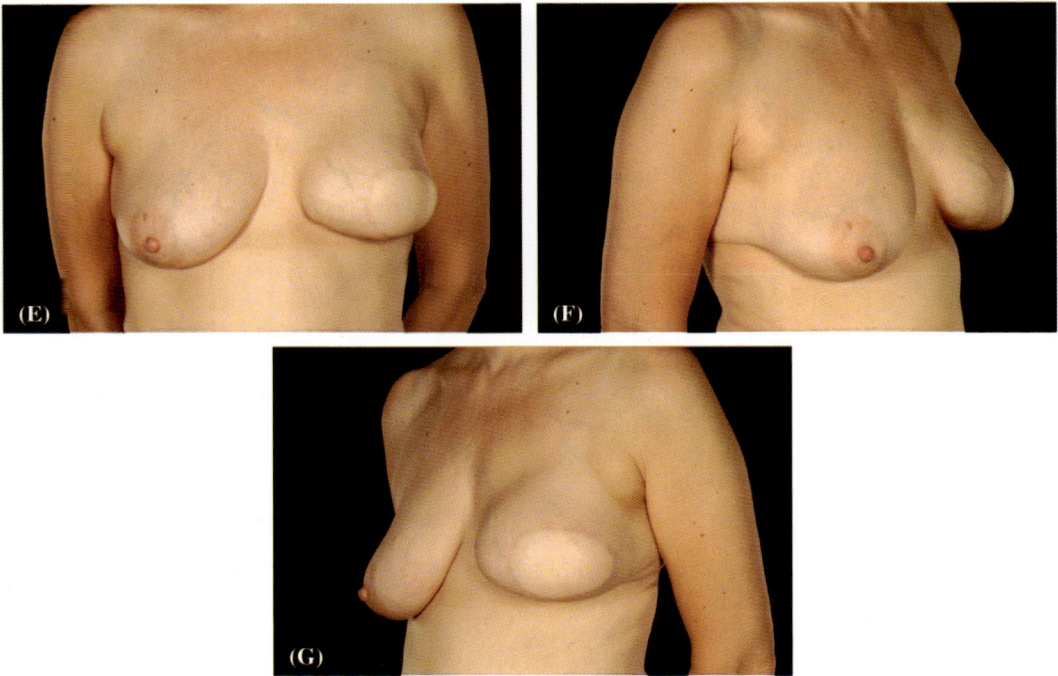

(E)

(F)

(G)

Figure 17   (*continued*)

upon completion of chemotherapy. Full
staging investigations (hepatic ultrasound
and bone scan) were requested and revealed
no evidence of metastatic disease.

Treatment and Progress

The patient proceeded to a course of FEC/
docetaxol with four cycles of 5-fluorouracil,
epirubicin, cyclophosphamide (FEC) followed by four cycles of docetaxel (see
Appendix III). This was well tolerated without any serious adverse effects and radiotherapy was commenced seven months following
surgery. The patient developed some edema
of the breast, but otherwise no acute sequelae from irradiation of the chest wall, reconstructed breast, and supraclavicular fossa.
This patient was considered to be at high
risk for relapse and was reviewed clinically on
a six-monthly basis (rather than annually).
Upon review at 18 months she was noted to
have a degree of capsular formation secondary to radiotherapy. This was not progressive
and did not lead to implant failure and
explantation. Nonetheless, the overall cosmetic outcome was slightly compromised by
these sequelae of radiotherapy (Fig. 17E–G).

Discussion

This patient presented with a relatively large
tumor with a clinically node-positive axilla.
Though she was managed with primary surgical treatment, a course of preoperative chemotherapy to downstage the tumor would
have been an alternative option. However,
whatever the degree of tumor response, mastectomy would still have been indicated on
the basis of central tumor location. An advantage of primary surgery is possession of maximum information on primary tumor
characteristics and nodal status prior to making any decision on adjuvant therapies. This
patient had involvement of >4 nodes and was
therefore a candidate for both chest wall and
supraclavicular irradiation (1). Furthermore,
the absolute nodal count influenced choice
of adjuvant systemic therapy, and this patient
received taxanes in addition to an anthracycline-based chemotherapy regimen (see
below). In theory, induction chemotherapy
could downstage nodal disease such that the
initial extent of involvement prechemotherapy is unknown. It is sometimes possible to
discern pathologically which nodes have been
"sterilized" by chemotherapy, but this is

unreliable. Similarly, ultrasound assessment of the axilla (with core biopsy) can provide histological evidence of nodal involvement, but does not yield information on the total number of nodes positive.

An increasing proportion of women are now requiring postmastectomy radiotherapy. Anticipation of chest wall radiation will influence the choice of reconstructive technique; an implant-only based technique (subpectoral implant) is generally avoided when there is a possibility of the patient requiring postoperative irradiation (2,3). All breast implants evoke a degree of fibrosis and scar tissue formation around the implant, and this occurs irrespective of whether reconstruction is carried out within an irradiated field or radiotherapy follows implant-based reconstruction (4). Excessive fibrosis with shrinkage of the scar tissue constitutes capsular contracture and results in distortion of the reconstruction. There is a high rate of capsular contracture under these circumstances, which may lead to implant failure. To some extent an implant can be protected from the adverse effects of radiation by an overlying latissimus dorsi myocutaneous flap. However, emerging data from several units suggests that even when placement of an implant is combined with transposition of a latissimus dorsi flap, there remains a significant risk of capsular contracture of up to 40% at four years (5,6). Other case series that involve both implant-only and implant-assisted latissiumus dorsi flap reconstruction confirm that postoperative radiotherapy worsens capsular contracture with rates varying from 0% to 40% without radiotherapy and 17% to 68% with radiotherapy (7,8). Moreover, severe capsular contracture is confined to the radiotherapy group and necessitates either capsulotomy (9–31.6%) or capsulectomy with implant exchange (1.2–11%). Most of these series involve a total radiation dose of 50 Gy given as 25 fractions (with or without a booster dose of 10–12 Gy to the scar). Nonetheless, despite these comments, when viewed from the other perspective, almost two-third of patients receiving radiotherapy after implant-assisted latissimus dorsi flap reconstruction do not develop clinically significant capsular formation and do not require exchange of implant.

Within the Cambridge Breast Unit, a different regimen is employed; a dose of 40 Gy is administered in 15 fractions over a three-week period. Among a group of 77 patients who underwent either implant-only (29 patients) or latissimus dorsi flap and implant (48 patients) reconstruction without radiotherapy, no cases of severe capsular contracture occurred. By contrast, five cases of severe contracture were found among a similar group who received radiotherapy postoperatively. These cases occurred in those with a latissimus dorsi flap and implant (35 patients), while no cases were documented among eight patients with an implant-only-based reconstruction. The actuarial rate of severe capsular contracture at four years was 28% (9). The potential problems of capsular contracture in this group of breast reconstruction patients receiving radiotherapy has led some surgeons to modify their surgical approach with a so-called "delayed immediate reconstruction" (10). A skin-sparing mastectomy can be undertaken initially with placement of a temporary tissue expander that acts as a scaffolding for the skin flaps (subpectoral or subcutaneous). Chest wall irradiation can then be given, and definitive reconstruction performed at a later stage (8–12 months). There are concerns about the viability of the mastectomy flaps after radiation, and it may be preferable overall to proceed with immediate reconstruction with latissimus dorsi flap and implant for all patients and undertake implant exchange if and when required. An extended autologous latissimus dorsi flap is not necessarily more tolerant of radiotherapy, and there is significant donor site morbidity. However, delayed immediate reconstruction is a method that can potentially preserve the aesthetic benefits of immediate breast reconstruction with preservation of the 3-D skin envelope. The decision for radiotherapy is made once the final histology is available and the temporary implant can be deflated prior to irradiation and re-inflated immediately afterward. This allows more accurate targeting of the tangential radiotherapy beams.

The taxanes are a new class of chemotherapeutic agents that are increasingly being employed in the adjuvant setting for treatment of those women at moderate and high risk of relapse. The two agents in current clinical usage are paclitaxel (Taxol) and docetaxel (taxotere). The taxanes have non-cross resistance with conventional agents, and their mechanism of action is to stabilize and prevent disaggregation of microtubules with disruption of the mitotic spindle. Paclitaxel was the first taxane to be investigated among node-positive patients with early-stage breast cancer. It was added to the sequential dose-dense regimen of doxorubicin and cyclophosphamide (AC) in the CALGB 9344 trial (11). The addition of four cycles of paclitaxel to four cycles of AC improved both disease-free (HR 0.83, $p = 0.0023$) and overall survival (HR 0.82, $p = 0.0064$). Dose escalation (density/total dose) for doxorubicin had no impact of these outcome parameters, and prolongation of therapy with taxanes led to only a modest increase in level of side effects. The NSABP B28 trial is of similar design and randomized node-positive patients to AC alone or AC followed by paclitaxel. Initial results showed benefits for relapse-free (HR 0.83, $p = 0.008$) but not overall survival (HR 0.94, $p = 0.46$) (12). Results were otherwise compatible with those of the CALGB 9344 trial.

Two trials have investigated the efficacy of the other taxane, docetaxel in node-positive patients. These have used more intensive anthracycline regimens; the BCIRG-01 trial compared six cycles of 5-fluorouracil, doxorubicin, and cyclophosphamide (FAC) with six cycles of docetaxel, doxorubicin, and cyclophosphamide (TAC) (13). The PACS-01 trial compared six cycles of 5-fluorouracil, epirubicin, and cyclophosphamide (FEC) with three cycles of FEC followed by three cycles of docetaxel. Both trials have shown statistically significant improvements in overall survival for taxane containing regimens (14).

This particular patient received an off-trial regimen similar to the PACS-01 protocol with four cycles of FEC followed by four cycles of docetaxel. It is current policy to offer FEC-taxotere as standard chemotherapy to all HER2-positive patients and those with ≥4 nodes positive. Provisional results from the TACT I trial involving 4000 patients suggest that there is minimal benefit in terms of disease-free and overall survival from adding four cycles of docetaxel to one of two standard antracycline-containing regimens (E-CMF × 8 cycles or FEC × 8 cycles) (15).

Related cases

Postmastectomy radiotherapy—*Case Studies 18, 22, 23, 25, 26, 27, and 28*

Irradiation of implants—*Case Studies 18 and 23*

Adjuvant chemotherapy—*Case Studies 2, 6, 11, 36, and 37*

Learning Points

1. At the time of mastectomy, plastic surgeons may opt to place an expander prosthesis beneath the pectoralis major muscle. This allows for expansion of skin overlying the muscle, and autogenous tissue reconstruction is undertaken after completion of systemic chemotherapy and postmastectomy radiotherapy.
2. Clinical trials have shown that there is no difference in survival between patients receiving pre- and postoperative systemic chemotherapy. However, preoperative chemotherapy is routinely administered to patients with inflammatory or locally advanced breast cancers and those with large tumors who are eager for BCT (preoperative chemotherapy may shrink the tumor, thereby making it amenable to BCT).
3. A sentinel node biopsy is contraindicated in patients who present with clinically suspicious axillary nodes. These patients should undergo a standard axillary lymph node dissection. However, some patients will develop palpable axillary nodes (reactive lymph nodes) following core biopsy of the breast tumor, and sentinel node biopsy is feasible in these cases. Therefore, in any patient with a suspicious breast mass, the axilla should be carefully examined, and the status of the axillary lymph nodes (clinically suspicious or not) is documented prior to core biopsy.
4. There is some retrospective evidence to suggest that the taxanes primarily

benefit patients with HER2-positive, ER-negative tumors, although patients with HER2-negative, ER-negative tumors may also derive significant absolute gains in disease-free and overall survival from taxanes (16).

References

1. Recht A, Edge SB, Solin SJ, et al. Post-mastectomy radiotherapy: clinical practice guidelines of the American Society of Clinical Oncology. J Clin Oncol 2001; 19:1539–1569.
2. Vandeweyer E, Deraemaecker R. Radiation therapy after immediate breast reconstruction with implants. Plast Reconstr Surg 2000; 106:56–58.
3. Evans G, Schusterman MA, Kroll SS, et al. Reconstruction and the irradiated breast: is there a role for implants? Plast Reconstr Surg 1995; 96:1111–1115.
4. Constant CM, van Geel AN, Van der Holt B, et al. Morbidity of immediate breast reconstruction after mastectomy by subpectorally placed silicone prosthesis: the adverse effect of radiotherapy. Eur J Surg Oncol 2000; 26:344–350.
5. Spear SL, Onyewu C. Staged breast reconstruction with saline-filled implants in the irradiated breast: recent trends and therapeutic implications. Plast Reconstr Surg 2000; 105:930–942.
6. Behranwala KA, Dua RS, Ross GM, et al. The influence of radiotherapy on capsule formation and aesthetic outcome after immediate breast reconstruction using biodimensional anatomical expander implants. J Plast Reconstr Aesthet Surg 2006; 59:1043–1051.
7. Halpern J, McNeese MD, Kroll SS, et al. Irradiation of prosthetically augmented breasts: a retrospective on toxicity and cosmetic results. Int J Radiat Oncol Biol Phys 1991; 21:339–344.
8. Cordiero PG, Pusic AL, Disa JJ, et al. Irradiation after immediate tissue expander/implant breast reconstruction:outcomes, complications, aesthetic results and satisfaction among 156 patients. Plast Reconstr Surg 2004; 113:877–881.
9. Whitfield GA, Horan G, Irwin MS, et al. Comparison of the incidence of severe capsular contracture following implant-based immediate breast reconstruction with or without postoperative chest wall radiotherapy using 40 Gy in 15 fractions. Eur J Cancer 2007; 5(3):23 (abstr 74).
10. Kronowitz S. Delayed-immediate reconstruction in patients who might require postmastectomy radiation therapy. Miami Breast Cancer Conference, Orlando, Florida, 2008.
11. Henderson IC, Berry DA, Demetri GD, et al. Improved outcomes from adding sequential paclitaxel but not from escalating doxorubicin dose in an adjuvant chemotherapy regimen for patients with node positive primary breast cancer. J Clin Oncol 2003; 21:976–983.
12. Mamounas EP, Bryant J, Lembersky B, et al. Paclitaxel after doxorubicin plus cyclophosphamide as adjuvant chemotherapy for node-positive breast cancer: results from NSABP B-28. J Clin Oncol 2005; 23:3686–3696.
13. Martin M, Pienkowski T, Mackey J, et al. Adjuvant docetaxol for node positive breast cancer. N Engl J Med 2005; 352:2302–2313.
14. Roche H, Fumoleau P, Spielman M, et al. Sequential adjuvant epirubicin based and docetaxel chemotherapy for node positive breast cancer patients: The FNCLCC PACS01 trial. J Clin Oncol 2006; 24:5664–5671.
15. Ellis PA, Barrett-Lee PJ, Bloomfield D, et al. Preliminary results of the UK Taxotere as Adjuvant Chemotherapy (TACT) trial. Breast Cancer Res Treat 2007; 106:S21 (abstr 78).
16. Hayes DF, Thor AD, Dressler LG, et al. HER2 and response to paclitaxel in node positive breast cancer. N Engl J Med 2002; 357:1496–1506.

CASE STUDY 4

History

A 72-year-old woman presented with a two-week history of a nontender lump in the left breast. There was no associated nipple discharge, and the patient had no previous breast problems. She had undergone regular screening mammography without recall. There was no family history of breast or ovarian cancer, and the patient had three children (eldest aged 40 years). She had never used the oral contraceptive pill or hormone replacement therapy.

Clinical Findings

Examination revealed a firm irregular 2-cm lump in the upper outer quadrant of the left breast. The lump was relatively close to the nipple, and the patient had small breasts. There was no associated axillary lymphadenopathy (E4) (Fig. 18).

Clinical Assessment

Clinically suspicious lump in the left breast (borderline conservable).

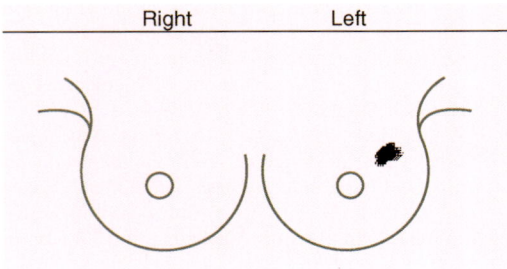

Figure 18

Investigations

Mammography

A spiculate opacity was seen in the upper outer quadrant of the left breast, which contained granular clustered microcalcification (R5) (Fig. 19A, B).

Breast Ultrasound

The palpable mass corresponded to a 12-mm isoechoic lesion without posterior enhancement or attenuation (Fig. 20A).

Core Biopsy

Ultrasound-guided core biopsy (16-gauge needle) confirmed the clinical and radiological impression of malignancy and showed an invasive ductal carcinoma (not graded, ER positive) (Fig. 20B) with papil-

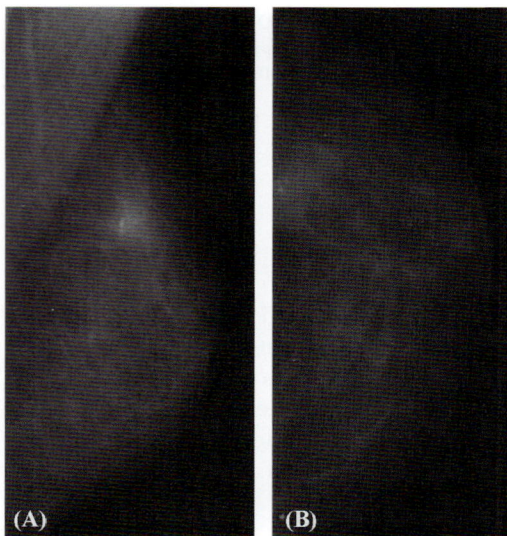

Figure 19

lary features (Fig. 20C). The lesion was borderline HER2 positive (Fig. 20D).

Diagnosis

Early-stage left breast cancer (T1N0)

Multidisciplinary Review 1

Following multidisciplinary discussion, it was recommended the patient undergo primary surgery with either wide local excision or mastectomy. The tumor was borderline conservable and surgical options should be discussed with the patient. It was unlikely that chest wall radiotherapy would be required in the event of mastectomy, and chemotherapy was a similarly improbable option (especially in view of the patient's age).

Treatment and Progress

The patient opted for mastectomy after fully informed consent that included discussion of issues such as the chance of further surgery after wide excision, cosmetic outcomes, the need for radiotherapy, and local recurrence rates. Despite her age, the patient expressed interest in immediate breast reconstruction and consulted with the plastic surgeons. She had relatively small breasts, and reconstruction with an implant-only-based technique was considered most appropriate in view of the patient's age and unlikely need for radiotherapy.

A left sentinel lymph node biopsy was undertaken in advance of definitive surgery and revealed no evidence of metastatic disease (3 nodes harvested) (Fig. 21). The patient proceeded with a left simple mastectomy (skin-sparing) via a periareolar incision. A subpectoral expander prosthesis was inserted at the time of extirpative surgery, and the patient was discharged home on the third postoperative day!

Definitive Histology

This revealed an invasive ductal carcinoma (grade II) measuring 12 mm in maximum

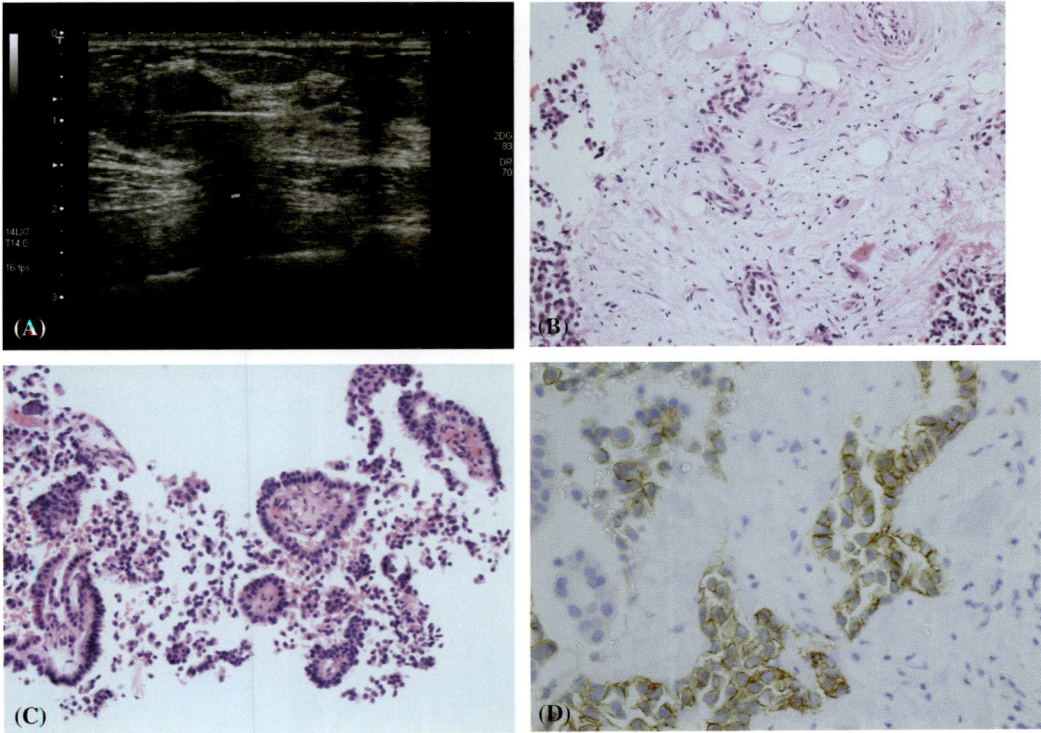

Figure 20

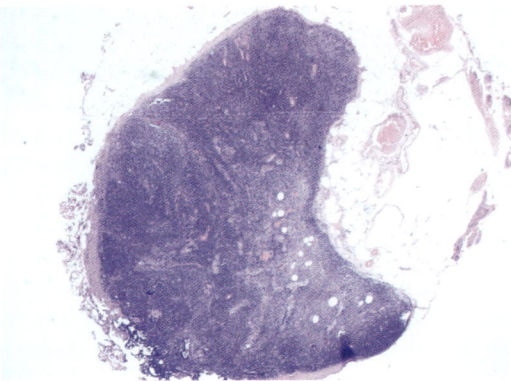

Figure 21

dimension (Fig. 22A, B). The tumor appeared to have arisen from a preexisting intracystic papillary carcinoma (Fig. 22C). There was no lymphovascular invasion and no in situ component.

Multidisciplinary Review 2

It was recommended that the patient initially be prescribed tamoxifen as adjuvant systemic hormonal therapy, and this might be switched to an aromatase inhibitor after two to three years in the light of emerging trial data.

Further Progress

The patient continued to make an excellent postoperative recovery and had adjustment of the implant size to achieve symmetry. She was reviewed annually in the clinic with follow-up contralateral mammography at two and four years postoperatively.

Discussion

This fit and active 72-year-old woman had a borderline conservable carcinoma of the left

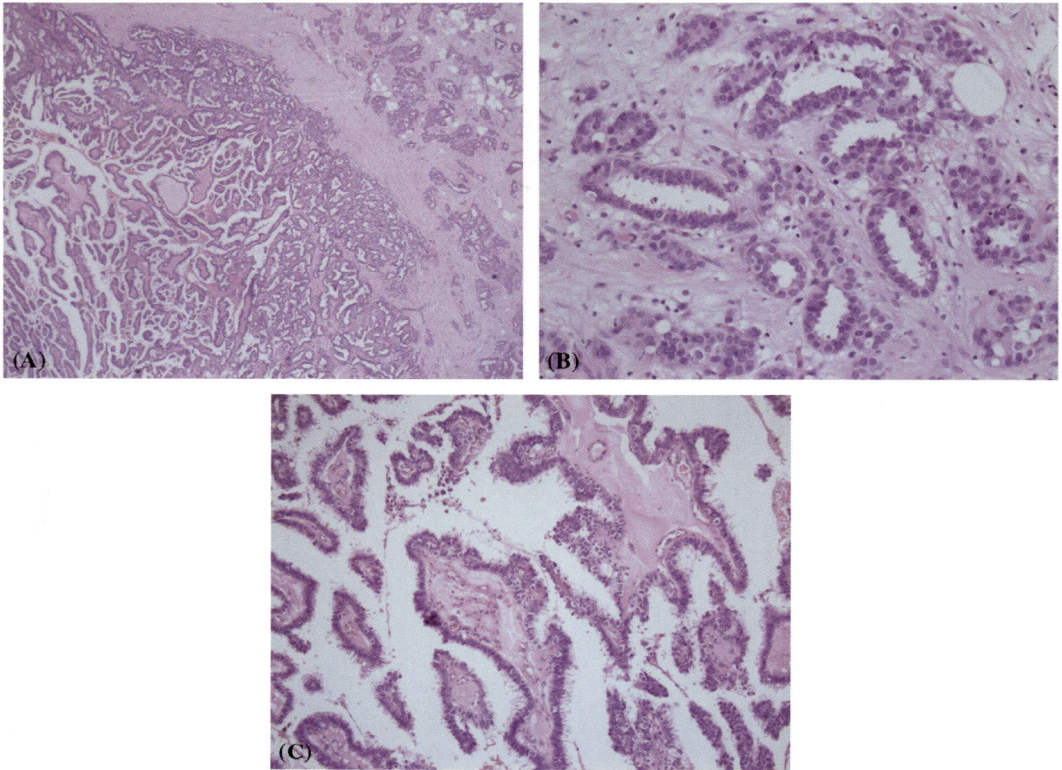

Figure 22

breast. Though the tumor measured only 12 mm on ultrasound (which corresponded exactly with the final pathological size), it lay relatively close to the nipple-areolar complex. Moreover, the patient had small breasts and was keen to avoid any second stage surgery (re-excision or completion mastectomy) and to minimize the chance of any local recurrence. After careful consideration she chose to undergo mastectomy with immediate breast reconstruction. Fortunately, her small breast size made her suitable for an implant-only-based technique. It is rather uncommon to offer reconstruction with autologous tissue transfer to patients over the age of 70 years, but there is no absolute upper age limit (1). It has been reported that older patients have a more attenuated and fragile chest wall musculature that can lead to increased rates of failure for reconstruction with a subpectoral

implant only (2). Furthermore, as this patient had a small non-high grade tumor, it was unlikely that chest wall radiotherapy would be indicated (3). Reconstruction with a sub-pectoral implant is usually avoided when radiotherapy is anticipated. Irradiation in these circumstances significantly increases the chance of capsular contracture and impairs the final cosmetic outcome. When chest wall radiotherapy is likely to be recommended, reconstruction with a latissimus dorsi flap and implant or an extended autologous latissimus dorsi flap is preferable. It is likely that this patient may have declined reconstruction had a relatively straightforward (implant only) procedure not been possible. She was discharged home on the third postoperative day and promptly resumed her regular daily activities including cycling! This patient had a low risk of relapse with an NPI of 3.24 [2 (grade II) + 1 (node negative) + 0.24]. She would have been ineligible for an aromatase inhibitor based on current unit guidelines for adjuvant hormonal therapy in hormonally responsive postmenopausal women.

This case illustrates the importance of patient choice in the decision-making process; some older patients will readily opt for mastectomy rather than breast-conserving surgery in order to reduce the chance of further surgery, local recurrence, and sometimes radiotherapy (to the breast). Within reason, patients should be managed according to physiological and not chronological age. The average life expectancy has increased and a fit 75-year-old woman may otherwise be expected to live for a further 10 years. Though restrictions may apply to chemotherapy and certain forms of reconstruction, older patients (>75 years) should otherwise be managed in a similar manner to their younger counterparts.

Related Cases

Immediate breast reconstruction—*Case Studies 3, 5, 18, 36, and 37*

Adjuvant hormonal therapy—*Case Studies 1, 2, 3, 9, 10, and 19*

Sentinel lymph node biopsy—*Case Studies 5, 7, 10, 11, 12, 13, 15, 16, 19, 24, 32, and 37*

Learning Points

1. A skin-sparing mastectomy involves removal of the breast and nipple-areolar complex, but leaves the skin overlying the breast intact. Breast reconstruction following skin-sparing mastectomy is associated with a better cosmetic outcome than reconstruction following standard mastectomy, which involves removal of the nipple-areolar complex, breast, and much of the overlying skin.

2. Although either tamoxifen or an aromatase inhibitor is appropriate endocrine agents in postmenopausal women with early-stage ER-positive tumors, the aromatase inhibitors have been gaining wider acceptance. The aromatase inhibitors are either administered alone for five years after surgery or in sequence with tamoxifen. Thus, patients can be switched to an aromatase inhibitor after two to three years of tamoxifen (completing a total of five years of endocrine therapy), or take five years of tamoxifen followed by five years of an aromatase inhibitor. The aromatase inhibitors are associated with an increased risk of fractures, osteoporosis, arthritis, and arthralgias.

References

1. Rosenqvist S, Sandelin K, Wickman M. Patients' psychological and cosmetic experience after immediate breast reconstruction. Eur J Surg Oncol 1996; 22:262–266.

2. Recht A, Edge SB, Solin SJ, et al. Post-mastectomy radiotherapy: clinical practice guidelines of the American Society of Clinical Oncology. J Clin Oncol 2001; 19:1539–1569.

3. Barreau-Pouhaer L, Le MG, Rietjens M, et al. Risk factors for failure of immediate breast reconstruction with prosthesis after mastectomy for breast cancer. Cancer 1992; 70:1145–1151.

CASE STUDY 5

History

A 58-year-old woman presented with a five-week history of a lump in the right breast. She reported no tenderness or nipple discharge and had undergone regular screening mammography since the age of 50 years and had never been recalled. There was otherwise no history of any previous breast investigations and no family history of breast or ovarian cancer. She gave birth to her only child at the relatively young age of 18 years and had never used any form of exogenous hormonal preparation.

Clinical Findings

Examination revealed a firm and rather ill-defined lump in the lower outer quadrant of the right breast, which was mobile with no tethering of the overlying skin. There was no axillary lymphadenopathy. The lump was relatively large (4 cm) and suspicious for malignancy (E4) (Fig. 23).

Clinical Assessment

The clinical impression was of a probable invasive carcinoma of the right breast

Investigations

Mammography

An irregular mass lesion was seen in the upper outer quadrant of the right breast

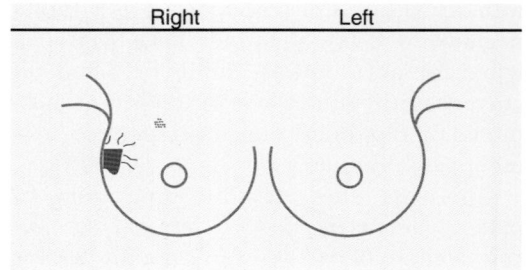

Figure 23

measuring 40 mm in maximum diameter (Fig. 24A, B). This contained fine granular cluster microcalcification that was not present on screening mammograms taken almost three years earlier.

Breast Ultrasound

The sonographic correlate of the mammographic abnormality was a hypoechoic mass lesion measuring 40 mm. The mass was heterogeneous and ill defined with a posterior

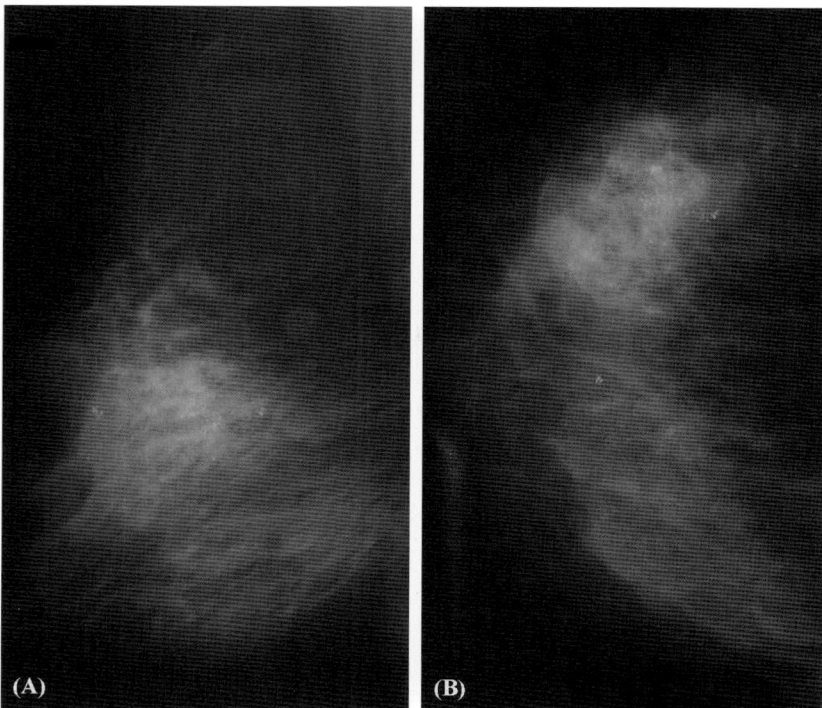

(A)   (B)

Figure 24

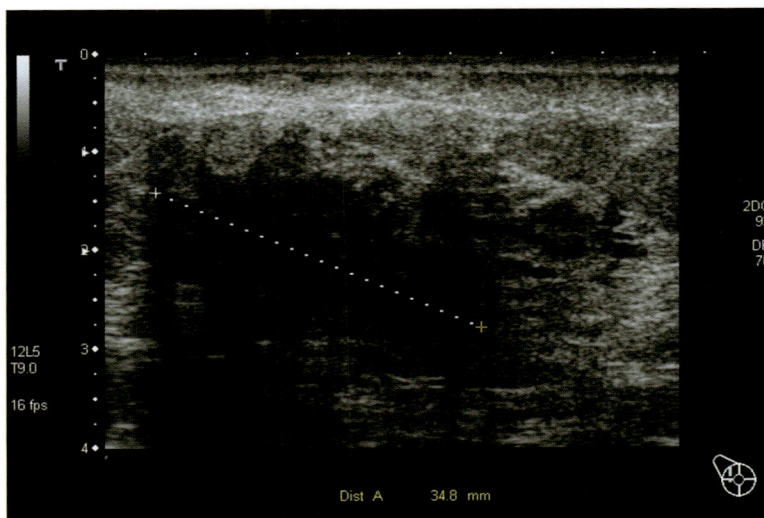

Figure 25

acoustic shadow highly suspicious for malignancy (U4) (Fig. 25).

Core Biopsy

Ultrasound-guided core biopsy of the right breast mass (16-gauge needle, 4 passes) revealed high nuclear grade DCIS only with no evidence of invasion (Fig. 26).

Diagnosis

Noninvasive cancer of the right breast presenting as a palpable mass (Tis).

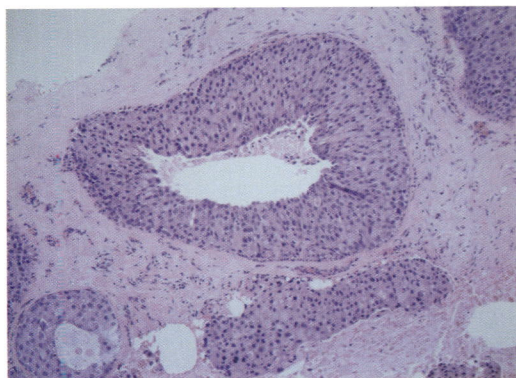

Figure 26

Multidisciplinary Review 1

The patient's mammogram was reviewed by the MDT team, and extensive microcalcification was noted in the right breast, which extended beyond the palpable mass and involved more than one quadrant. It was recommended that the patient undergo a right simple mastectomy with sentinel lymph node biopsy. It was commented that invasive cancer was likely to be found on definitive histology in the presence of a palpable mass. However, further core biopsies of the mass in an attempt to establish a preoperative diagnosis of invasion were not considered appropriate.

Treatment and Progress

Despite her age, the patient was keen to pursue immediate breast reconstruction and was referred to the plastic surgeons for discussion of reconstructive options. A right sentinel lymph node biopsy was undertaken in advance of mastectomy and reconstruction and revealed no evidence of tumor in any of the nine "sentinel" nodes removed (Fig. 27). The patient proceeded to definitive surgery approximately eight weeks after initial

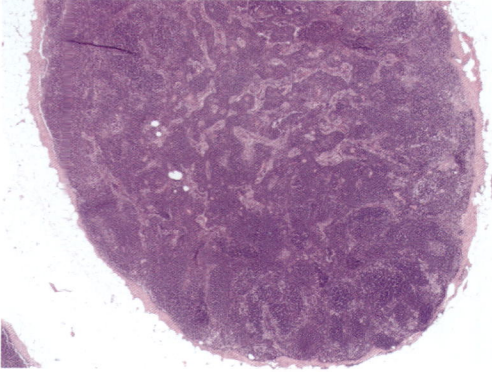

Figure 27

presentation to the breast unit. No further axillary surgery was indicated, and reconstruction was undertaken with a latissimus dorsi flap and implant. An extended periareolar incision was employed with a skin-sparing technique. The patient made an uneventful recovery and was discharged home on the sixth postoperative day.

Definitive Histology

This revealed extensive high nuclear grade DCIS measuring at least 50 mm with comedo necrosis (Fig. 28). There was no evidence of invasive tumor, and a single node within the axillary tail was normal.

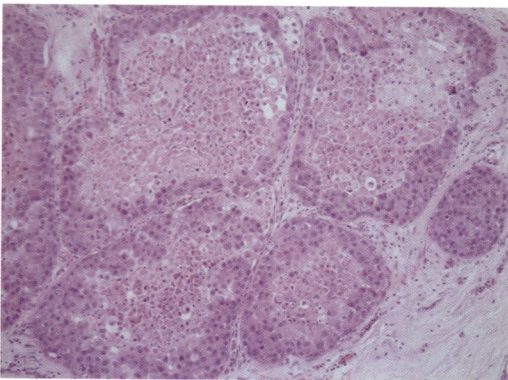

Figure 28

Multidisciplinary Review 2

In the absence of invasion, the patient had received a potentially curative treatment for DCIS and required no further treatment. She was offered entry into a patient-led follow-up program and would receive contralateral mammography at two and four years posttreatment.

Treatment and Progress

Despite initial satisfaction with the cosmetic results of immediate breast reconstruction, the patient became increasingly conscious of the disparity in size of the two breasts. She finally opted to undergo an implant exchange two years later with replacement of the original expander implant with a larger sized prosthesis to achieve better symmetry.

Discussion

Despite undergoing regular screening within the NHS Breast Screening Programme, this patient presented with an interval cancer that was not evident retrospectively (i.e., was not a missed cancer) on previous screening films. It is unusual for a symptomatic interval cancer to represent pure "DCIS" with no invasive component. Fewer than 5% of palpable cancers are exclusively DCIS, and suspicion of invasion may prompt a repeat core biopsy (1). Prior to sentinel lymph node biopsy, it was not appropriate to perform axillary dissection without histological confirmation of invasion (2). Sentinel node biopsy can be justified for extensive high nuclear grade DCIS, which mandates mastectomy and for a palpable mass (whatever type of breast surgery).

This patient had a mass lesion measuring 40 mm on both mammography and ultrasound. For cases of DCIS associated with calcification only, some surgeons would attempt wide excision for lesions of this size. However, even if adequate surgical clearance is achieved, these patients will require radiotherapy to the breast, which can impair the final cosmetic result. Moreover, there is a finite rate of local recurrence (<10% at 5 years), and half of these will be invasive disease. Therefore, the opportunity to "cure" a patient may be sacrificed when conservation surgery is chosen for in situ disease. For borderline cases, it may be preferable to undertake skin-sparing mastectomy via a periareolar incision with immediate breast reconstruction. This patient underwent sentinel lymph node biopsy in advance of definitive mastectomy and immediate breast reconstruction. A relatively large number of "sentinel" nodes (9 in total) were harvested at the time of surgery, but this was within the range that is commonly cited in the literature (1–10) (3). None of these contained metastases, which was consistent with the absence of invasion on definitive histology. In one of the author's own series of 33 patients undergoing mastectomy for extensive DCIS, 8 (27%) had invasive carcinoma on final histology. A total of four patients had a positive sentinel node (14%) of whom three had invasive disease with foci measuring between 1.5 and 12 mm (mean 5.5 mm). Despite intensive pathological examination, only a small focus of microinvasion (<1 mm) could be found in one of these node-positive cases who had extensive DCIS measuring in excess of 100 mm. There were no cases of metastases in the sentinel node without evidence of macro- or microinvasion on final pathology. Furthermore, all four node-positive cases involved a single node only (3 micrometastases, 1 micrometastasis).

It has been suggested that sentinel node biopsy for extensive DCIS could serve as a surrogate diagnostic test for invasion; if metastases are found in the sentinel node, there must be a focus of invasion somewhere in the breast (4). The chance of finding these very small areas of invasion depends on the thoroughness and diligence of the pathologist. Usually, such deposits can be found upon retrospective examination in those rare cases of node positivity for "pure" DCIS.

This patient required no systemic adjuvant hormonal therapy; in the absence of invasion (or nodal involvement), the recurrence risk at 5 to 10 years is approximately 1%. The risk of contralateral disease is 4% to 5% for DCIS and 2% to 3% for invasive breast cancer (1). Tamoxifen would act in a prophylactic capacity for the opposite breast but would yield minimal absolute benefit for the ipsilateral breast. A patient, therefore, has an accepted risk of at least 5% by not opting for bilateral prophylactic mastectomy.

Related Cases

DCIS—*Case Studies 5, 12, 13, 15, 16, 17, 18, and 21*

DCIS and sentinel lymph node biopsy—*Case Study 12*

Breast reconstruction—*Case Studies 3, 17, 18, 36, and 37*

Learning Points

1. Ductal carcinoma in situ (DCIS) is rarely palpable and generally presents as a mammographic finding. In countries where mammography screening is widely utilized, DCIS constitutes 8% to 25% of all breast cancer cases diagnosed annually. However, DCIS is much less commonly diagnosed in countries that do no have systematic mammography screening programs.

2. DCIS is generally treated with wide local excision and radiotherapy. Patients with ER-positive DCIS (the vast majority) are then usually treated with tamoxifen 20 mg/day for five years.

3. Axillary lymph node surgery is generally not indicated for DCIS. However, many surgeons advocate a sentinel node biopsy if a mastectomy is performed for DCIS. In such instances, an axillary assessment proves useful if invasive cancer is ultimately discovered in the mastectomy specimen. A mastectomy is indicated for multicentric DCIS (DCIS in more than one quadrant of the breast).

References

1. Hwang ES, Esserman LJ. Management of ductal carcinoma in situ. Surg Clin North Am 1999; 79(5): 1007–1030.
2. Winchester DP, Menck HR, Osteen RT, et al. Treatment trends for ductal carcinoma in situ of the breast. Ann Surg Oncol 1995; 2:207–213.
3. Benson JR, Querci della Rovere G. Management of the axilla in women with breast cancer. Lancet Oncol 2007; 8:331–348.
4. Cox CE, Nguyen K, Gray RJ, et al. Importance of lymphatic mapping in ductal carcinoma in situ (DCIS): Why map DCIS? Am Surg 2001; 67:513–519.

Part II: Breast Conservation Therapy

CASE STUDY 6

History

A 38-year-old woman presented with a two-week history of a nontender lump in the right breast. She reported no change in size of the lump and no associated nipple discharge. She had no previous breast problems and no family history of breast or ovarian cancer. The patient had two children (eldest aged 11 years) and had used the oral contraceptive pill briefly for a period of 18 months.

Clinical Findings

There was an area of focal nodularity in the upper inner quadrant of the right breast but no dominant lump was palpable. There was no axillary lymphadenopathy (E2) (Fig. 29).

Clinical Assessment

There were no clinically suspicious features on examination, and in particular no discrete lump was apparent. The area of focal nodularity was considered most likely to represent an area of fibrocystic change.

Investigations

Mammography

The mammographic interpretation of both breasts was normal but revealed dense breast parenchyma (Fig. 30A, B).

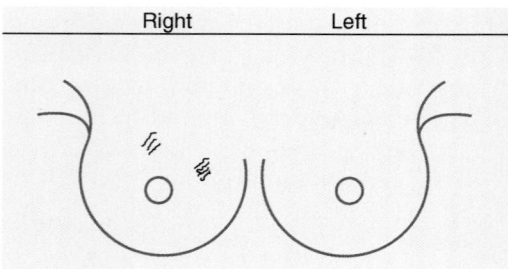

Figure 29

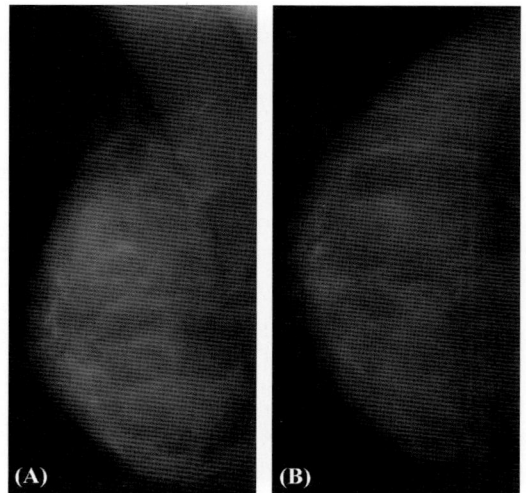

Figure 30

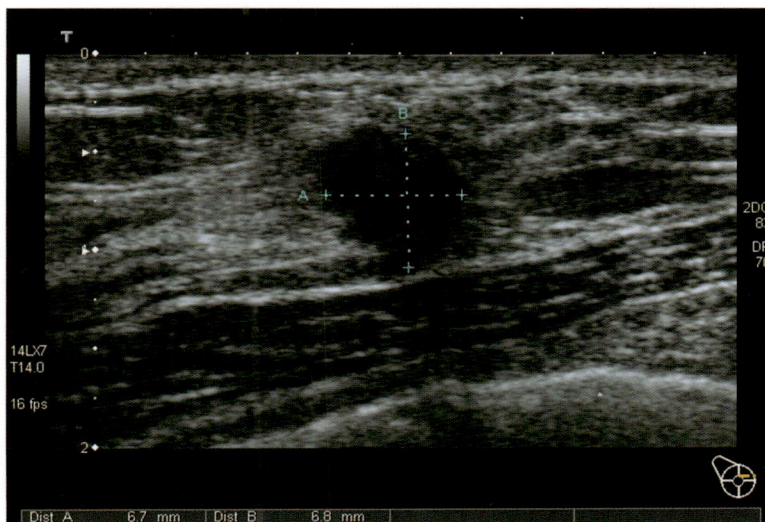

Figure 31

Breast Ultrasound

Ultrasound examination showed a focal mass lesion within the area of clinical nodularity measuring 8 mm in maximum diameter. The mass was ill defined and hypoechoic with posterior acoustic shadowing. The appearances were suggestive of a small carcinoma (U4) (Fig. 31).

Core Biopsy

Ultrasound-guided core biopsy of this small breast mass (16-gauge needle, 3 passes) confirmed an invasive ductal carcinoma (grade II, ER positive, HER2 negative) with associated intermediate nuclear grade DCIS of solid type [Fig. 32A (magnification 10×), B (magnification 20×)]. Routine ER measurements were not done on core biopsies at the time, and the axilla was not interrogated sonographically.

Diagnosis

Small early-stage cancer of the right breast (T1bN0)

Multidisciplinary Review 1

In view of the cancer being mammographically occult, it was recommended that further radiological evaluation be undertaken

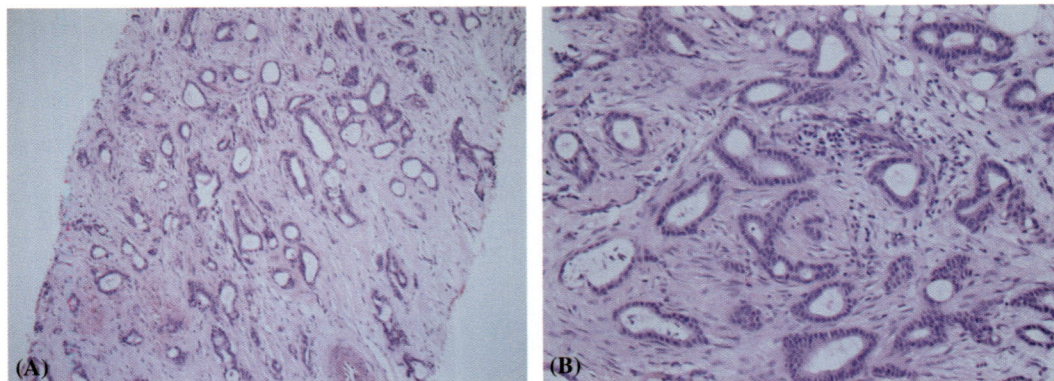

Figure 32

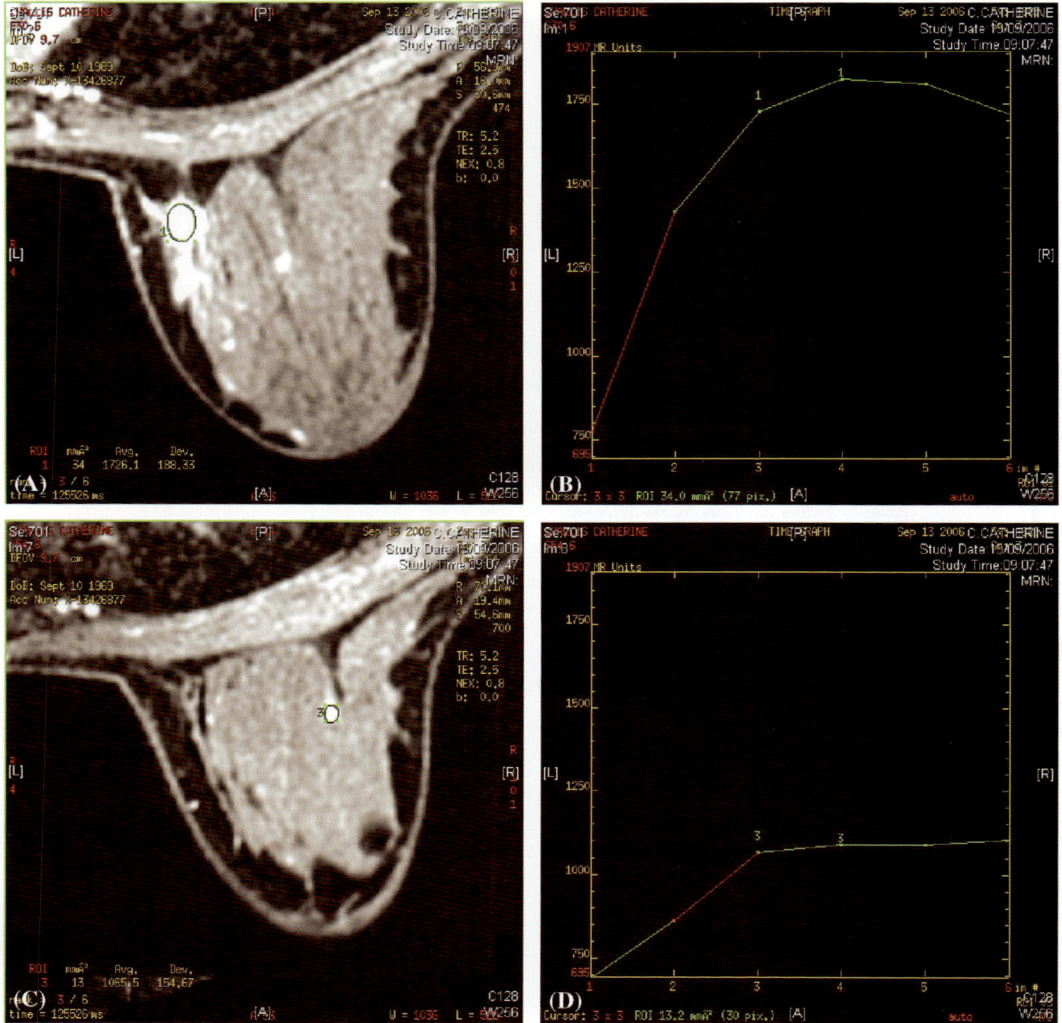

Figure 33

with MRI of the breasts. Should this confirm a unifocal lesion of the estimated dimensions, this would be amenable to wide local excision and sentinel lymph node biopsy.

Further Investigations

MRI Breasts

This confirmed a primary lesion measuring 10 mm in the upper inner quadrant of the right breast (Fig. 33A) with a time-intensity enhancement curve consistent with malignancy (Fig. 33B). A possible second tumor focus was seen inferior to the right nipple (Fig. 33C). The latter measured 6 mm and warranted tissue biopsy, though did not

display a malignant type enhancement curve (Fig. 33D). The patient was informed that in the event a second focus of malignancy was found, then mastectomy (+/− reconstruction) would be indicated.

Core Biopsy

Core biopsy of this second focal abnormality after ultrasound localization revealed a fibroadenoma only (Fig. 34A).

Treatment and Progress

The patient proceeded to a right wide local excision and sentinel node biopsy (no

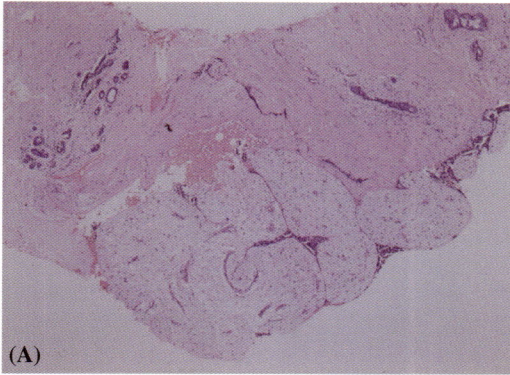

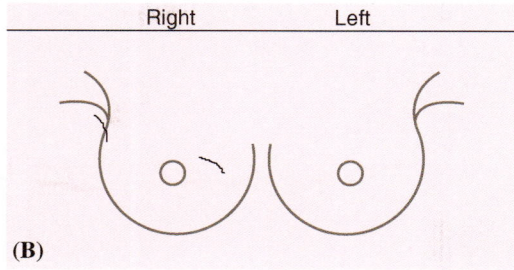

Figure 34

evidence of multifocality from second core biopsy result) (Fig. 34B). A preoperative skin marker was applied to assist surgical identification. A single hot and blue sentinel node was identified and removed. The patient made an uneventful recovery and was discharged home one day after surgery. She had a very good cosmetic result on subsequent follow-up at 12 months (Fig. 35A, B).

Definitive Histology

This confirmed an invasive ductal carcinoma (grade I) measuring 9 mm in maximum diameter [Fig. 36A (low power), B (high power)]. The tumor was excised with clear surgical margins (>5 mm), but the single sentinel lymph node retrieved contained a 6 mm macroscopic tumor deposit (Fig. 36C).

Multidisciplinary Review 2

Following multidisciplinary discussion, it was recommended that the patient undergo a

right completion axillary lymph node dissection. The final nodal status would inform the decision on systemic therapy. On the basis of a single node positive for macrometastasis and the patient's relatively young age, she would likely derive significant benefit from chemotherapy despite having a small (<1 cm) grade I tumor.

Treatment and Progress

The patient underwent a right completion axillary lymph node dissection four weeks after the initial surgery. She made an uneventful recovery and was discharged home the following day with a drain in situ. This was subsequently removed by the district nurse. Histology of the nonsentinel lymph nodes showed a further micrometastatic deposit in 1 out of 17 nodes giving an overall nodal status of 2 out of 18 (2/18) (Fig. 37). Despite further axillary surgery, the patient ultimately had a discrete scar in the right axilla (Fig. 38A, B).

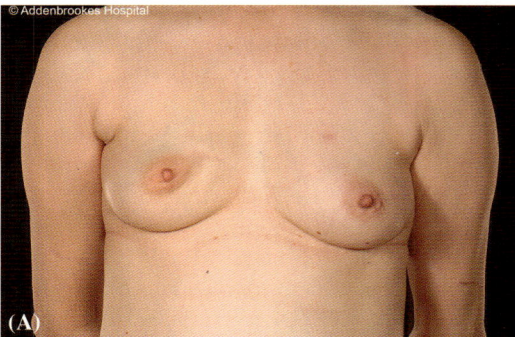

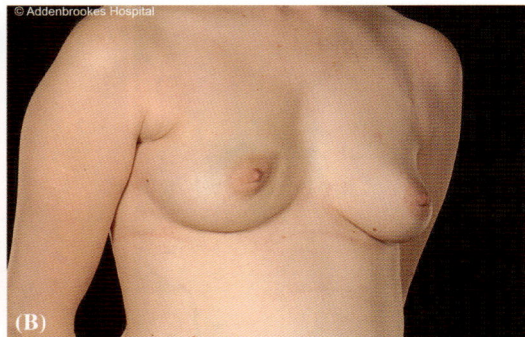

Figure 35

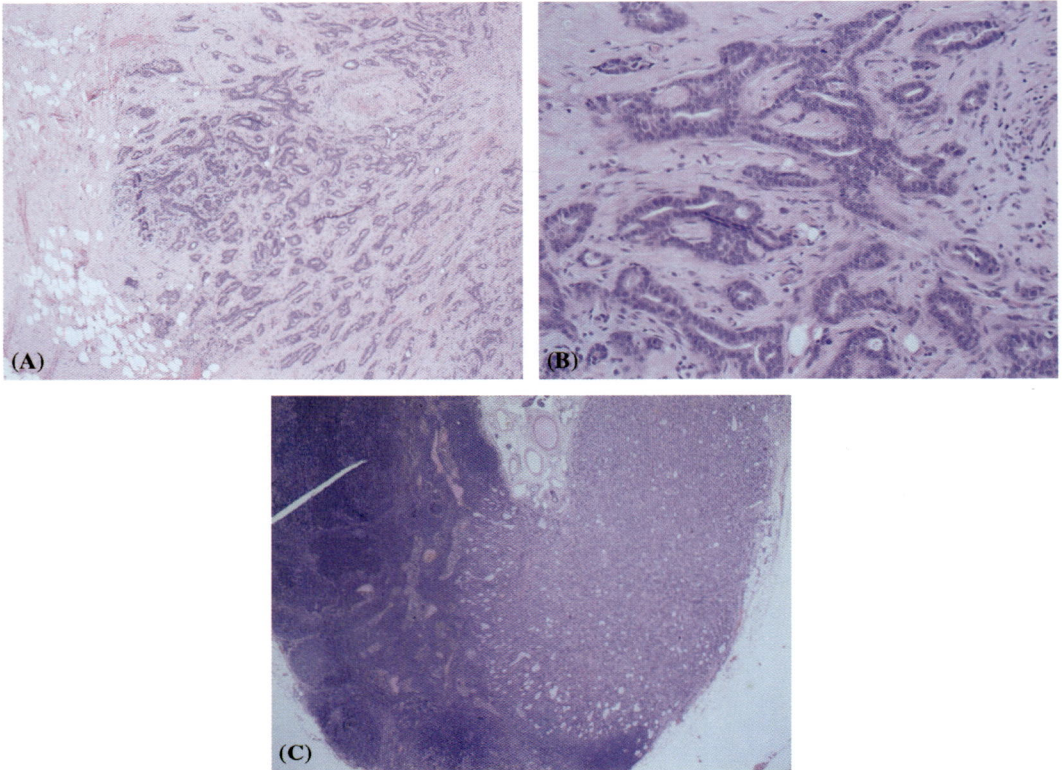

Figure 36

Multidisciplinary Review 3

Following further multidisciplinary review, the patient was offered adjuvant chemotherapy on the basis of an estimated absolute benefit of approximately 2% to 3% (adjuvantonline.

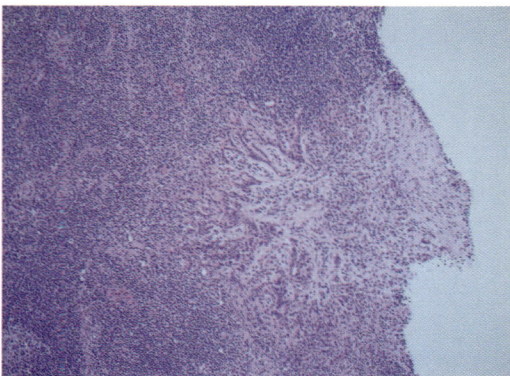

Figure 37

com). She was eligible for ovarian suppression, having a strongly ER-positive tumor with an Allred score of 8/8.

Treatment and Progress

The patient was initially reluctant to undergo a course of chemotherapy and considered the absolute benefits to be modest (2–3%). However, following further discussion and consideration of her age, she agreed to enter the TACT II trial that evaluates accelerated adjuvant chemotherapy with capecitabine in early breast cancer. Patients with operable disease are randomized to one of the following four arms: (*i*) four cycles of epirubicin (3 weekly) followed by four cycles of classical CMF, (*ii*) four cycles of epirubicin (2 weekly) with GCSF support followed by four cycles of classical

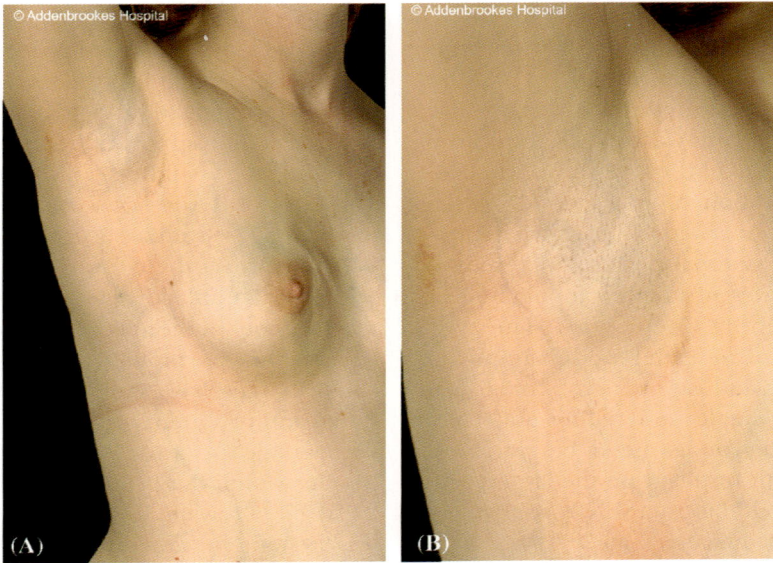

Figure 38

CMF, (*iii*) four cycles of epirubicin (3 weekly) followed by four cycles of oral capecitabine, and (*iv*) four cycles of epirubicin (2 weekly) with GCSF support followed by four cycles of oral capecitabine (see Appendix III). After completion of chemotherapy, the patient proceeded to ovarian suppression with a laparoscopic oophorectomy. She received tamoxifen (20 mg daily) as an additional component of adjuvant hormonal therapy. The patient received a standard schedule of radiotherapy to the right breast after completion of chemotherapy. This consisted of a total dose of 40 Gy delivered in 15 fractions over a three-week period. The patient remains well and disease-free at routine two-year follow-up.

Discussion

This patient presented with a clinically obscure lesion in the right breast, which manifest as an area of focal nodularity with no suspicious features (E2). Moreover, there was no mammographic correlate, and the tumor was initially detected on ultrasound assessment. MRI examination has greater sensitivity than mammography for imaging the breasts of younger women, which are more dense and can conceal a focal mass lesion mammographically. Benign lesions such as fibroadenomas can exhibit a "malignant-type" curve on MRI due to their intrinsic blood flow. This can generate false-positive results, which subsequently require biopsy to exclude a (further) focus of cancer. Nonetheless, MRI is very helpful in clarifying the extent of a tumor and confirming unifocality prior to breast-conservation surgery (1). It could be argued that ideally all such patients should undergo breast MRI that will also assess the contralateral breast (2). However, there is emerging evidence that breast cancer patients evaluated with MRI are more likely to undergo (unnecessary) mastectomy instead of BCS. Current rates of ipsilateral breast tumor recurrence (IBTR) are relatively low, and additional lesions detected by MRI might be adequately treated with adjuvant therapies (3).

An ultrasound-guided skin marker is a useful preoperative aid for lesions that have ill-defined margins clinically but that are just palpable and do not require formal wire localization. Care should be taken when placing scars in the upper inner quadrants of the breast; these should lie below the bra-line whenever possible and be curvilinear and follow the natural skin crease lines (Kreislers lines). Adequate subcutaneous tissue should be preserved to optimize the final cosmetic result and avoid an unsightly scar with an obvious depression.

Dual localization methods with both dye (Patent Blue) and isotope (technetium 99 nanocolloid, 20 MBq) permit more confident identification of the sentinel lymph node and are associated with a shorter learning curve and optimal performance indicators such as rates of identification (>90%) and false negativity (5–10%) (4). The average number of sentinel nodes removed using both dye and isotope is 2.9 to 3.0 (4). In theory, if a single node is hot and blue, then no further nodes need be retrieved. However, recent results from the largest sentinel lymph node biopsy (SLNB) trial reveal an overall false-negative rate of 9.8% with higher rates when only a single sentinel node is removed as opposed to two to three nodes (5). It is perhaps surprising that the sentinel node contained a macrometastatic deposit (6 mm) when the primary tumor was of such favorable size and grade. Moreover, one of the nonsentinel nodes contained a metastatic deposit yielding an overall status of 2/18 nodes positive. This together with the patient's relatively young age conferred a higher risk of distant relapse and increased the absolute benefits from chemotherapy in terms of mortality reduction. It was considered appropriate to complete axillary surgery prior to chemotherapy as this provided maximum information on nodal status (the patient would still be eligible for chemotherapy with a single sentinel node containing a macrometastasis). In circumstances where completion mastectomy with immediate breast reconstruction is indicated, further surgery can be deferred until after chemotherapy. Planning of breast reconstruction (particularly as a joint procedure with the plastic surgeons) can incur significant time delays (6–8 weeks). When patients are deemed at higher risk for distant metastases, it is preferable to commence chemotherapy as soon as possible after initial surgery. This can sometime render subsequent axillary surgery more difficult technically.

This patient had a strongly ER-positive tumor with a so-called Allred score of 8/8. The Allred system has been developed to more accurately define ER expression to predict response to endocrine treatments. Tumors are assigned an intensity score (1–3) and a frequency score (0–5), and ER levels are based on an aggregate score from 0 (no expression) to 8 (strong expression) (6). Ovarian ablation has long been known to improve outcomes in premenopausal women with hormonally responsive disease. Clinical trials have confirmed that proportional improvements in overall survival are comparable for ovarian ablation and chemotherapy within this group of women (24% vs. 27%) (7). Ovarian ablation appears to be of less benefit in women who have received chemotherapy (8%), which is most likely attributable to a "chemical castration." Menstrual activity is more likely to resume in women under the age of 40 years at the time of chemotherapy, and these women should be considered for ovarian suppression. Indeed, up to 80% of women under 35 years of age retain or regain menstrual function after chemotherapy compared with 30% of women over the age of 39 years (8). The latter is most commonly achieved by either laparoscopic oophorectomy or use of an LHRH receptor agonist. Surgical ablation causes an immediate fall in hormone levels, whereas LHRH agonists (and ovarian radiation) suppress ovarian function more gradually. An advantage of LHRH agonists is their potentially reversible effects upon cessation of treatment (2 years). This may allow subsequent conception that is increasingly an issue as more women are being diagnosed with breast cancer before they have started a family. There have been reports of the use of LHRH agonists concurrently with chemotherapy in patients under the age of 40 years in an attempt to preserve fertility (9).

Trials of LHRH agonists are currently seeking to answer two crucial questions (10–12):

1. Can LHRH agonists (with or without tamoxifen) provide an alternative to

chemotherapy in patients with ER-positive disease?

2. Do LHRH agonists confer any additional benefit when combined with standard treatment (surgery $+/-$ radiotherapy $+/-$ tamoxifen $+/-$ chemotherapy)?

A recent update of the GROCTA trial has confirmed that after more prolonged follow-up (median 12 years) the combination of tamoxifen and ovarian suppression is as effective as conventional CMF chemotherapy in premenopausal estrogen receptor–positive tumors. There was no statistically significant difference in progression-free or overall survival ($p = 0.7$), and multivariate analysis showed that neither tumor grade nor nodal status were independent predictors of recurrence and mortality (12).

The typical schedule for whole breast irradiation is delivery of a total dosage of 50 Gy over a period of five weeks in 25 daily fractions. Each fraction is 2 Gy and patients must attend Monday to Friday for a five-week period. This can represent a considerable burden for those patients with limited mobility and who live some distance from the radiotherapy center. In certain geographical locations, the latter can pose a significant problem (e.g., highlands of Scotland and parts of rural Australia). Accelerated hypofractionated whole breast irradiation (AHWBI) is being investigated as a means for reducing overall treatment times and making radiotherapy more readily available in some parts of the world. The principle of AHWBI is to deliver radiotherapy in fewer fractions of larger dosage. The standardization of breast radiotherapy (START) trial is investigating the use of larger fraction sizes (>2 Gy) and evaluates both efficacy and side effects (which may be greater with larger fraction sizes). One arm of this trial compares the standard regimen of 50 Gy in 25 fractions with a total dosage of 40 Gy delivered in 15 fractions over a three-week period. Despite an average fraction size of 2.67 Gy, rates of local control and late-normal tissue effects are similar to the standard regimen. The majority of patients within the Cambridge area now receive AHWBI with 40 Gy delivered over three weeks. This applies to both breast and chest wall irradiation. A radiation boost can be delivered to the tumor bed to minimize the chance of local recurrence (13,14).

Related Cases

Positive sentinel lymph node biopsy—*Case Studies 10, 11, 24, and 37*

Ovarian suppression—*Case Studies 1, 8, 23, 27, and 37*

Adjuvant chemotherapy—*Case Studies 1, 3, 8, 11, 36, and 37*

Preoperative MRI—*Case Studies 8, 24, and 37*

Breast radiotherapy—*Case Studies 8, 9, 10, 13, 14, 15, and 19*

Learning Points

1. The false-negative rate for mammography is about 10%. Lobular cancers, in particular, are often difficult to discern on mammography. Thus, a tissue diagnosis is warranted for any suspicious breast mass, even if the mammogram reported it as benign.

2. The use of breast MRI is increasing, but remains controversial. Recently, it has been suggested that a breast MRI should be obtained prior to surgery in all women with newly diagnosed breast cancers. MRI may reveal additional cancer foci in the ipsilateral or contralateral breast that are not evident on mammography and clinical examination. MRI may therefore result in an increase in mastectomy (and even bilateral mastectomy) rates. Yet, the clinical relevance of the additional lesions detected on MRI is not clear, and some have argued that these lesions could be adequately treated with radiotherapy and/or systemic therapy.

3. LHRH agonists can be used to induce ovarian suppression. In premenopausal women with ER-positive tumors, these agents reduce rates of recurrence and of death following relapse when administered together with tamoxifen, chemotherapy, or both.

References

1. DeMartini W, Lehman C, Partridge S. Breast MRI for cancer detection and characterization: a review of evidence-based clinical applications. Acad Radiol 2008; 15:408–416.
2. Warren R. Is breast MRI mature enough to be recommended for general use? Lancet 2001; 358:1745–1746.
3. Morrow M. Magnetic resonance imaging in the breast cancer patient: curb your enthusiasm. J Clin Oncol 2008; 26:352–353.
4. Lyman GH, Guiliano AE, Somerfield MR, et al. The Americal Society of Clinical Oncology Guideline Recommendations for sentinel lymph node biopsy in early stage breast cancer. J Clin Oncol 2005; 23:7703–7720.
5. Krag DN, Anderson SJ, Julian TB, et al. Technical outcomes of sentinel-lymph node resection and conventional axillary lymph node dissection in patients with clinically node negative breast cancer: results from the NSABP B-32 randomised phase III trial. Lancet Oncol 2007; 8:881–888.
6. Allred DC, Harvey JM, Berardo M, et al. Prognostic and predictive factors in breast cancer by immunohistochemical analysis. Mod Pathol 1998; 11:155–168.
7. Early Breast Cancer Trialists Collaborative Group. Ovarian ablation in early breast cancer: overview of the randomized trials. Lancet 1996; 348:1189–1196.
8. Petrek JA, Naughton MJ, Case LD, et al. Incidence, time course and determinants of menstrual bleeding after breast cancer treatment: a prospective study. J Clin Oncol 2006; 24:1045–1051.
9. Recchia F, Sica G, de Filippis S, et al. Ovarian protection with goserelin during chemotherapy for early breast cancer: long term results of a phase II study. Proc Am Soc Clin Oncol 2002; 21 (abstr 62).
10. Jakesz R, Hausmaninger H, Samonigg E, et al. Comparison of adjuvant therapy with tamoxifen and goserilin versus CMF in premenopausal stage I and II hormone responsive breast cancer patients: four-year results of Austrian Breast Cancer Study Group (ABCSG) Trial 5. Proc Am Soc Clin Oncol 1999; 18:67a (abstr 250).
11. Jakesz R, Hausmaninger H, Samonigg E, et al. Complete endocrine blockade with tamoxifen and goserelin is superior to CMF in the adjuvant treatment of premenopausal, lymph node positive and negative patients with hormone responsive breast cancer. Breast 2001; 10(suppl):S10 (abstr S26).
12. Boccardo F, Rubagotti P, Guglielmini D, et al. Ovarian suppression and tamoxifen as an alternative to chemotherapy in early breast cancer. Long term results of the GROCTA02 trial. Eur J Cancer 2007; 5:2.
13. Venables K, Winfield E, Deighton A, et al. The START trial—measurements in semi-anatomical breast and chest wall phantoms. Phys Med Biol 2001; 46:1937–1948.
14. The START trialists' Group. The UK Standardisation of Breast Radiotherapy (START) Trail A of radiotherapy hypofractionation for treatment of early breast cancer: a randomized trial. Lancet Oncol 2008; 9:331–41.

CASE STUDY 7

History

A 68-year-old woman was found to have an opacity in the lower inner quadrant of the left breast on routine screening mammography. The patient had undergone regular screening within the NHS Breast Screening Programme and had never been recalled. She had no family history of breast cancer and had four children (eldest aged 44 years). She had no significant usage of the oral contraceptive pill but had taken hormone replacement therapy for a total period of 14 years.

Clinical findings

Clinical examination was normal and revealed no discrete lumps or areas of focal nodularity in either breast (E1).

Clinical assessment

Screen-detected abnormality of the left breast in an asymptomatic patient

Investigations

Mammography (screening)

A rounded opacity associated with microcalcification was seen in the lower inner quadrant of the left breast (Fig. 39A, B), which was more evident on paddle and compression views (Fig. 39C, D).

Breast Ultrasound–

The sonographic correlate of this mammographic abnormality was an 11-mm hypoechoic lesion with the appearances of a small cancer (U5) (Fig. 40).

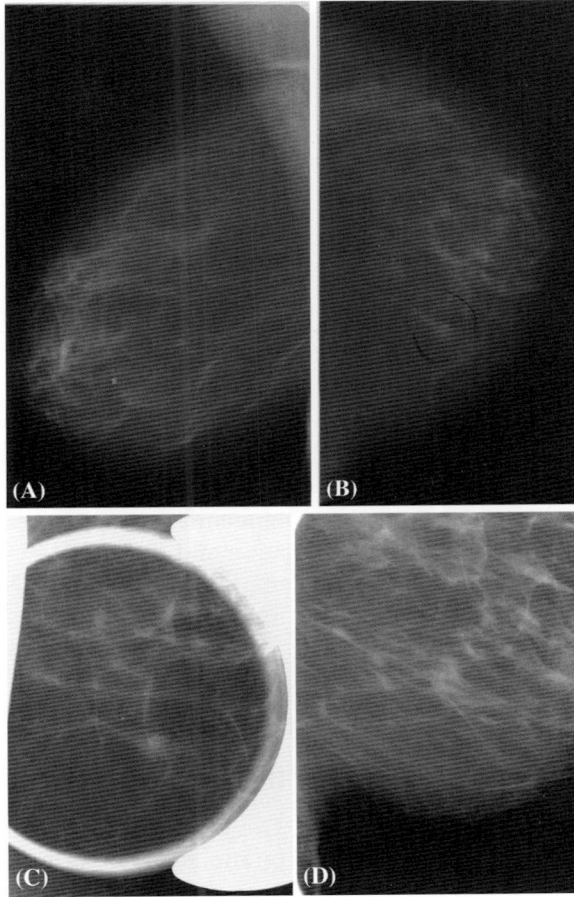

Figure 39

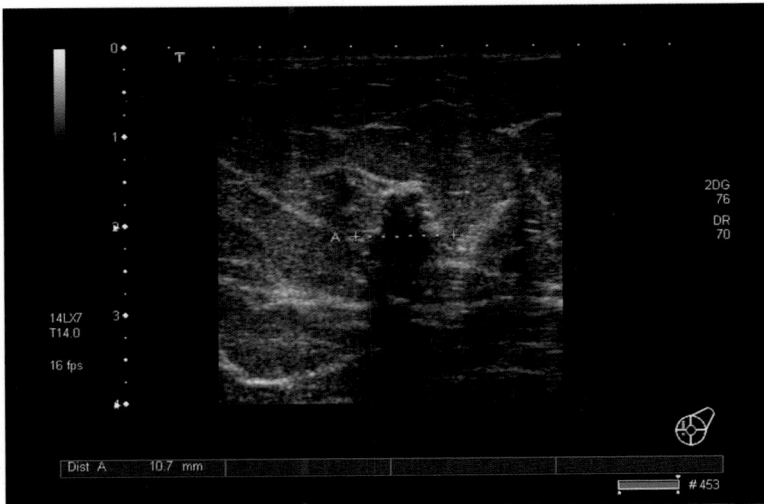

Figure 40

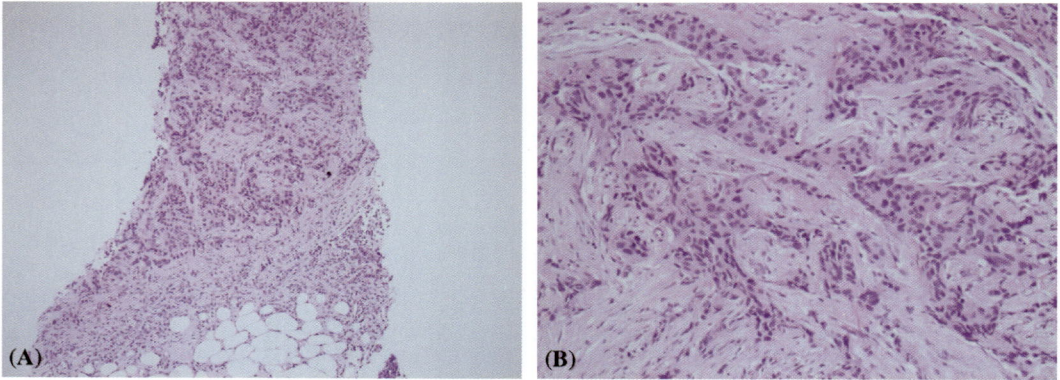

Figure 41

Core Biopsy–

Ultrasound-guided core biopsy confirmed an invasive carcinoma (grade II, ER positive) with no associated in situ component [Fig. 41A (low power), B (high power)].

Diagnosis

Screen-detected left breast cancer (T1N0)

Multidisciplinary Review 1

Following multidisciplinary review, it was recommended that the patient undergo a left guidewire localized wide local excision and sentinel lymph node biopsy.

Treatment and Progress

The decision of the multidisciplinary team was communicated to the patient who suffered from spinal stenosis with chronic back pain and restricted mobility. In particular, she was dependent on crutches and expressed some concern about any morbidity from sentinel lymph node biopsy. The patient was reassured that there is minimal morbidity from this form of targeted axillary sampling, and the likelihood of nodal involvement (necessitating subsequent axillary dissection) was very low. The patient proceeded to surgery one week later, having requested an early operation (Fig. 42). Two

blue and hot nodes were identified at operation and the lesion lay close to the anterior margin on specimen X ray, but appeared well clear of other margins radiologically.

The patient made an uneventful recovery and was discharged home on the second postoperative day.

Definitive Histology

This confirmed an invasive ductal carcinoma (grade III) measuring 8 mm in maximum diameter with associated high nuclear grade DCIS. The latter was of solid type with central necrosis and extended beyond the invasive component to yield an overall tumor diameter of 19 mm [Fig. 43A (low power); B (higher power)]. DCIS extended to within 1 mm of the superior margin (Fig. 43C) but was clear of all other radial margins by >5 mm. Lymphovascular space invasion was

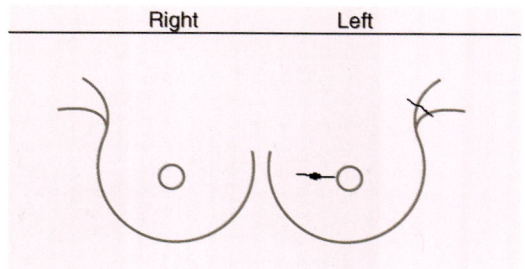

Figure 42

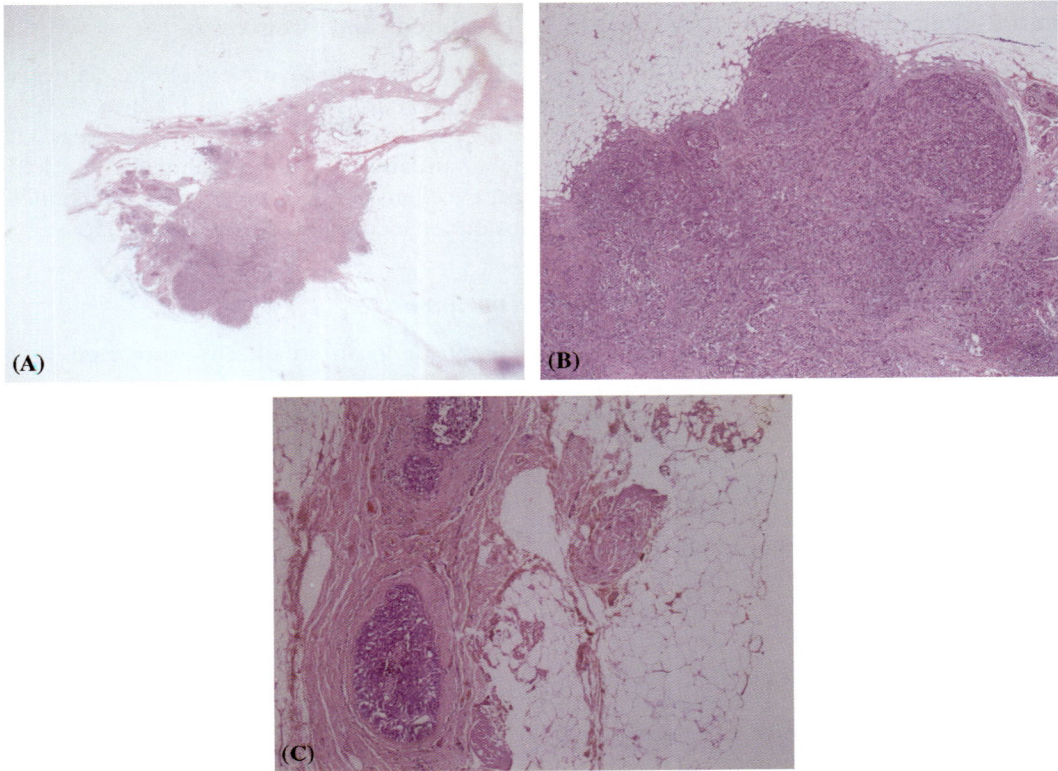

Figure 43

present but neither of the two sentinel nodes contained metastases.

Multidisciplinary Review 2

Following multidisciplinary review, it was recommended the patient undergo re-excision of the superior margin and thereafter receive radiotherapy to the breast and tamoxifen for five years as adjuvant systemic hormonal therapy.

Treatment and Progress

Further surgery was arranged within the next few days and a 2-cm thickness of tissue was re-excised from the superior margin of the surgical cavity. Histopathological evaluation revealed residual high–nuclear grade DCIS measuring 10 mm in maximum dimension and extending to the *new* superior margin (Fig. 44A, B).

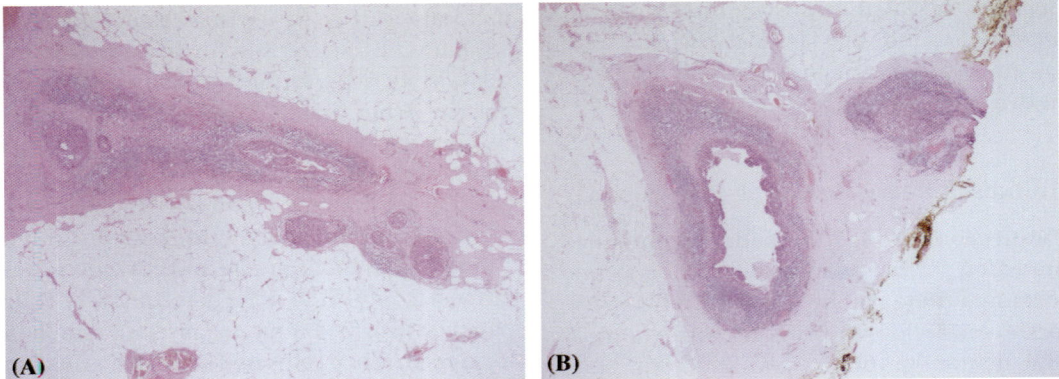

Figure 44

Multidisciplinary Review 3

In view of the DCIS being present at the new superior margin, further surgery was indicated. However, the aggregate diameter of the tumor (invasive and noninvasive) was less than 30 mm, and it was considered appropriate by members of the multidisciplinary team to offer further re-excision in the first instance. The patient should be warned that completion mastectomy may be necessary for adequate surgical management of the DCIS.

Treatment and Progress

The patient expressed concerns about the possible need for radiotherapy in the event of a further re-excision achieving satisfactory margins. The patient was specifically worried about lying flat on the radiotherapy table for any prolonged period of time. She visited the radiotherapy unit and discussed these issues in more detail with the oncology nurses. She found the prospect of radiotherapy very distressing and did not feel able to cope with a standard three-week course of radiotherapy. Furthermore, she wished to minimize her chances of any recurrent disease and therefore finally opted for a left completion mastectomy. This was carried out within the next 10 days and the patient was encouraged to mobilize as much as possible postoperatively.

Definitive Histology

Examination of the completion mastectomy specimen revealed extensive fibrosis and fat necrosis around the surgical cavity. There was no evidence of any residual DCIS or invasive malignancy.

Multidisciplinary Review 4

It was recommended the patient commence tamoxifen for five years as adjuvant systemic hormonal therapy. She was entered into the patient-led follow-up program with contralateral mammography at two and four years postoperatively.

Treatment and Progress

The patient made an excellent recovery from her final surgery and adjusted very well psychologically to loss of her breast. It was emphasized to the patient that she had an excellent prognosis with minimal chance of either locoregional or distant relapse.

Discussion

Despite a localized opacity associated with microcalcification on routine screening, this patient had extensive high–nuclear grade DCIS that was not evident radiologically. About one-quarter of invasive carcinomas have a coexistent in situ component that may extend beyond the limits of the invasive tumor (1,2). Where this has no clinical nor radiological correlate, attainment of clear surgical resection margins can be challenging. There has been lack of uniformity in definition of a positive resection margin and this in turn has compounded issues relating to microscopically negative margins and degrees of surgical clearance—how wide must a negative margin be to result in acceptable rates of local recurrence (3)? According to the NSABP protocol B-17 positivity implies tumor cells (invasive or in situ) present at the resection margin (4). Hence, negative margins could be associated with tumor cells at a distance of only 1 mm from the edge of the specimen. Many American surgeons consider a margin clearance of 2 to 3 mm to be appropriate and this echoes the view of the British Association of Surgical Oncologists. Approximately 30% of breast units in Europe strive for a radial margin clearance of 5 mm that can lead to re-excision rates of up to 50%. It is unusual to find further tumor when re-excision is performed to achieve a wider margin rather than a negative margin per se. By contrast, further disease will be found in about 40% to 50% of cases undergoing re-excision for "positive" margins. Singletary has provided a useful analysis; for patients with a 1-mm negative margin, local recurrence rates ranged from 0% to 7% (median 3%), while patients with a 2-mm negative margin had local recurrence rates of 3% to 10% (median 6%). However, those patients with margins that were just clear (no tumor cells within 1 microscopic field of the cut edge) had the lowest rates of local recurrence, ranging from 2% to 4% (median 2%). Thus although rates of recurrence are determined by negative margin status, no direct relationship exists between margin width and rates of local recurrence (5).

This patient had a small invasive carcinoma measuring only 8 mm in diameter, but associated in situ disease that extended well beyond the invasive component. The initial excision revealed an aggregate tumor diameter of 19 mm with in situ disease present within 1 mm of the superior margin (other radial margins >5 mm). This mandated re-excision, which confirmed further DCIS that extended to the new superior resection margin. When the first re-excision fails to achieve surgical clearance, mastectomy is often indicated. However, American guidelines for breast-conservation therapy state that mastectomy is indicated if margins remain positive after a "reasonable" number of surgical attempts (6). Second and third attempts are less common but may be considered acceptable if the breast has a satisfactory cosmetic appearance and the patient is keen to preserve her breast. In this particular case, the total extent of tumor (invasive + in situ) remained <30 mm, and it was once again the superior margin that was positive. DCIS could therefore still be confined to one area (quadrant) of the breast and a further re-excision of the superior margin could be offered. When re-excisions are undertaken they should be confined to the margins that are positive in order to minimize the amount of normal tissue that is excised.

Interestingly, the patient herself had strong views on her management and was closely involved in shared decision making. She was adamant that she could not tolerate lying flat on a radiotherapy couch and for this reason opted for mastectomy (to avoid radiotherapy). At an earlier stage in the clinical pathway, the patient had expressed a great abhorrence at the thought of mastectomy. However, her views and perspective had evolved with the pathological findings. It was perhaps fortunate that she was sentinel

node negative and did not requ tion axillary lymph node disse emphasizes the potential benefi node biopsy for patients with musculoskeletal comorbidities.

Though this patient ultimately underwent mastectomy, her long-term prognosis was excellent.

Related Cases

Re-excision after breast conserving surgery—*Case studies 11, 16, and 19*
Sentinel lymph node biopsy—*Case studies 5, 6, 7, 8, 10, 11, 12, 13, 15, 16, 24, 32, and 37*

Learning Points

1. Randomized clinical trials have shown that, in women over the age of 50, mammography screening reduces breast cancer mortality by about 25%. In younger women, the benefit of mammography screening is disputed.
2. If a patient with a screen-detected (nonpalpable) cancer opts for breast-conserving surgery, then needle localization is required. The radiologist localizes the breast lesion with a wire, and the surgeon excises a margin of breast tissue around it. A specimen mammogram is obtained (of the breast tissue and the wire within) to confirm that the screen-detected cancer has been excised.
3. There is considerable debate as to what constitutes an adequate margin of resection around a breast tumor at the microscopic level. To minimize the risk of local recurrence, many surgeons recommend at least a 2-mm margin around DCIS.
4. If a surgeon is not able to obtain clear margins after repeated attempts at excising the breast tumor, then mastectomy is indicated.

References

1. Salam S, Jader SN, Benson JR. Invasive breast carcinoma. In: Querci della Rovere G, Warren R, Benson JR, eds. Early Breast Cancer. London and New York: Taylor and Francis, 2006:286–318.

2. Holland R, Connolly JL, Gelman R, et al. The presence of an extensive intraductal component following a limited excision correlates with prominent residual disease in the remainder of the breast. J Clin Oncol 1990; 8:113–118.
3. Taghian A, Mohiuddin M, Jagsi R, et al. Current perceptions regarding surgical margin status after breast conserving therapy: results of a survey. Ann Surg 2005; 241:629–639.
4. Fisher ER, Costantino J, Fisher B, et al. Pathologic findings from the National Surgical Adjuvant Breast and Bowel Project. Protocol B-17. Cancer 1995; 75:1310–1319.
5. Singletary SE. Surgical margins in patients with early stage breast cancer treated with breast conservation therapy. Am J Surg 2002; 184:383–393.
6. Morrow M, Harris JR. Practice guidelines for breast conserving therapy in the management of invasive breast cancer. J Am Coll Surg 2007; 205:362–376.

CASE STUDY 8

History

A 35-year-old woman presented with a two-week history of a lump in the left breast. The lump had not changed in size and was non-tender with no associated nipple discharge. The patient had no previous problems and no family history of breast or ovarian cancer. She had two children (3 pregnancies) both of whom were breast-fed and gave birth to her first child at the age of 32 years. There had been brief usage of the oral contraceptive pill in the past prior to pregnancy.

Clinical Findings

There was a smooth, round mobile mass in the upper outer quadrant of the left breast measuring 3 cm in maximum diameter. This was clinically benign with no suspicious features (E2) (Fig. 45).

Clinical Assessment

Probable cyst or fibroadenoma of the left breast. There was no index of suspicion, and the patient was reassured accordingly following clinical assessment.

Investigations

Mammography

Bilateral mammography showed an ill-defined mass lesion in the superolateral aspect of the left breast. A possible smaller lesion was seen in the retroareolar region on the right side, but this disappeared on compression views (Fig. 46A, B).

Breast Ultrasound

The sonographic correlate of the mammographic opacity was an irregular hypoechoic lesion measuring 2.1 cm in maximum diameter, and this corresponded to the palpable abnormality (U5) (Fig. 47A). There was no evidence of enlarged axillary nodes on ultrasound assessment (Fig. 47B).

Breast MRI

An MRI examination was recommended to clarify the radiological extent of the left breast lesion that had the appearances of a carcinoma (R5). This confirmed a unifocal lesion in the upper outer quadrant of the left breast with slightly larger dimensions (2.7 cm) than the sonographic estimate (2.1 cm). No other significant lesions were identified in either the left or right breasts (Fig. 48).

Core Biopsy

Ultrasound-guided core biopsy (14-gauge needle) of the left breast mass confirmed

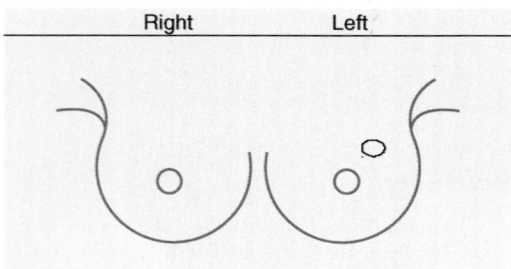

Figure 45

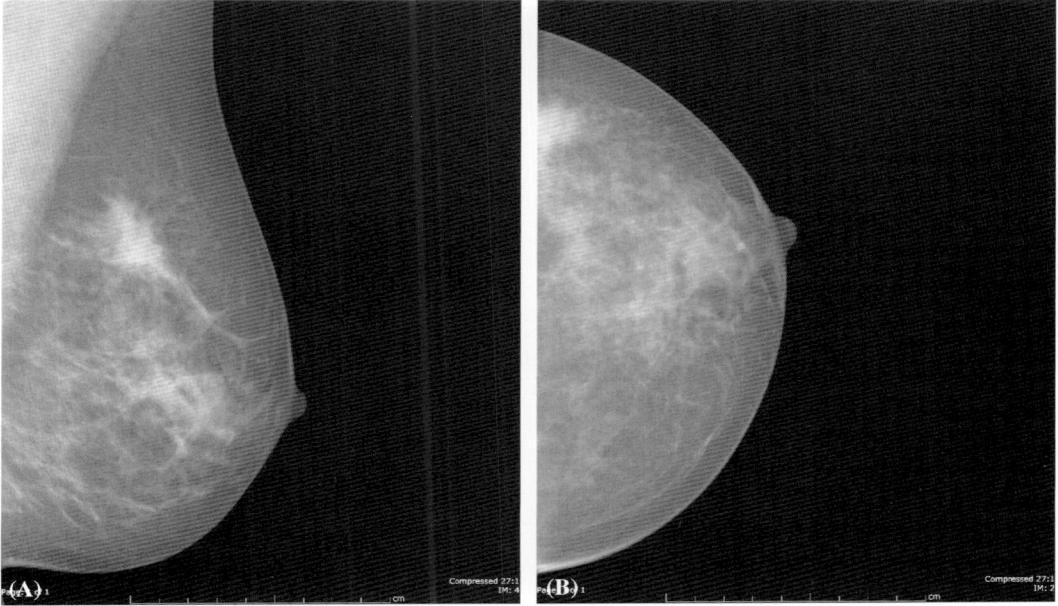

Figure 46

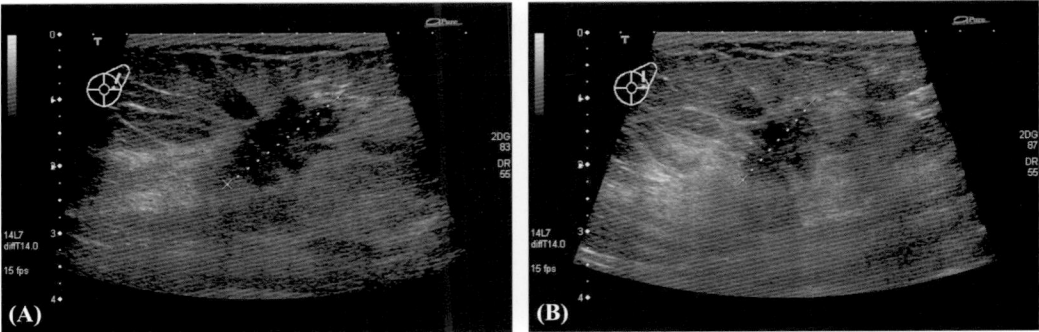

Figure 47

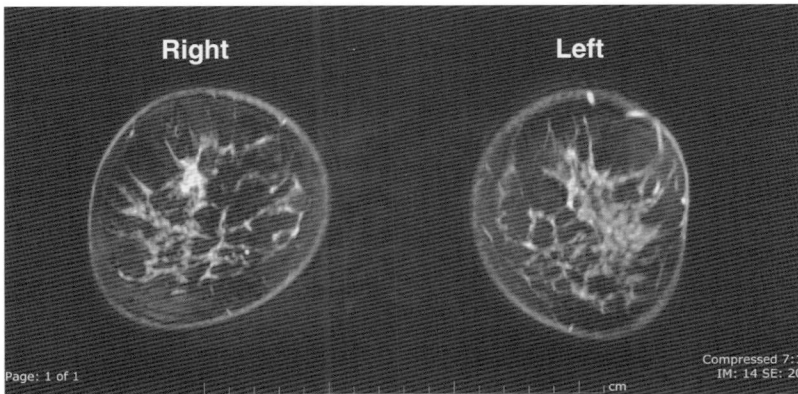

Figure 48

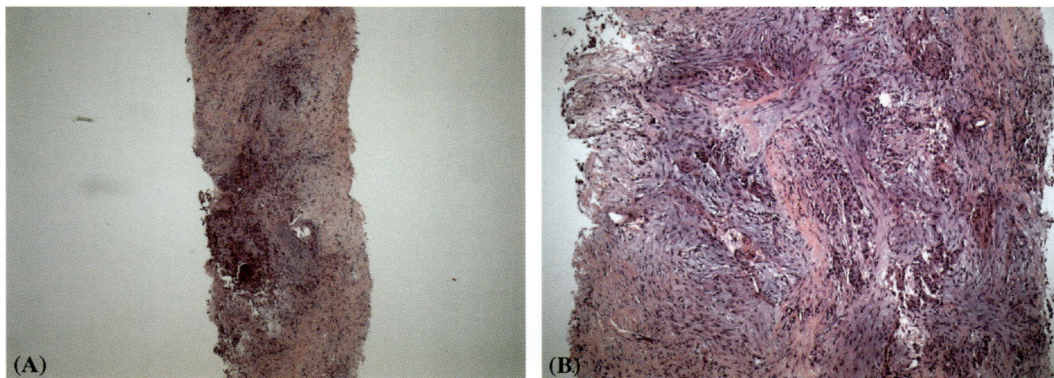

Figure 49

an invasive carcinoma (grade II, ER positive) with no in situ component seen. [Fig. 49A (low power), B (high power)].

Diagnosis

Early-stage left breast cancer (T2N0)

Multidisciplinary Review 1

The cancer in the upper outer quadrant of the left breast was considered amenable to breast-conservation surgery. It measured <3 cm in size, was more than 2 cm from the nipple-areolar complex, and there was no evidence of any satellite foci/multifocality on further interrogation with MRI examination. Moreover, in the absence of any sonographically suspicious nodes, it was appropriate to undertake node sampling in the first instance rather than formal axillary dissection. Radioisotope facilities were not available in the unit where surgery was to be carried out and therefore a blue dye–assisted node sampling (BDANS) was recommended rather than sentinel node biopsy with dual localization (dye and isotope).

Treatment and Progress

The patient underwent a quadrantic style resection with a radial incision and removal of a narrow ellipse of skin (Fig. 50). The BDANS was carried out through the lateral part of the incision (and not a separate axillary incision). Two large blue nodes

were identified together with several non-blue nodes, which were palpably suspicious and therefore removed. The patient made an uneventful recovery from surgery.

Definitive Histology

This revealed an invasive ductal carcinoma (grade III) measuring 30 mm in maximum diameter. There was associated high nuclear grade DCIS that did not extend beyond the invasive component and lymphovascular invasion was seen [Fig. 51A (magnification 20×)]. Tumor extended to the inferior margin, but a cavity shave was taken at the time of surgery (9-mm thickness) resulting in all radial margins being clear (≥5 mm)—indeed the minimal radial margin was 9 mm. Rather surprisingly, all six nodes sampled (blue and nonblue) contained metastatic carcinoma (macrometastases > 2 mm) yielding an NPI of $(0.2 \times 3.0) + 3 + 3 = 6.6$ (Fig. 51B).

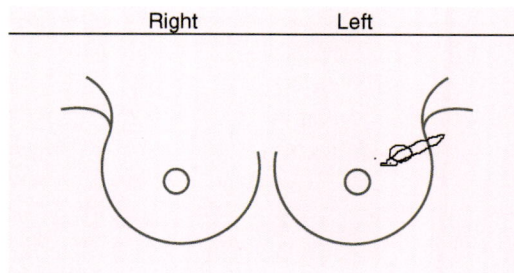

Figure 50

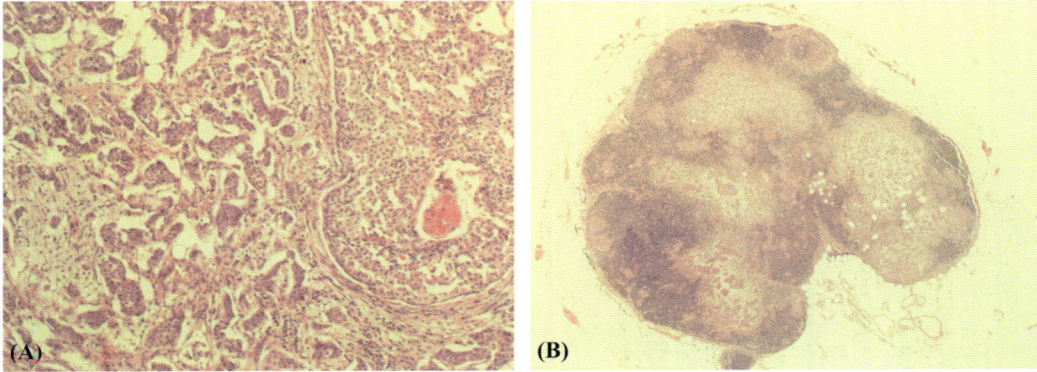

Figure 51

Multidisciplinary Review 2

Following multidisciplinary discussion, it was recommended that the patient undergo chemotherapy (taxane containing regimen) before completion axillary lymph node dissection. The patient would also require radiotherapy to the breast with a booster dose and irradiation of the supraclavicular fossa (≥ 4 nodes positive on sampling alone). Further systemic therapy would include ovarian suppression (oophorectomy or LHRH analogue) and tamoxifen. Additional investigations were requested including

1. Chest X-ray
2. Hepatic ultrasound—1.5 cm echogenic lesion in the right lobe with appearances of hemangioma (confirmed with triple-phase CT scan of the liver)
3. Isotope bone scan—no conclusive evidence of metastatic bone disease (Fig. 52).
4. HER2/neu status—positive

Treatment and Progress

The patient proceeded to chemotherapy with four cycles of epirubicin and cyclophosphamide (EC) followed by four cycles of docetaxel (see Appendix III). This was well tolerated and a completion axillary lymph node dissection was undertaken three weeks after the final cycle of taxane. Herceptin was commenced after second-stage axillary surgery and continued during radiotherapy to the breast and left supraclavicular fossa (40 Gy in 15 fractions over 3 weeks with a 9 Gy in 3 fraction boost to the tumor bed).

The patient's treatment program was completed with endocrine manipulation; she requested laparoscopic oophorectomy and this was carried out approximately 12 months from the time of the initial diagnosis of breast cancer. The patient was prescribed zoladex for an interim period of two months prior to surgical ablation of the ovaries. Tamoxifen was subsequently commenced for a period of five years (followed by letrozole for 2.5 years).

Discussion

This young woman presented with a clinically benign lump in the left breast, which was consistent with a cyst or fibroadenoma. However, triple assessment combining radiological imaging and biopsy with clinical examination revealed the lesion to be a cancer. The case demonstrates the important principle of triple assessment for the complete evaluation of a discrete breast lump; reliance cannot be placed on clinical findings alone (1). Same-day imaging and biopsy (one-stop clinic) ensues that significant delays are not incurred along the diagnostic pathway. It is inevitable that some patients will be falsely reassured immediately after the clinical assessment and subsequently be informed that the lesion has suspicious features on mammography and ultrasound, which are confirmed on biopsy. Phased information giving is useful in these circumstances

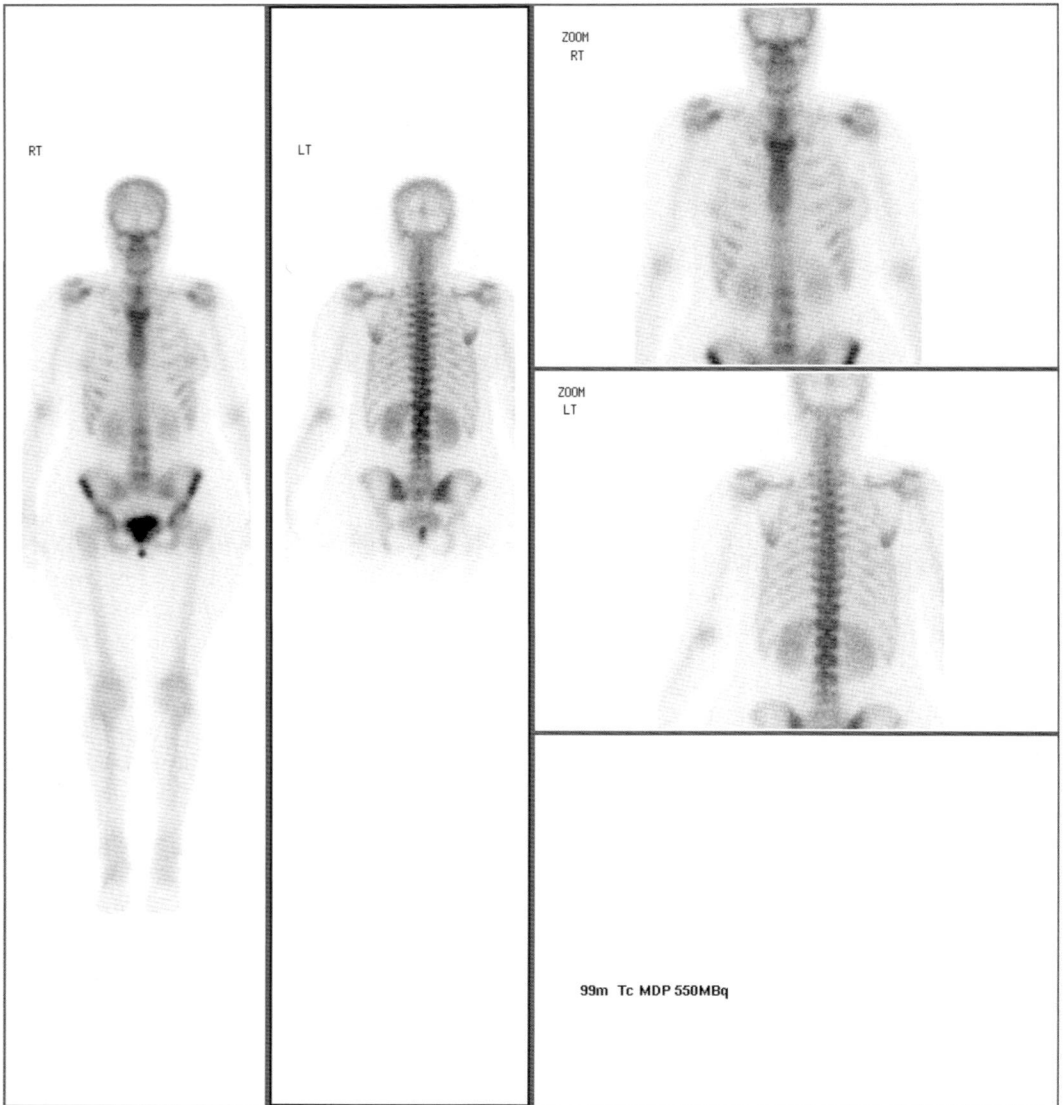

Figure 52

and is one advantage of the "two-stop" clinic when patients must return within a few days for the results of core biopsy.

In younger patients with relatively dense breast tissue, MRI is a useful adjunct radiologically to confirm unifocality and exclude any additional foci of tumor either in the same or a different quadrant (2,3). The latter would normally mandate mastectomy but breast conservation may be feasible when satellite lesions are present in the vicinity of the index lesion and are confined to one quadrant of the breast. MRI examination also has an important role in screening the contralateral breast, though there is no convincing evidence that any "earlier" detection of recurrence has any impact on overall survival (4). In particular, younger women may opt for a prophylactic procedure when there is evidence of any proliferative changes in the other breast. Between 4% and 8% of women with recently diagnosed breast cancer will be found to have an unsuspected occult cancer in the contralateral breast.

Some clinicians have advocated MRI examination in all (younger) women in whom breast-conservation surgery is comtemplated. However, this mode of investigation can generate false-positive results, and a degree of "over call" may have inadvertently increased rates of mastectomy in recent years. A recent analysis of local recurrence rates at eight years among breast-conservation patients with or without preoperative MRI imaging revealed minimal differences—3% and 4%, respectively (5). Indeed, with modern methods of breast surgery and radiotherapy, rates of local recurrence are already <5% at 10 years.

This patient underwent a quadrantic style resection with a single radial incision. This can produce excellent cosmetic results for tumors located in the upper outer quadrant and allows the cancer to be removed in continuity with the lymphatic vessels and axillary lymph nodes (intervening tissue between tumor and nodes is removed). This technique is best suited to small/moderate-sized breasts in which the distance between the tumor and axilla is not excessive. Scar contracture can sometimes compromise the final cosmetic outcome following breast irradiation. Despite a high tumor load, preoperative axillary ultrasound failed to identify any suspicious nodes that warranted biopsy. Axillary ultrasound (+/− core biopsy or fine-needle aspiration cytology) has been shown to identify up to 50% of node-positive cases (with macrometastases) overall and 75% to 90% of those with ≥3 nodes positive (6). This can potentially avoid two-stage axillary surgery in a substantial number of cases. Those patients with a "negative" axillary ultrasound examination can proceed to sentinel lymph node biopsy, though an axillary dissection is probably advisable for patients with tumors >5 cm in size (even when undergoing primary systemic therapy with potential downstaging of nodal status).

The optimal method for staging the axilla is sentinel lymph node biopsy using dual localization techniques (7). The use of technetium[99] requires a special ARSAC license that is not possessed by all breast units within the United Kingdom. This had limited the use of radiocolloid as a tracer agent for sentinel lymph node biopsy. The use of BDANS has evolved from the original blind sampling technique and permits a degree of targeting that reduces the chance of a false-negative result. With the technique of BDNAS, the surgeon aims to remove four to five nodes as opposed to two to three nodes. Clearly, this is a matter of degree and some surgeons routinely perform "sentinel lymph node biopsy" using blue dye alone (8,9). Techniques for axillary staging remain variable and standardization of methodology is ongoing. Axillary relapse rates of 0.12% among a group of more than 2000 sentinel node-negative patients have been reported by the Memorial Sloan-Kettering group at three years follow-up (10). Other reports involve smaller numbers of patients but reveal comparably low rates of axillary relapse varying between 0% or 1.4% with relatively short follow-up periods of less than two years. It is essential that rates of axillary relapse following sentinel lymph node biopsy for node-negative disease do not exceed those for axillary lymph node dissection that is the "gold standard" for axillary management (0.8–2.5%). However, A recent short communication reveals an actual recurrence rate of 5% at a median follow-up of 6.5 years with a prediction that up to 10% of patients may ultimately develop isolated axillary recurrence after a negative sentinel lymph node biopsy (11). Any residual disease within the axillary nodes will be low volume, and a longer follow-up period may be required for clinical manifestation.

Completion axillary dissection was carried out following chemotherapy; this patient was at high risk for distant relapse and likely to have micrometastatic disease at presentation. Commencement of adjuvant systemic therapy was therefore considered a priority. It was already confirmed that >4 axillary nodes were involved histologically, and knowledge of any additional nodal disease would not have altered adjuvant therapies (e.g., chemotherapy or radiotherapy to the supraclavicular fossa). In circumstances where axillary staging has shown macro- or micrometastatic disease in a single node, then complete information on nodal status from axillary dissection may be desirable prior to planning further management. This patient received an anthracycline-containing regimen with the addition of taxanes based on the extent of nodal involvement (≥ 4 nodes positive) and positive HER2 status. This was a modified regimen similar to four cycles of doxorubicin and cyclophosphamide followed by four cycles of paclitaxel (AC—paclitaxel rather than EC—docetaxel), which is a more widely used combination based on results of the CALGB 9344 and NSAPB B28 trials (12,13).

Ovarian suppression is usually offered to premenopausal women with hormone-sensitive tumors (irrespective of age and menstrual activity postchemotherapy) (14). The additional benefits of ovarian ablation in absolute terms remains controversial, and there are concerns about the longer-term sequelae of estrogen deprivation in younger women (15). The SOFT study specifically investigates whether the combination of ovarian ablation with chemotherapy in premenopausal women offers any additional benefit to chemotherapy alone. This patient was adamant about laparoscopic oophorectomy and was fortunate to have completed her family; for those premenopausal women diagnosed with breast cancer prior to conception, LHRH analogues offer an alternative form of ovarian suppression that may preserve fertility (16). Once rendered postmenopausal, patients can be prescribed aromatase inhibitors as adjuvant systemic hormonal therapy. The current policy of the Cambridge Breast Unit is to commence treatment with tamoxifen for two to three years with an early switch to an aromatase inhibitor (arimidex or exemestane) for patients at moderate risk (NPI ≥ 4.4). Some units use an aromatase inhibitor upfront in patients considered to be at high risk of locoregional relapse on the basis of primary tumor parameters and nodal status.

Herceptin was commenced after completion of chemotherapy. There can be potential compound toxicity from Herceptin and anthracyclines with no clear difference in oncological efficacy between concomitant and sequential regimens.

Related Cases

Fertility issues—*Case Studies 23, 27, 35, and 37*

Adjuvant hormonal therapy—*Case Studies 1, 9, 10, 15, and 19*

Herceptin—*Case Studies 11 and 26*

Breast-conservation surgery—*Case Studies 6, 7, 9, 14, 15, and 19*

Adjuvant chemotherapy—*Case Studies 2, 3, 11, 36, and 37*

Learning Points

1. Sentinel nodes are identified using either blue dye and/or radioactive colloid. Additionally, any nodes that appear clinically suspicious should be removed and submitted for histological assessment.
2. The status of the sentinel nodes might also be determined intraoperatively, using either touch prep (cytology) or frozen section. If either indicates the presence of metastatic disease in the sentinel node, then an axillary dissection should be undertaken at the time of the sentinel node biopsy. However, intraoperative assessment is occasionally associated with false-negative results. Thus, a second procedure (delayed axillary dissection) would be required if intraoperative assessment reveals no evidence of metastasis in the sentinel node, but metastasis is uncovered on permanent histology.
3. Patients with breast cancer in which HER2 is amplified or overexpressed will benefit from adjuvant trastuzumab (Herceptin) and chemotherapy. Clinical trials indicate that Herceptin reduces the risk of recurrence in these patients by about 50%.

References

1. Scott S, Morrow M. Breast cancer–making the diagnosis. Surg Clin North Am 1999; 79:991–1005.
2. Kumar NA, Schnall MD. MR imaging: its current and potential utility in the diagnosis and management of breast cancer. Magn Reson Imaging Clin N Am 2000; 8:715–728.
3. Mumtaz H, Hall-Craggs MA, Davidson T, et al. Staging of symptomatic primary breast cancer with MR imaging. Am J Roentgenol 1997; 169:417–424.

4. Lehman CD, Gatsonis C, Kuhl CK, et al. MRI evaluation of the contralateral breast in women with recently diagnosed breast cancer. N Engl J Med 2007; 356:1295–1303.

5. Solin L, Orel S, Hwang W, et al. The relationship of breast magnetic resonance imaging to outcome after breast conserving treatment with radiation for women with early stage invasive breast carcinoma or ductal carcinoma in situ. J Clin Oncol 2008; 26:386–391.

6. MacMillan RD, Blamey RW. The case for axillary sampling. Adv Breast Cancer 2004; 1:9–10.

7. Lyman GH, Guiliano AE, Somerfield MR, et al. The American Society of Clinical Oncology Guideline Recommendations for sentinel lymph node biopsy in early stage breast cancer. J Clin Oncol 2005; 23:7703–7720.

8. Purushotham AD, MacMillan RD, Wishart G. Advances in axillary surgery for breast cancer—time for a tailored approach. Eur J Surg Oncol 2005; 31:929–931.

9. Benson JR, Querci della Rovere G. Management of the axilla in women with breast cancer. Lancet Oncol 2007; 8:331–348.

10. Naik AM, Fey J, Gemignani M, et al. The risk of axillary relapse after sentinel lymph node biopsy for breast cancer is comparable with that of axillary lymph node dissection. Ann Surg 2004; 240:462–471.

11. Kujit GP, Roumen RMH. Second thoughts on sentinel lymph node biopsy in node negative breast cancer. Br J Surg 2008; 95:310–311.

12. Henderson IC, Berry DA, Demetri GD, et al. Improved outcomes from adding sequential paclitaxel but not from escalating doxorubicin dose in an adjuvant chemotherapy regimen for patients with node positive primary breast cancer. J Clin Oncol 2003; 21:976–983.

13. Mamounas EP, Bryant J, Lembersky BC, et al. Paclitaxel (T) following doxorubicin/cyclophosphamide (AC) as adjuvant chemotherapy for node positive breast cancer: results from NSABP B-28. Proc Am Soc Clin Oncol 2003; 22: (abstr 12).

14. Early Breast Cancer Trialists Collaborative Group. Ovarian ablation in early breast cancer: overview of the randomized trials. Lancet 1996; 348:1189–1196.

15. Davidson N, O'Neill A, Vukov A, et al. Effect of chemohormonal therapy in premenopausal, node positive, receptor positive breast cancer: an Eastern Cooperative Oncology Group phase III Intergroup trial (E5188 INT-0101). Breast 1999; 8:232–233.

16. Recchia F, Sica G, de Filippis S, et al. Ovarian protection with goserilin during chemotherapy for early breast cancer: long term results of a phase II study. Proc Am Soc Clin Oncol 2002; 21: (abstr 62).

CASE STUDY 9

History

A 60-year-old woman presented with a three-week history of a nontender lump in the left breast. The patient had undergone a normal screening mammogram two years earlier. She had no family history of breast cancer and had never used any form of exogenous hormones.

Clinical Findings

A rather hard discrete lump was palpable immediately superior to the left nipple-areolar complex. This measured approximately 1 cm and was associated with subtle skin tethering but no indrawing of the nipple. There was no axillary lymphadenopathy (E4) (Fig. 53)

Clinical Assessment

The clinical findings were suggestive of a small cancer of the left breast lying in close proximity to the nipple.

Investigations

Mammography

No focal mass lesion or any other abnormality could be seen in either the left breast (Fig. 54A, B) or the right breast (Fig. 54C, D). Previous screening films were requested for review and comparison with current films and no new lesion was apparent upon review of the most recent left (Fig. 55A and B) and right (Fig. 55C, D) screening mammograms.

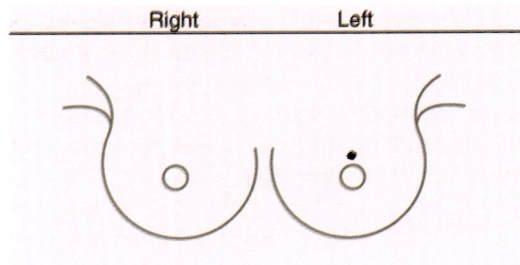

Figure 53

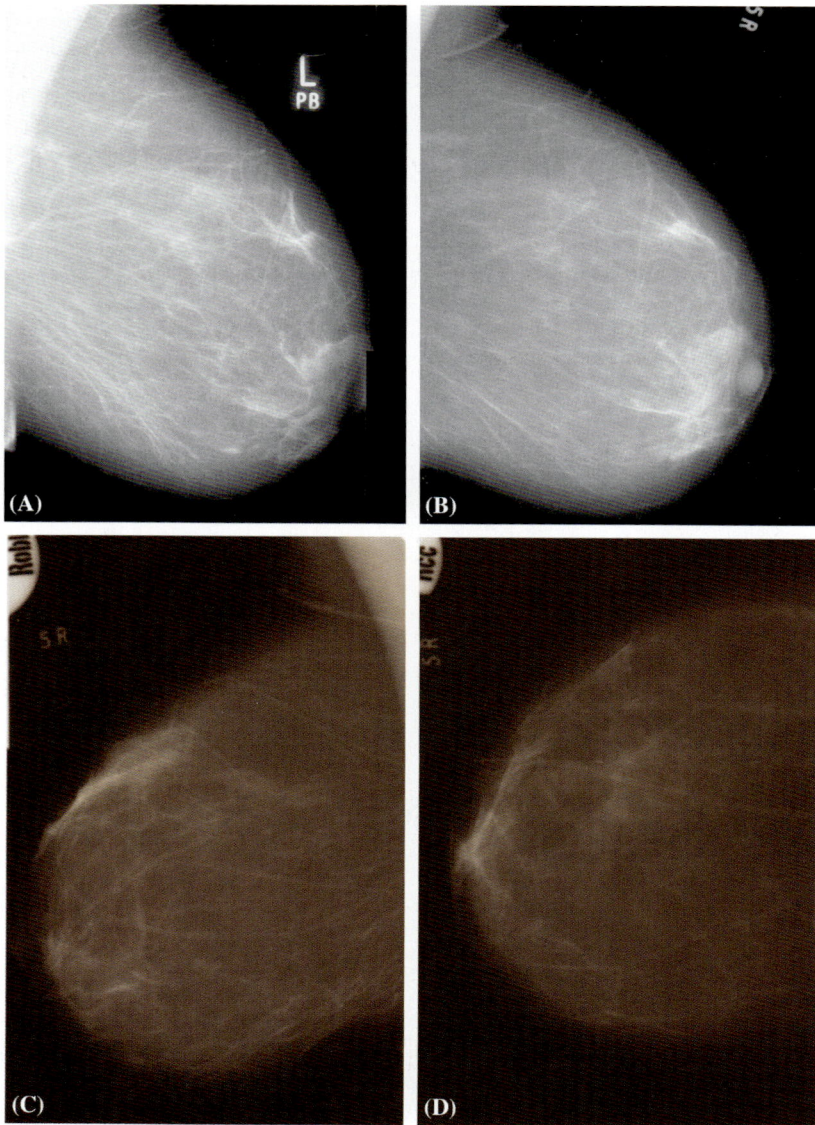

Figure 54

Breast Ultrasound

An ill-defined hypoechoic mass lesion with posterior acoustic shadowing and measuring 1.1 cm was found in the left breast at 12 o'oclock (corresponding to the palpable abnormality). The radiological appearances were consistent with a small carcinoma, though inflammatory changes could not be excluded (U4) (Fig. 56).

Core Biopsy

Ultrasound-guided core biopsy (14-gauge needle) of the left breast mass confirmed an invasive carcinoma (grade II) with mixed ductal and lobular features [Fig. 57A (low power), B (high power)]. The tumor was ER positive, but HER2 testing was not routinely performed on core biopsies at that time.

Diagnosis

Small, early-stage cancer of central left breast (T2N1).

Multidisciplinary review 1

The cancer was of small size in relation to the overall size of the patient's breast (large

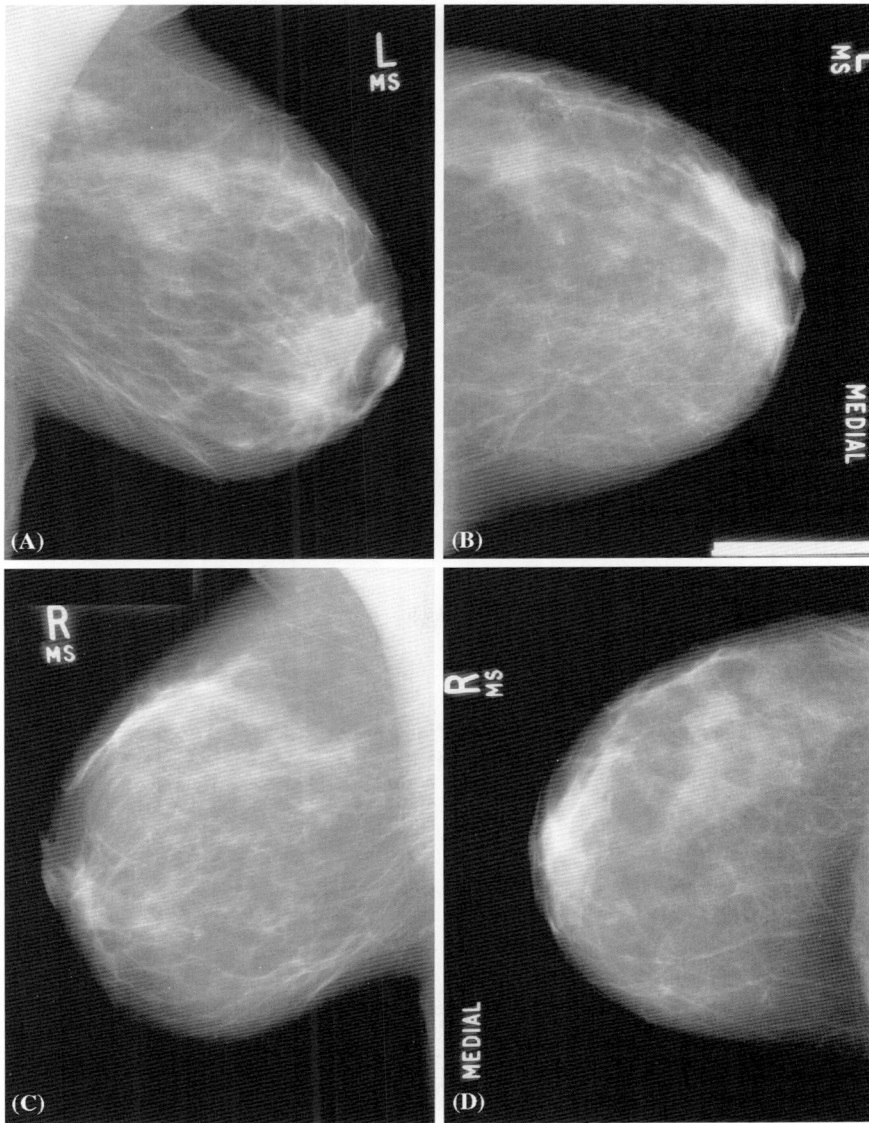

Figure 55

and pendulous). The lesion was amenable to central segmental resection with wide excision of the tumor including the nipple-areolar complex. It was considered that this procedure would yield a satisfactory cosmetic result and preserve much of the volume and shape of the breast. A contralateral mastopexy could be carried out at a later date were there to be any marked disparity in size between the breasts. This central segmental mastectomy was combined with a level II axillary lymph node dissection (standard axillary staging procedure at the time).

Treatment and Progress

The patient was very keen to preserve her breast and in the event of mastectomy being advised, she would have insisted on immediate breast reconstruction. She was not concerned about the loss of her nipple and understood that irradiation of the breast would be indicated postoperatively. She proceeded with a central segmental resection and at operation a generous wide excision was performed with removal of a central skin ellipse (11 cm × 3 cm), the nipple-areolar complex, tumor, and surrounding normal

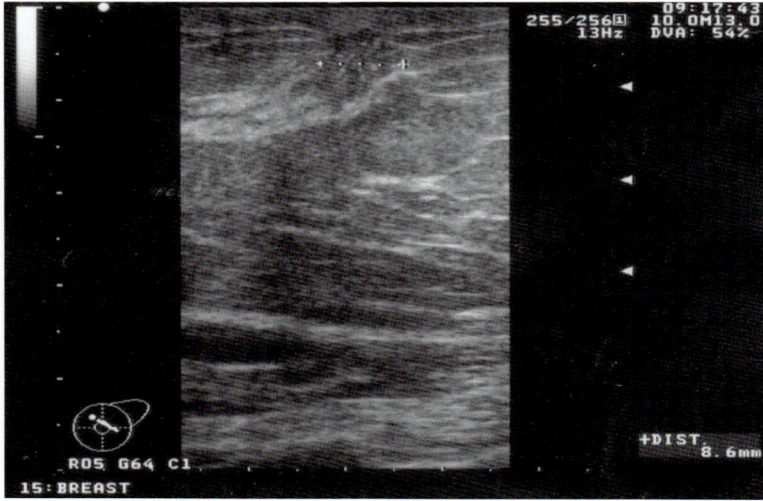

Figure 56

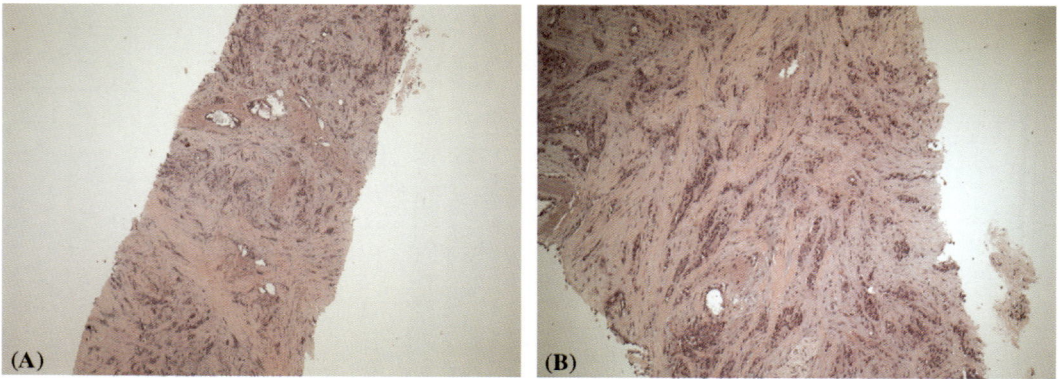

(A)   **(B)**

Figure 57

breast tissue en masse (180 g) (Fig. 58). The breast was reconstituted and closed with a linear horizontal wound and deep supporting sutures. The patient made an uneventful recovery and was very pleased with the cosmetic result.

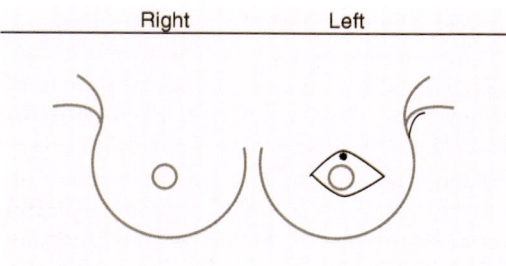

Figure 58

Definitive Histology

This revealed a grade II invasive ductal carcinoma measuring 9 mm in maximum diameter. There was no associated in situ component and tumor was clear of all resection margins by >5 mm [Fig. 59A (magnification 10×), B (magnification 20×)]. None of the nine lymph nodes contained metastatic carcinoma.

Multidisciplinary Review 2

It was recommended the patient receive radiotherapy to the left breast and tamoxifen for five years as adjuvant systemic hormonal therapy. She required no further surgery and the tumor was excised with a good margin of clearance.

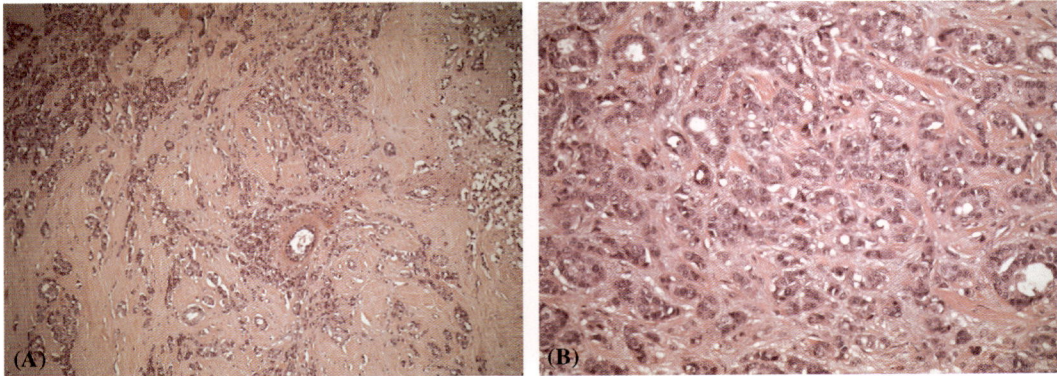

Figure 59

Treatment and Progress

The patient commenced breast radiotherapy two months after completion of surgery. She developed some acute radiation sequelae and experienced intermittent episodes of shooting pains in the left breast, which were self-limiting. A follow-up mammogram of the ipsilateral breast at 12 months revealed an area of fat necrosis (confirmed on fine-needle aspiration cytology) but otherwise the patient had an excellent cosmetic result (Fig. 60). The patient also had troublesome hot flashes and was switched from tamoxifen to the aromatase inhibitor Arimidex. She was in a favorable prognostic group with an NPI < 4.4 and was ineligible for a routine early switch from tamoxifen to an aromatase inhibitor after two to three years.

Discussion

This patient had a small (1 cm) tumor situated close to the nipple-areolar complex in a

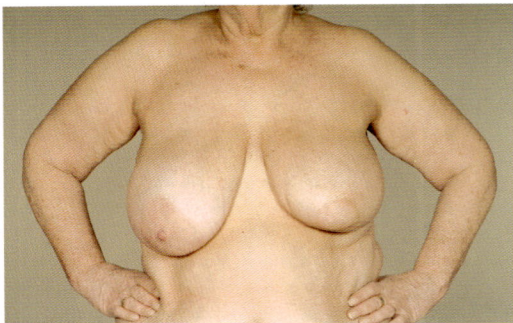

Figure 60

relatively large pendulous breast. Conventional wide local excision is precluded due to proximity of the tumor to the nipple and problems of surgical clearance without devascularization or subsequent cosmetic distortion of the nipple-areolar complex. A central segmental resection can produce an excellent result in these circumstances combining wide excision of the tumor with an acceptable cosmetic outcome. Despite sacrifice of the nipple-areolar complex, much of the breast volume is preserved together with the natural ptosis of the breast. A complete mastectomy without reconstruction would leave a large-breasted patient rather lop-sided. Occasionally, tumor excision can be incorporated into a reduction mammoplasty or therapeutic mammoplasty (1). This technique removes the tumor with a wide margin of clearance and refashions the breast that is smaller in overall size. A contralateral symmetrization procedure is usually required, and there may be problems with re-excision when margins are positive or the width of clearance is inadequate. There are specific oncoplastic procedures that can preserve the nipple-areolar complex (e.g., Grisotti flap), but careful patient selection and explanation is essential (2–4). A potential advantage of breast reduction is minimization of dose inhomogeneity with radiotherapy (5). This can lead to areas of fat necrosis in larger breasts when focal areas receive an excessive dose of radiotherapy.

There is some evidence that radiotherapy could be omitted in some older women (≥50 years) with a small favorable tumor that has been excised with clear surgical margins. This patient had a small (9 mm) grade II tumor that was widely excised as part of a central breast excision. Clinical trials involving this subgroup of patients confirm that IBTR is significantly decreased with radiotherapy from about 8% to 1% at five years. The absolute numbers of recurrences are small in both groups and disease-free survival is 76% without radiotherapy compared to 82% with irradiation (1.4% difference in disease-free events) (6–8). It is important to distinguish between statistical and clinical significance; the benefits of local control for radiotherapy may not be clinically significant in women aged >70 years with comorbidities and limited life expectancy.

At the time this patient underwent surgery, sentinel lymph node biopsy was not routinely offered and a standard level II axillary lymph node dissection was therefore performed. Such a patient has a low probability of nodal involvement and is ideally suited to axillary staging with sentinel node biopsy. Where radioisotope facilities are not available, an alternative staging option is BDANS (9).

This patient had a low risk of relapse and was initially prescribed tamoxifen only as adjuvant systemic hormonal therapy. Hot flashes are a relatively common side effect of tamoxifen and are an indication for switching to an aromatase inhibitor. When patients are switched from tamoxifen on account of adverse side effects, Arimidex is usually the aromatase inhibitor of choice. By contrast, when switched after two to three years as part of an "early switch" regimen, exemestane is the preferred agent.

Related Cases

Adjuvant hormonal therapy—*Case Studies 1, 4, 10, 15, and 19*

Breast-conservation surgery—*Case Studies 6, 7, 8, 14, 15, and 19*

Axillary staging—*Case Studies 6, 8, 10, and 24*

Learning Points

1. There have been six randomized prospective trials that have compared mastectomy to BCT in the treatment of primary breast cancer. These two treatment options are associated with similar survival rates, but locoregional recurrence is slightly greater among women who undergo BCT.

2. For centrally located tumors, resection of the nipple-areolar complex is feasible, and the wound should be closed with horizontal approximation of the tissue edges. Alternatively, if the tumor is adjacent to the nipple-areolar complex but not immediately beneath it, then an area around the nipple-areolar complex can be de-epithelialized. The tumor can then be excised through this de-epithelialized area, the dermis closed, and the skin re-attached to the nipple-areolar complex with a running stitch.

3. There is some evidence suggesting that some women who are aged 70 or older might safely avoid radiotherapy after lumpectomy. Although this puts these women at a small increased risk for locoregional recurrence, this might not be clinically significant.

4. In patients with positive sentinel nodes (or those who do not undergo sentinel node biopsy), dissection should include both levels I and II of the axilla. These levels refer to the relationship of the axillary tissue to the pectoralis minor muscle. Thus, a level I dissection refers to extirpation of tissue lateral to the pectoralis minor muscle, level II refers to removal of tissue posterior to the muscle, and level III indicates dissection medial to the muscle.

References

1. McCulley SJ, Durani P, Macmillan RD. Therapeutic mammoplasty or centrally located breast tumours. Plast Reconstr Surg 2006; 117:366–373.
2. Grissotti A. Immediate reconstruction after partial mastectomy. *Oper Tech Plastic Reconstr Surg* 1994; 1:1–12.
3. Galimberti V, Zurrida S, Zanini V, et al. Central small size breast cancer: how to overcome the problem of nipple and areolar involvement. Eur J Cancer 1993; 29:1093–1096.
4. Benelli LC. Periareolar Benelli mastopexy and reduction: the round block. In: Scott L. Spear, ed.,

The Breast. Philadelphia and New York: Lippincott-Raven, 1998.

5. Kestin LL, Sharpe MB, Frazier RC, et al. Intensity modulation to improve dose uniformity with tangential breast radiotherapy: initial clinical experience. Int J Radiat Oncol Biol Phys 2000; 48:1559–1568.

6. Lim M, Bellon J, Gelman R, et al. A prospective study of conservative surgery without radiation therapy in selected patients with stage I breast cancer. Int J Radiat Oncol Biol Phys 2006; 65:1149–1154.

7. Fyles A, McCready D, Manchul L, et al. Tamoxifen with or without breast irradiation in women 50 years of age or older with early breast cancer. N Engl J Med 2004; 351:963–970.

8. Hughes K, Schnaper L, Berry D, et al. Lumpectomy plus tamoxifen with or without irradiation in women 70 years of age or older with early breast cancer. N Engl J Med 2004; 351:971–977.

9. Purushotham AD, MacMillan RD, Wishart G. Advances in axillary surgery for breast cancer—time for a tailored approach. Eur J Surg Oncol 2005; 31:929–931.

CASE STUDY 10

History

A 79-year-old woman presented with a three-week history of a nontender lump in the right breast. There was no associated nipple discharge and the patient had no previous breast problems. She had undergone a screening mammogram more than 10 years earlier and had no family history of breast or ovarian cancer. There was previous usage of hormone replacement therapy for a period not exceeding five years.

Clinical Findings

A 2-cm firm ill-defined lump was palpable in the upper outer quadrant of the right breast. There was subtle skin dimpling immediately below the inferior aspect of the mass but no indrawing of the nipple and no axillary lymphadenopathy (E5) (Fig. 61).

Clinical Assessment

Clinically suspicious right breast lump in an elderly patient consistent with cancer (conservable)

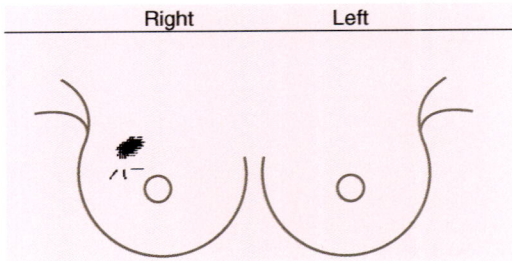

Figure 61

Investigations

Mammography

A spiculate mass was seen in the upper outer quadrant of the right breast measuring 15 mm in maximum diameter. The appearances were of a small carcinoma (R5) (Fig. 62A, B).

Breast Ultrasound

The mammographic abnormality corresponded to a 17-mm hypoechoic mass lesion with posterior acoustic attenuation (U5) (Fig. 63).

Core Biopsy

Ultrasound-guided core biopsy (16-gauge needle, 3 passes) of the right breast mass confirmed the clinical and radiological impression of malignancy and showed an invasive carcinoma (grade II, ER positive, HER2 negative) [Fig. 64A (magnification 10×), B (magnification 20×)].

Diagnosis

Early-stage right breast cancer (T2N1).

Multidisciplinary Review 1

Following multidisciplinary discussion, it was recommended the patient undergo a right wide local excision and sentinel lymph node biopsy. The lesion was unifocal, 3 cm in size,

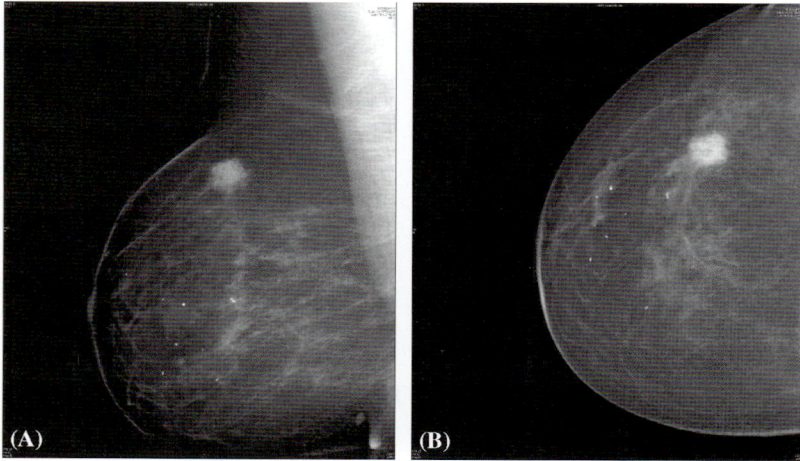

Figure 62

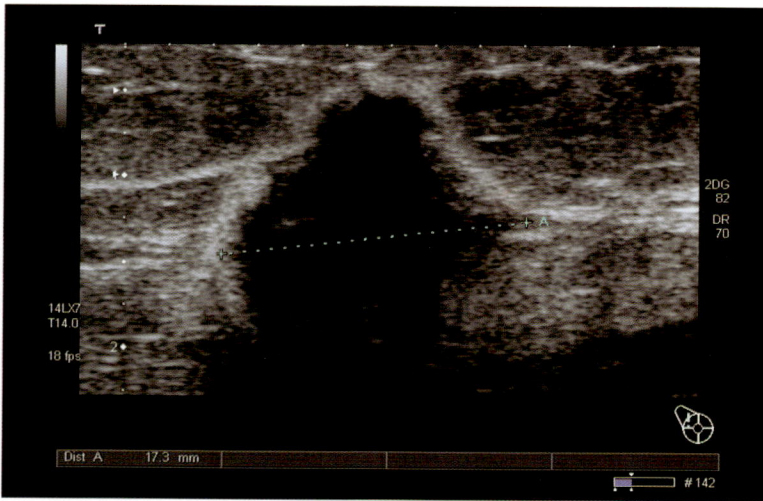

Figure 63

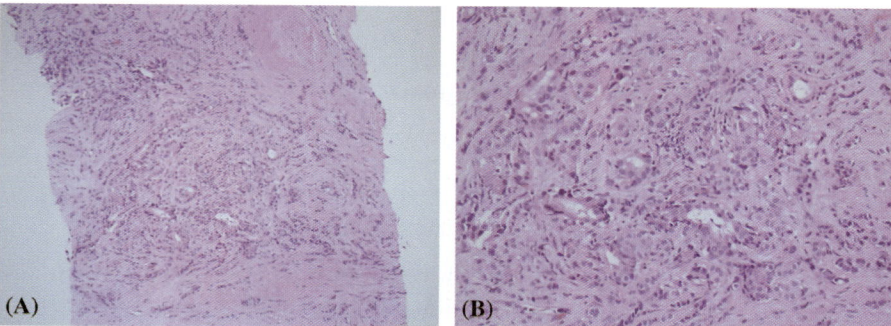

Figure 64

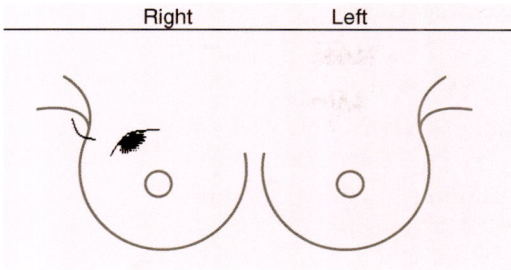

Figure 65

and situated well away from the nipple. The skin dimpling was confined to the area immediately adjacent to the tumor and did not involve the nipple.

Treatment and Progress

The patient was admitted for surgery within the next four weeks. At operation the tumor was widely excised and no more tissue was present either superior or lateral to the surgical cavity (Fig. 65). Sentinel node biopsy was carried out via a separate axillary incision and yielded several blue, though cold nodes. The patient made an uneventful recovery and was discharged home the following day.

Definitive Histology

This confirmed an invasive ductal carcinoma (grade II) measuring 19 mm in maximum diameter. Excision was clear of all radial margins but one out of four sentinel nodes contained micrometastases (1/4) with extracapsular spread [Fig. 66A (low power), B (high power)]. Several foci of lymphovascular invasion were seen in the primary tumor [Fig. 66C (low power), D (high power)].

Multidisciplinary Review 2

It was considered appropriate to offer this patient a completion axillary lymph node dissection as this was the unit policy for micrometastases in the sentinel node. This

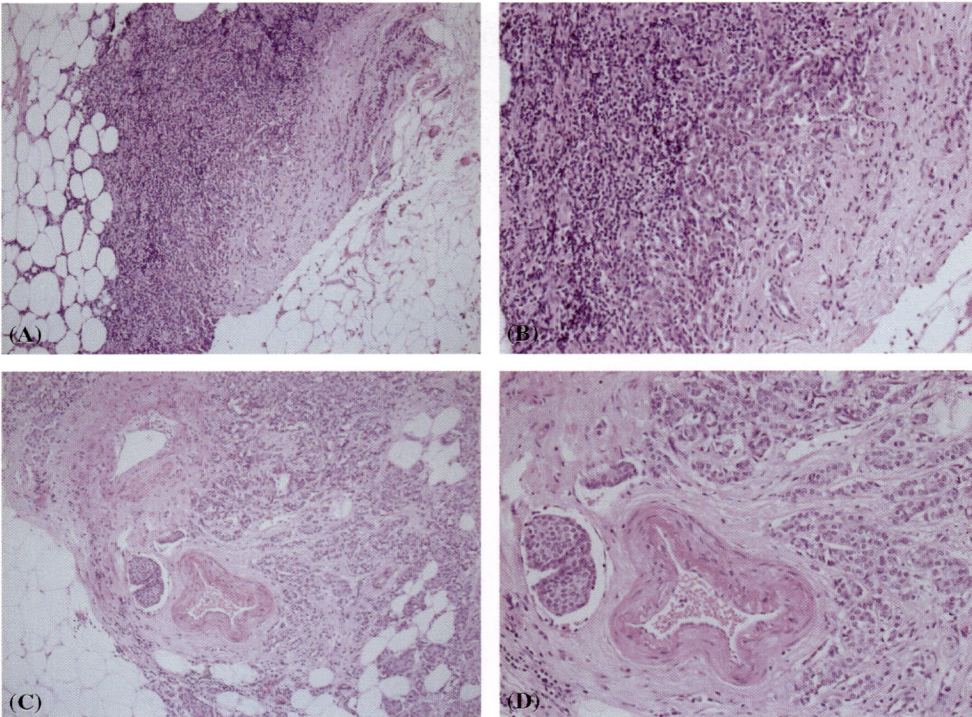

Figure 66

should be followed by radiotherapy to the breast and tamoxifen for two to three years with an early switch to an aromatase inhibitor as adjuvant systemic hormonal therapy [NPI: $(0.2 \times 1.9) + 2 + 2 = 4.38$].

Treatment and Progress

It was explained to the patient that she had a 10% to 12% chance of further disease in the nonsentinel lymph nodes and was unlikely to develop any regional recurrence in her remaining lifetime. After careful consideration of these and related issues such as potential morbidity from further axillary surgery, the patient adamantly declined any completion axillary dissection. She felt she had made an excellent recovery from primary surgery and did not wish to incur any significant morbidity from further axillary surgery. Arrangements were therefore made for radiotherapy planning and the patient commenced on tamoxifen.

Discussion

This is another example of an older patient declining completion axillary lymph node dissection when fully informed of the risks and benefits of this procedure. This patient was 79 years of age with a 19-mm grade II invasive ductal carcinoma for which one out of four sentinel nodes contained a single micrometastatic deposit. For patients in whom fewer than half the nodes retrieved contain micrometastases, the chance of disease in the remaining nonsentinel nodes is about 10% (1–3). There is therefore a 90% chance that no further disease will be found, but the patient may suffer significant morbidity from additional axillary surgery. Indeed, there is evidence that the morbidity from initial sentinel node biopsy followed by delayed axillary dissection may be greater than routine level II axillary dissection performed at the outset. It is unlikely that this patient would have any residual axillary disease that would cause problems with regional recurrence or compromise survival expectations (4,5).

Related Cases

Completion axillary dissection—*Case Studies 13 and 24*

Breast-conservation surgery—*Case Studies 6, 7, 8, 14, 15, and 19*

Adjuvant hormonal therapy—*Case Studies 1, 4, 9, 15, and 19*

Learning Points

1. In a clinically node-negative patient, the axilla can be treated with either surgery (sentinel node biopsy/axillary dissection) or radiotherapy alone.
2. Either surgery or radiotherapy reduces the risk of local recurrence in the axilla by about 90%. However, the stage of the breast cancer cannot be determined if the axilla is treated with radiotherapy alone.
3. It should also be emphasized that patients with clinically suspicious axillary nodes cannot be treated with axillary radiotherapy alone. These patients should be managed with axillary surgery.

References

1. Rescigno J, Taylor LA, Aziz MS, et al. Predicting negative axillary lymph node dissection in patients with positive sentinel lymph node biopsy: can a subset of patients be spared axillary dissection? Breast Cancer Res Treat 2005; 94:S35.
2. Benson JR, Wishart GC, Forouhi P, et al. The incidence of nodal involvement following completion axillary dissection for sentinel node positive disease. Eur J Cancer 2007; 5:21.
3. Dabbs DJ, Fung M, Landsittel D, et al. Sentinel lymph node micrometastases as a predictor of axillary tumour burden. Breast J 2004; 10:101–105.
4. Naik AM, Fey J, Gemignani M, et al. The risk of axillary relapse after sentinel lymph node biopsy for breast cancer is comparable with that of axillary lymph node dissection: a follow up study of 4008 procedures. Ann Surg 2004; 240:462–471.
5. Benson JR, Querci della Rovere G. Management of the axilla in women with breast cancer. Lancet Oncol 2007; 8:331–348.

CASE STUDY 11

History

A 51-year-old woman presented with a nine-month history of a lump in the left breast. Despite the patient's age, she remained pre-menopausal and the mass did not fluctuate in size with the menstrual cycle. There was no associated tenderness or nipple discharge and the patient had no previous breast problems. There was no family history of either breast or ovarian cancer. The patient had one daughter who was breast-fed. She gave birth to her first child at the age of 38 years and had used the oral contraceptive pill for a cumulative duration in excess of 20 years.

Clinical Findings

Examination revealed a firm, ill-defined mass in the extreme upper outer quadrant of the left breast. This measured 2 cm in maximum diameter and was clinically suspicious. There was no axillary lymphadenopathy (E4) (Fig. 67).

Clinical Assessment

Probable carcinoma of the left breast that appeared unifocal and potentially conservable

Investigations

Mammography

Bilateral mammography revealed an asymmetric density in the upper outer quadrant of the left breast measuring 25 mm in diameter (Fig. 68A, B). This was radiologically suspicious for a left breast cancer (R4).

Breast Ultrasound

The sonographic correlate of this density was a 24-mm hypoechoic mass lesion without posterior acoustic enhancement or attenuation (U5) (Fig. 69).

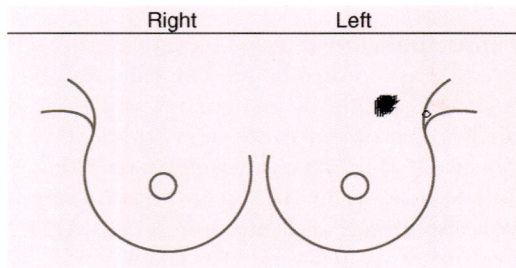

Figure 67

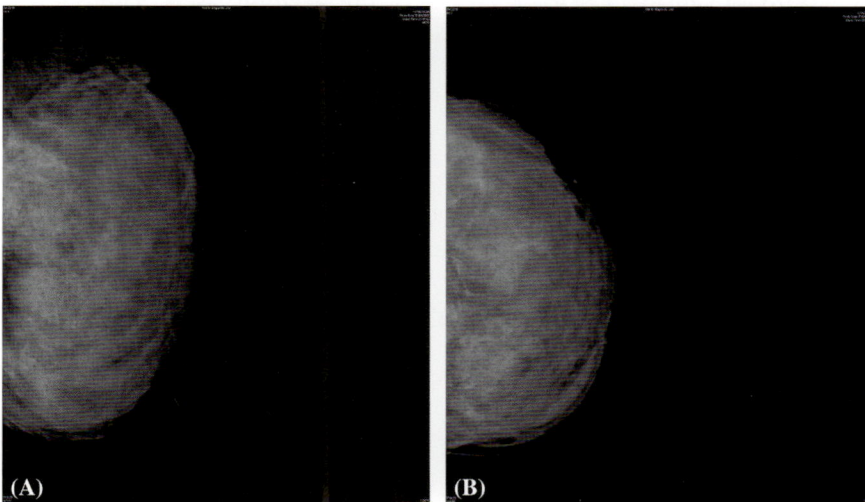

(A) (B)

Figure 68

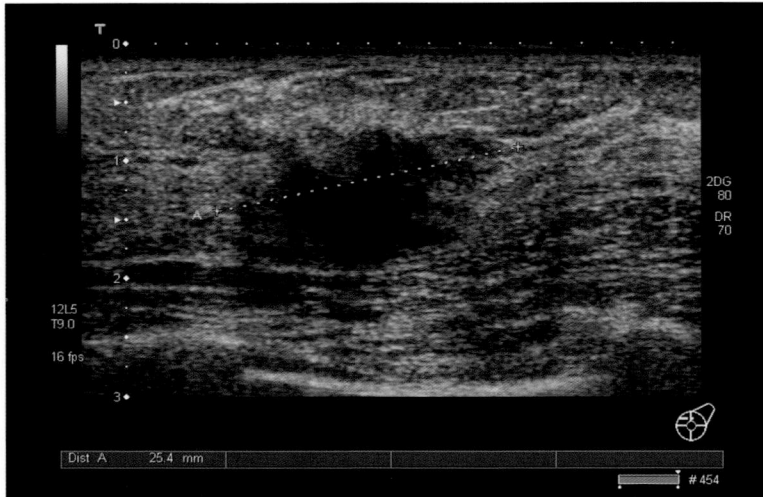

Figure 69

Core Biopsy

Ultrasound-guided core biopsy of the left breast mass confirmed the clinical and radiological suspicion of malignancy and showed an invasive ductal carcinoma (grade II, ER positive[b]) [Fig. 70A (magnification 10×), B (magnification 20×)]. No in situ component was identified and the tumor was HER2 positive on core biopsy (Fig. 70C).

Diagnosis

Early-stage left breast cancer (T2N0)

Multidisciplinary Review 1

Following multidisciplinary review, it was recommended that the patient undergo a left wide local excision and sentinel lymph node biopsy. It was not considered necessary to perform breast MRI to exclude multifocality. Axillary ultrasound assessment (+/− core biopsy) was requested prior to any axillary surgery. This was carried out at the next clinic attendance and revealed no evidence of metastatic disease on core biopsy.

Treatment and Progress

The patient underwent the proposed surgery two weeks following tissue diagnosis using a curvilinear incision in the upper outer quadrant of the left breast combined with a transverse axillary incision (Fig. 71). At operation a single large blue and hot node was identified together with two further blue and cold nodes. All three nodes were removed and there was no residual activity in the axilla. A wide excision of the breast mass was performed down to the level of the pectoral fascia. There was no further tissue to excise superiorly. The patient made an uneventful postoperative recovery.

Definitive Histology

This confirmed an invasive ductal carcinoma (grade II) measuring 24 mm in maximum diameter [Fig. 72A (magnification 10×), B (magnification 20×)]. There was associated high nuclear grade DCIS with a solid growth pattern (no necrosis). The aggregate diameter (invasive component and DCIS) reached 48 mm and DCIS was transected at

---

[b]Allred score 8/8

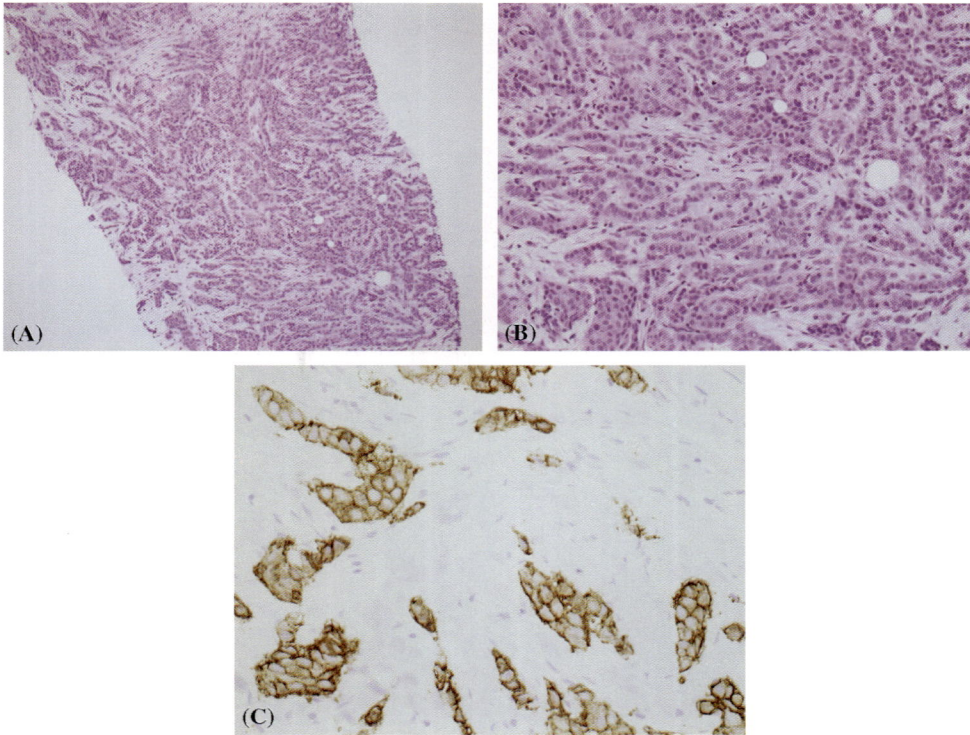

Figure 70

the inferior margin (Fig. 72C). All other margins were clear of any cancer cells by >5 mm. Four sentinel nodes were identified and one of these contained a macrometa-static focus (>2 mm) (Fig. 72D). A further nonsentinel node showed focal fat necrosis and a fibroblastic reaction consistent with the site of previous biopsy.

Multidisciplinary Review 1

Following further multidisciplinary review, it was recommended that the patient undergo re-excision of the inferior cavity margin

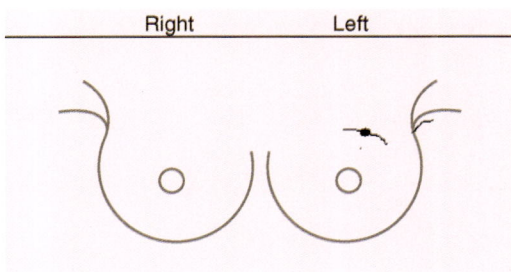

Figure 71

together with a completion axillary dissec-tion. In terms of adjuvant therapy, the patient would require radiotherapy to the breast (conditional upon adequate clear-ance on re-excision) and chemotherapy together with Herceptin (HER2 positive). It was considered appropriate to offer this patient chemotherapy prior to any further surgery in view of the documented node involvement and HER2 positivity, which con-fers a worse prognosis with higher risk of distant relapse.

Treatment and Progress

The patient proceeded to systemic therapy with six cycles of FEC/docetaxol together with Herceptin (see Appendix III). This was well tolerated, though the patient developed a port-site thrombosis that required reposi-tioning of the port and anticoagulant ther-apy. The patient attended for further surgical review after the fifth cycle of chemotherapy. At this stage, she was informed that although DCIS involved only the inferior margin of resection, the total documented tumor

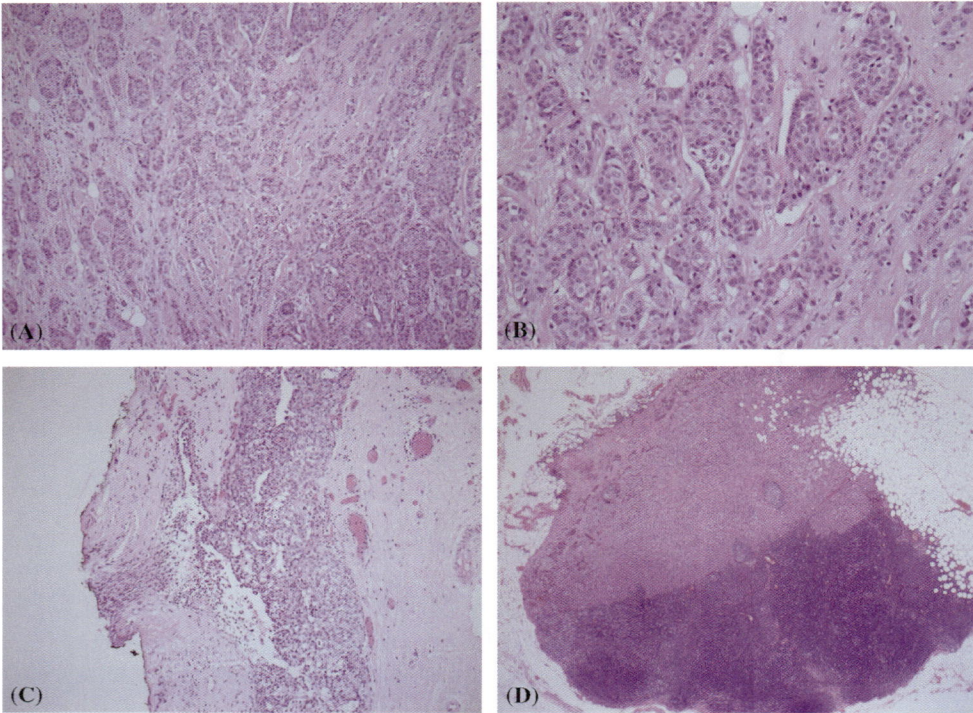

Figure 72

diameter was 48 mm; in the event of extensive involvement of the re-excision specimen, the overall extent of DCIS might mandate mastectomy (even if the new inferior margin was clear). The patient was keen to proceed with re-excision in the first instance with the understanding that mastectomy may yet be indicated. A left cavity re-excision and completion axillary dissection was undertaken five weeks following the final cycle of chemotherapy (clexane at a therapeutic dosage of 100 mg daily was discontinued five days preoperatively). Despite the tumor lying in the superior aspect of the left breast, further re-excision did not impair the final cosmetic result (Fig. 73A, B).

Definitive Histology

The inferior cavity shave was submitted in entirety and revealed no residual DCIS or invasive carcinoma. The surgical cavity contained fibrous scar tissue and foamy macrophages with foreign body giant cells. None of the 10 lymph nodes retrieved contained any tumor, and there was no evidence of any nodes that had been downstaged by chemotherapy (final nodal status 1/14).

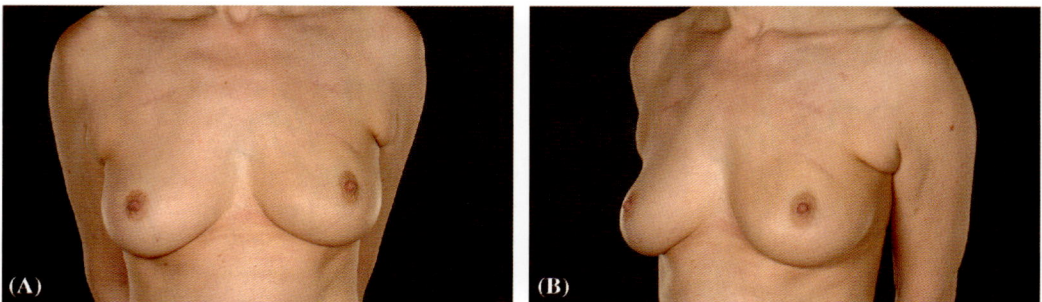

Figure 73

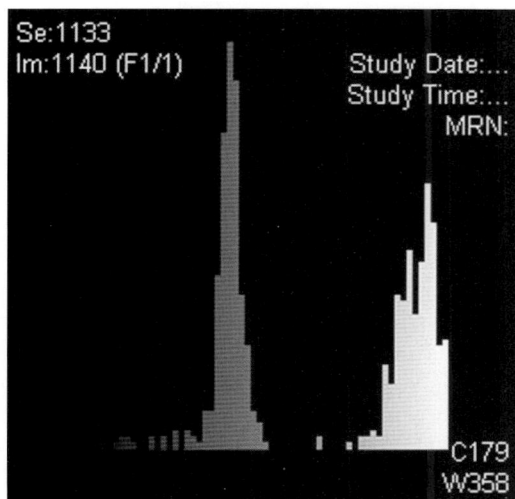

Figure 74

Multidisciplinary Review 2

Satisfactory margin clearance had been achieved, and it was therefore recommended the patient proceed to breast radiotherapy for completion of locoregional treatment. In view of the history of port-site thrombosis, an aromatase inhibitor was the agent of choice for adjuvant systemic hormonal therapy (the patient had been rendered amenorrheic by chemotherapy). Herceptin was continued perioperatively, but temporarily discontinued after a MUGA scan revealed a fall in left ventricular ejection fraction (LVEF) from 70% to 49% at 12 weeks. A MUGA scan was repeated after a one-month break from Herceptin (Fig. 74).

Discussion

Though the patient had a unifocal invasive carcinoma measuring <3 cm, there was extensive associated DCIS yielding an aggregate diameter after initial excision of 48 mm. The invasive component had been excised with good clearance, and DCIS was present at one margin only (inferior). The other margins ranged from 4 (superior—no further tissue to take) to 10 mm medially. On the basis of the modified Van Nuys Prognostic Index (VNPI) (see page 90, case study 16),

this patient would have the following score (1):

$$[3(\text{size } 48\,\text{mm}) + 2(\text{margins } 1 - 9\,\text{mm}) + 3$$
$$(\text{high grade with necrosis}) + 2$$
$$(\text{age } 51\,\text{years})] = 10$$

According to the Van Nuys database, this patient would be at a relatively high risk for relapse even with breast radiotherapy; mastectomy is usually recommended for scores of 10, 11, and 12 (5- and 10-year recurrence-free survival of 54% and 37%, respectively) (2). This patient was very keen to preserve her breast and requested re-excision in the first instance. She was warned that the presence of further DCIS in the re-excision specimen might mandate mastectomy whatever the new inferior margin clearance. This patient was at the lower end of the 10 to 12 VNPI category, and fortunately no residual tumor was found after re-excision.

This patient was advised to have chemotherapy first in order to avoid any delays with systemic therapy. She definitely required the latter on the basis of macrometastases in one of the sentinel nodes. However, this patient was not at an exceptionally high risk for distant relapse and could have undergone further surgery immediately. Sometimes theatre scheduling issues can influence the decision on the timing of further surgery. Moreover, there was a possibility that this patient may have required a mastectomy after re-excision and would have demanded immediate breast reconstruction. Therefore, completion of all surgery before commencing chemotherapy could have potentially led to significant delays with systemic treatments. It could be argued that this patient might have benefited from completion of locoregional treatment (i.e., radiotherapy to the breast) within a 12- to 16-week interval from initial surgery. There is currently no clear evidence that breast-conservation patients undergoing delayed radiotherapy (postchemotherapy) have higher rates of local relapse. Systemic therapies (chemotherapy/hormonal) themselves reduce local recurrence by about one-third (3).

Herceptin or trastuzumab is a humanized monoclonal antibody directed against the extracellular domain of the HER2/neu growth factor receptor (coded by the cerbB2 gene). Overexpression of HER2/neu occurs in approximately 30% of invasive breast cancers and is associated with a worse prognosis (4). When combined with taxane-based chemotherapy for management of advanced breast cancer, Herceptin improved time to disease progression (4.6 months vs. 7.4 months) (5). This was the first example of a specific oncogene pathway being targeted for breast cancer treatment. Though Herceptin has been widely used in the United Kingdom for treatment of metastatic disease since 2001, its use in the adjuvant setting is much more recent and was officially approved by the National Institute for Clinical Excellence (NICE) in 2006. Prior to this, adjuvant Herceptin was only used for management of high-risk HER2-positive women, defined as those with an absolute survival benefit in excess of 8%—often ≥4 nodes positive. Adjuvant Herceptin is given as a slow intravenous infusion every three weeks for one year. Clinical trials have confirmed improvements in both disease-free and overall survival. The two American trials (NSABP B31 and the Intergroup) reported a reduction in risk of recurrence of about 50% (HR 0.48, $p = 0.0000000003$) and have shown an early survival benefit favoring Herceptin at two years (HR 0.67, $p = 0.015$) (6). The European trial (HERA) showed similar reductions in risk of recurrence (HR 0.54, $p < 0.00001$) but no overall survival advantage (HR 0.76, $p = 0.26$) (7). In those patients analyzed in the American trials, Herceptin was given concurrently with an anthracycline based chemotherapy (4 cycles of AC followed by paclitaxel), while in the European trial Herceptin was prescribed only after completion all chemotherapy (any regimen of ≥ 4 cycles). The principle side effect of Herceptin is cardiotoxicity that is potentially greater when the drug is combined with chemotherapy than given sequentially (clinically significant heart failure 4% vs. 0.5%). Overall, between 2% and 4% of patients receiving Herceptin will have significant cardiotoxicity within the first three to six months. There appears to be no evidence for any delayed cardiac effects (e.g., late myocardial infarction). The value of left ventricular ejection fraction (LVEF) on completion of AC and age >50 years are risk factors for cardiotoxicity and a fall in LVEF that mandates temporary cessation of Herceptin. About 3% of patients on Herceptin will develop congestive cardiac failure and this can be managed with β-blockers and ACE inhibitors (may be difficult to subsequently get patients off medication).

This patient received Herceptin concurrently with an anthracycline-based chemotherapy regimen (FEC/taxotere). Though there was a fall in LVEF from 70% to 49%, this was not manifest clinically, and Herceptin was resumed after recovery of cardiac function. Trials are currently ongoing to assess whether there are benefits in continuing Herceptin for a total duration of two years. This will involve a careful analysis of cost-effectiveness, and results on the optimal duration of Herceptin usage should be available by 2008. Herceptin has been approved by the U.S. Food and Drug Administration for the treatment of node-positive, HER2-positive early-stage breast cancer and will be given with the non-anthracycline component of chemotherapy for a duration of one year (8). The optimal duration of Herceptin is unknown, though at present one year is the favored period of treatment. Patients should receive at least nine weeks of therapy and a three-weekly schedule is more convenient than a weekly course (though of comparable efficacy). The HERA study is investigating 1 versus 2 years of treatment with Herceptin, while a major French trial is addressing 6 months versus 12 months of treatment.

Related Cases

Re-excision after breast-conservation surgery—*Case Studies 7, 16, and 19*

Positive sentinel lymph node—*Case Studies 6, 10, 24, and 37*

Taxane-based adjuvant chemotherapy—*Case Studies 3 and 8*

Herceptin—*Case Studies 8, 25, 26, and 27*

Learning Points

1. A diagnostic bilateral mammogram should be obtained in any patient who presents with a clinically suspicious breast mass. Ideally, the mammogram should be obtained prior to tissue biopsy. However, even if the mammogram reported it as benign, the surgeon should proceed with a tissue biopsy (the false-negative rate for mammography is about 10%). The mammogram is essential for evaluating both breasts for occult lesions, as this could potentially influence the choice of local therapy.

2. Most patients with early-stage breast cancer are suitable candidates for BCT. However, there are a few contraindications to BCT: multicentric cancers, early pregnancy (patients require radiotherapy after BCT), previous radiotherapy to the breast, collagen vascular disease, and large tumors (although tumors can be downstaged with preoperative systemic therapy).

3. Women are at greatest risk for recurrence and death during the first three years following surgery for early-breast cancer (peak in the hazard curve). In patients with HER2-positive tumors, adjuvant therapy with Herceptin reduces that risk by half.

References

1. Silverstein MJ. USC/Van Nuys Prognostic Index. In: Silverstein MJ, ed. Ductal Carcinoma in Situ of the Breast. 2nd ed. Philadelphia: Lippincott, Williams and Wilkins, 2002.
2. Woo CS, Skinner KA, Silverstein MJ. Ductal carcinoma in situ: clinical studies and controversies in treatment. In: Querci della Rovere G, Warren R, Benson JR, eds. Early Breast Cancer.London and New York: Taylor and Francis, 2006:349–374.
3. Early Breast Cancer Trialists Collaborative Group. Effects of radiotherapy and of differences in the extent of surgery for early breast cancer on local recurrence and 15 year survival: an overview of the randomized trials. Lancet 2005; 366:2087–2106.
4. Slamon DJ, Clark GM, Wong SG, et al. Human breast cancer: correlation of relapse and survival with amplication of the HER-2/neu oncogene. Science 1987; 235:177–182.
5. Slamon DJ, Leyland-Jones B, Shak S, et al. Use of chemotherapy plus a monoclonal antibody against HER2 for metastatic breast cancer overexpresses HER2. N Engl J Med 2001; 344:783–792.
6. Romond EH, Perez EA, Bryant J, et al. Trastuzumab plus adjuvant chemotherapy for operable HER2 positive breast cancer. N Engl J Med 2005; 353:1659–1684.
7. Piccart-Gebhart MJ, Procter M, Leyland-Jones B, et al. 2 year follow up of trastuzumab after adjuvant chemotherapy in HER2 positive breast cancer. N Engl J Med 2005; 353:1659–1672.
8. FDA Approvals: Herceptin, Eloxatin, Extended-Release Venlafaxine HCI. Medscape Medical News. Available on http://www.medscape.com/viewarticle/575596.

Screen-Detected Breast Cancer

2

Part I: Mastectomy

CASE STUDY 12

History

A 52-year-old woman was recalled from a first-round screening mammogram for further evaluation of an area of extensive microcalcification in the right breast. There was no family history either of breast or of ovarian cancer. The patient was asymptomatic and reported no lumps in either breast, no areas of tenderness, and no nipple discharge.

Clinical Findings

No discrete mass lesion or areas of focal nodularity were evident in either breast, though there was a degree of generalized lumpiness (E2).

Clinical Assessment

Asymptomatic screen-detected microcalcification of the right breast.

Investigations

Mammography (Screening)

This showed extensive fine granular microcalcification within the right breast, which was suspicious for DCIS (R5) (Fig. 1A, B).

Breast Ultrasound

No sonographic assessment of the breast was undertaken.

Mammotome Biopsy

Mammotome biopsy using an 11-gauge needle was performed, and all cores showed microcalcification on specimen radiography. Histopathological examination confirmed the high radiological index of suspicion with areas of microcalcification associated with high–nuclear grade DCIS of cribriform architecture and comedo necrosis. There was no definite evidence of invasion (B5) [Fig. 2A (magnification 10×), B (magnification 20×)].

Diagnosis

Screen-detected extensive DCIS of the right breast (Tis)

Multidisciplinary Review 1

It was recommended that the patient undergo a right simple mastectomy and sentinel lymph node biopsy. The latter would

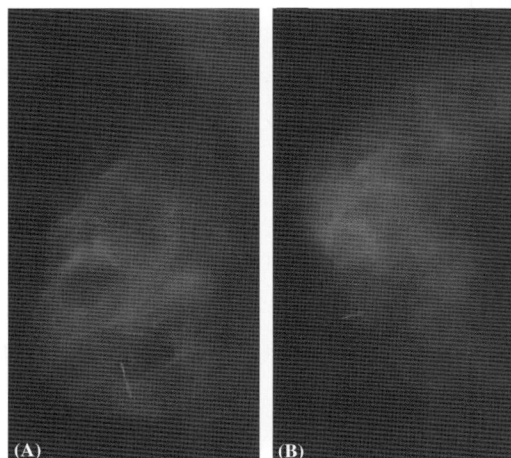

Figure 1

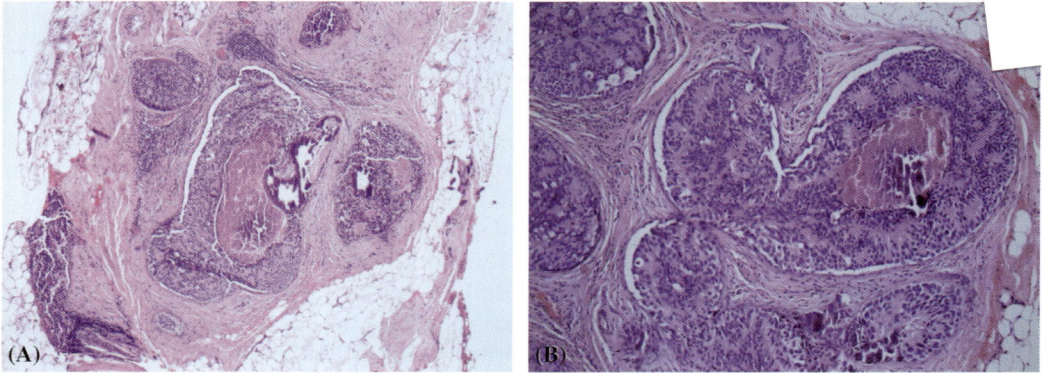

Figure 2

provide valuable axillary staging information in the event of an incidental finding of invasive disease on definitive histology (up to 20% chance).

Treatment and Progress

The patient proceeded with the planned surgery within four weeks of tissue diagnosis (mammotome biopsy). Sentinel lymph node biopsy on this occasion was performed through a separate axillary incision, though it can be done using the lateral aspect of the mastectomy incision (Fig. 3). When the mastectomy incision is placed horizontally, a separate axillary incision is more likely to gain access to level I nodes. A dual localization technique was employed to identify three sentinel nodes with patent blue dye (2.5%) and technetium 99m nanocolloid. Two milliliters of the former was used diluted to 5 mL in total; more recently,

only 1 mL of undiluted blue dye has been used as a tracer with similar rates of identification of the sentinel node(s). The patient made an uneventful recovery and was discharged home with two suction drains in situ (to be removed by a trained district nurse).

Definitive Histology

This revealed extensive high–nuclear grade DCIS with central necrosis extending over an area of 53 mm. There was no evidence of either microinvasion or invasive carcinoma [Fig. 4 (magnification 2.5×)]. None of the three sentinel nodes contained metastatic carcinoma (0/3 nodes).

Multidisciplinary Review 2

In the absence of any invasive component, the patient had undergone a potentially curative surgical procedure and required

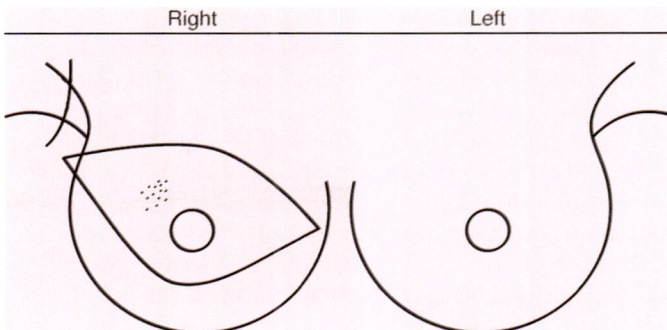

Figure 3

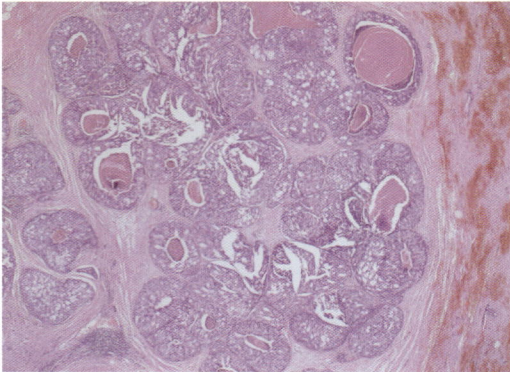

Figure 4

no further treatment. She was entered into a patient-led follow-up program with contralateral mammography at two and four years postoperatively.

Discussion

With the advent of breast-screening programs, the diagnosis of DCIS has increased dramatically and now constitutes between 20% and 25% of all new breast cancer diagnoses. Indeed, within a screened population alone, this figure rises to 40% (1,2). Usually, DCIS is manifest as a localized cluster of microcalcification, but sometimes calcification is extensive and extends throughout a high proportion of the breast. Such cases must be managed with simple mastectomy, which is potentially curative (>98%) in the absence of detectable invasion. Longer-term follow-up at eight years reveals that only 1.5% of patients with DCIS within the NSABP B-17 trial have died of metastatic breast cancer (3). An incidental invasive component is found in up to 20% of cases in which mastectomy is the choice of operation and extensive DCIS is a risk factor for invasion from historical studies (4). It is now acknowledged that extensive high–nuclear grade DCIS on imaging, which mandates mastectomy (or DCIS presenting as a palpable lesion), is an indication for sentinel lymph node biopsy. Up to 10% of cases with microinvasion will be sentinel lymph node positive (5), and one of the authors (JRB) has reported a sentinel node positivity

rate of 14% in patients undergoing mastectomy for extensive high–nuclear grade DCIS (6). This is likely to incur minimal additional morbidity, and not infrequently some level I nodes are inadvertently removed during a simple mastectomy. Such a policy avoids any subsequent potential dilemma of axillary staging for small foci of invasive disease. Sentinel lymph node biopsy cannot be undertaken as a delayed procedure post mastectomy and staging would otherwise involve either full dissection or blind sampling (which can be technically challenging if immediate breast reconstruction has been carried out). Sentinel lymph node biopsy must be done prior to removal of breast tissue. The axilla can be approached either through an incision in the lateral aspect of the mastectomy incision or via a separate transverse axillary incision. The latter may be more appropriate when a horizontal rather than an oblique mastectomy incision has been used.

There was no evidence of any invasive component within the mastectomy specimen, and none of the three sentinel nodes contained metastases. The patient had an excellent long-term outlook with an estimated risk of local recurrence and mortality of approximately 0.9% and 1.1%, respectively (7). In the absence of invasion, there is no indication for tamoxifen treatment in terms of ipsilateral DCIS managed with mastectomy. The latter minimizes the chance of local recurrence, and this is not further reduced by tamoxifen by any clinically meaningful degree. However, tamoxifen would act in a chemopreventive capacity to reduce the chance of contralateral disease (by about 40%).

Drain policies are highly variable; all the district nurses within the immediate catchment area of a hospital can be trained to remove drains. This allows patients to be discharged with drains in situ—usually on the first postoperative day (unless elderly or reluctant to go home with drains). Our current policy is to remove drains when the volume is <40 to 50 mL in the preceding 24 hours or at 72 hours, i.e., all drains are out at 72 hours. It is important that patients do not feel compelled to go home with drains in situ; drain management is best discussed at the time of pre-clerking so that the patient knows in advance what to expect.

Related Cases

Screen-detected cancer—*Case Studies 13, 14, 15, 16, and 17*

DCIS and sentinel node biopsy—*Case Study 5*

Learning Points

1. DCIS is considered a preinvasive lesion, but not all cases progress to invasive breast cancer. In fact, it has been suggested that only one out of every four or five cases of DCIS would develop into invasive cancer. DCIS is usually found on mammography, and its incidence has increased dramatically since the advent of mammographic screening.
2. DCIS is generally treated with wide local excision. Adjuvant radiotherapy and tamoxifen should also be considered in the management of DCIS. Following wide local excision alone, the risk of recurrence is 25%. However, the risk is 13% with excision + radiotherapy and only 8% with excision + radiotherapy + tamoxifen. Half of the recurrences will be DCIS, and the other half invasive cancers.
3. If the mammogram reveals diffuse (multicentric) DCIS, then mastectomy is indicated.

4. For localized DCIS treated with wide local excision, a sentinel node biopsy is not indicated. However, for multicentric DCIS treated with mastectomy, a sentinel node biopsy should be considered, as there is a much greater likelihood of finding invasive cancer.

References

1. Sickles EA. Mammographic features of 300 consecutive nonpalpable breast cancers. AJR Am J Roentgenol 1986; 146:661–663.
2. Silverstein MJ, Gamagami P, Colburn WJ, et al. Nonpalpable breast lesions: diagnosis with slightly overpenetrated screen-film mammography and hook wire-detected biopsy in 1014 cases. Radiology 1989; 171:633–638.
3. Fisher B, Dignam J, Wolmark N, et al. Lumpectomy and radiation therapy for the treatment of intraductal breast cancer: findings from National Surgical Adjuvant Breast and Bowel Project B-17. J Clin Oncol 1998; 16:441–452.
4. Meyer JE, Smith DN, Lester SC, et al. Larger-core needle biopsy of impalpable lesions. JAMA 1999; 281:1638–1164.
5. Intra M, Zurrida S, Maffini F, et al. Sentinel lymph node metastasis in microinvasive breast cancer. Ann Surg Oncol 2003; 10:1160–1165.
6. Benson JR, Wishart GC, Forouhi P, et al. The role of sentinel node biopsy in patients with a preoperative diagnosis of ductal carcinoma in situ. Eur J Cancer 2003; 5(3):22.
7. Woo CS, Skinner KA, Silverstein MJ. Ductal carcinoma in situ: clinical studies and controversies in treatment. In: Querci della Rovere G, Warren R, Benson JR, eds. Early Breast Cancer. London and New York: Taylor and Francis, 2006:357.

Part II: Breast Conservation Therapy

CASE STUDY 13

History

A 70-year-old woman was recalled from routine breast screening with a spiculate lesion in the right breast. She had previously undergone regular screening mammography and never been recalled. There was no family history of breast or ovarian cancer. The patient was asymptomatic and reported no lumps in either breast, no areas of tenderness and no nipple discharge. She was nulliparous and had never used exogenous hormones.

Clinical Findings

On examination of the right breast, a discrete *lump* in the breast was just palpable in the upper outer quadrant (E3).

Clinical Assessment

Screen-detected palpable carcinoma of the right breast

Investigations

Mammography (Screening)

A spiculate opacity was seen in the upper outer quadrant of the right breast, which was suspicious for a small carcinoma (Fig. 5A, B).

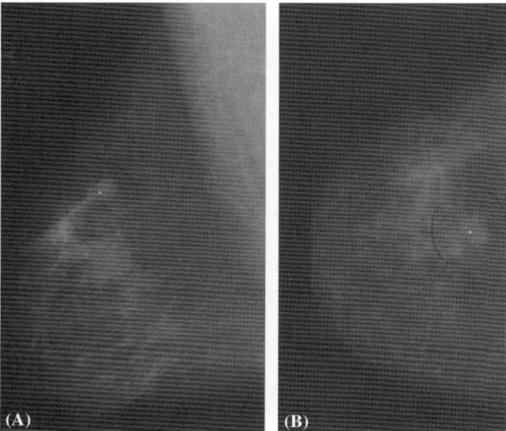

(A)   (B)

Figure 5

Breast Ultrasound

The sonographic correlate of the mammographic abnormality was a 16-mm hypoechoic lesion with posterior acoustic shadowing (Fig. 6).

Core Biopsy

Ultrasound-guided core biopsy confirmed an invasive ductal carcinoma (grade II; ER positive; HER2 negative) [Fig. 7A (low power), B (high power)].

Diagnosis

Early-stage screen-detected right breast cancer (T1N0)

Multidisciplinary Review 1

Following multidisciplinary review, it was recommended that the patient be offered a right guide wire–localized wide local excision and sentinel lymph node biopsy. Despite the lesion being just palpable, it was considered appropriate to localize with both a wire and an ultrasonic skin marker.

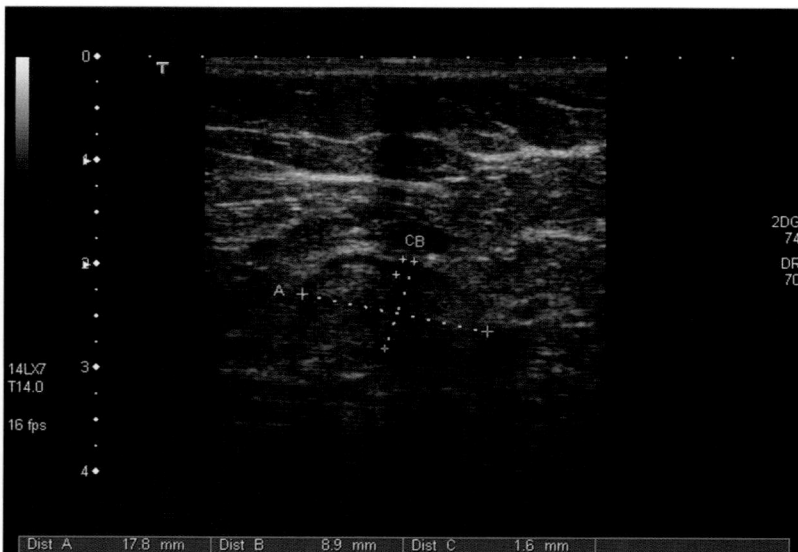

Figure 6

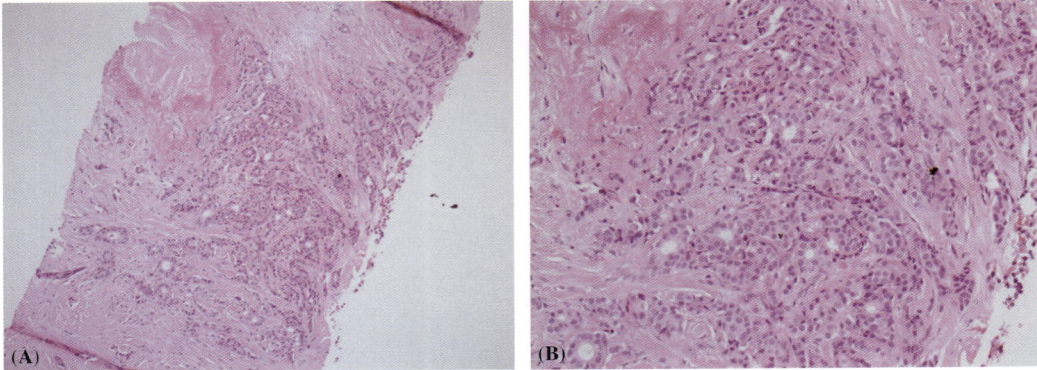

Figure 7

Treatment and Progress

An ultrasound-guided core biopsy of a right axillary lymph node was performed as part of a study and revealed no evidence of malignancy. The patient therefore proceeded with the planned surgery, including sentinel lymph node biopsy.

A curvilinear incision was made in the breast centered on the ultrasound skin marker (Fig. 8). The specimen radiograph was satisfactory and confirmed that the mammographic lesion had been excised with a good margin of surrounding tissue. Two hot and blue sentinel nodes were removed at surgery. The patient made an uneventful recovery and was discharged home the following day.

Definitive Histology

This revealed an invasive ductal carcinoma (grade II) measuring 22 mm in maximum diameter [Fig. 9A (magnification 2.5×), B (magnification 40×)]. There was a minor component of high–nuclear grade DCIS within the invasive tumor, which was clear of all radial margins by >5 mm. One of the

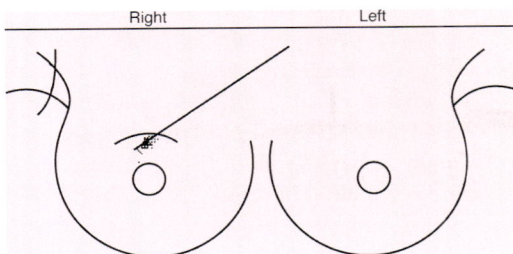

Figure 8

two sentinel nodes contained a micrometastatic focus measuring <2 mm, which was seen on both H and E sections (Fig. 9C) and immunohistochemistry (Fig. 9D).

Multidisciplinary Review

Because of the presence of tumor in one of the sentinel nodes, it was recommended that the patient undergo a level II axillary lymph node dissection. She would require radiotherapy to the right breast, and systemic adjuvant therapy would be decided after the final nodal status was known.

Treatment and Progress

An axillary lymph node dissection was carried out as a delayed or second-stage procedure one month following the initial surgery. At the time of surgery, several fleshy nodes were found, but these were probably reactive. Histology revealed presence of metastases in one of seven non-sentinel nodes, giving an overall nodal status of two out of nine. The patient proceeded to irradiation of the right breast and received adjuvant hormonal therapy with tamoxifen for two to three years followed by an early switch to an aromatase inhibitor.

Discussion

This patient was at the upper age limit for routine NHS breast screening and was found to have a typical spiculate opacity corresponding to a 2-cm tumor, which was just palpable. The ultrasound measurement had

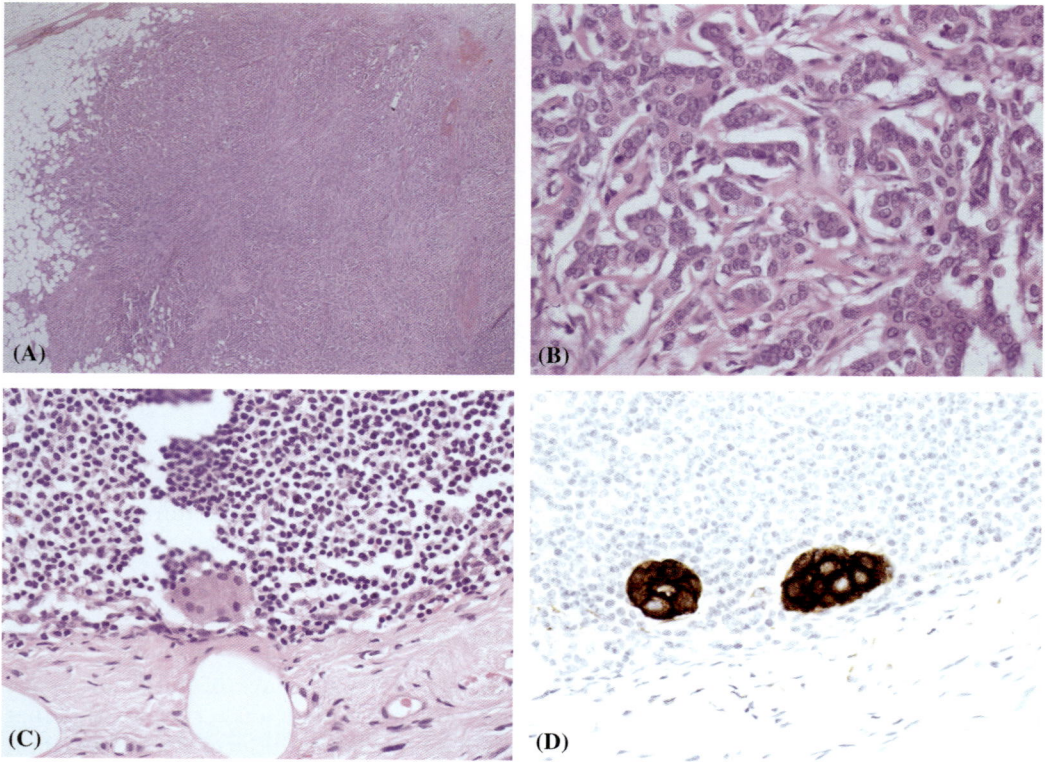

Figure 9

slightly underestimated the final pathological size. Nonetheless, the tumor was excised with clear radial margins in excess of 5 mm. One of the two sentinel nodes contained a micrometastasis, and a further metastasis was found in one of the non-sentinel nodes. However, this did not affect choice of systemic therapy, and it is unclear whether completion axillary lymph node dissection is always indicated for older patients with a positive sentinel node (1). This patient only had two nodes harvested, one of which contained a micrometastasis. The chance of non-sentinel lymph node involvement is significantly higher when macrometastases are present in the sentinel node and when the proportion of nodes harvested containing metastases is high (e.g., one out of two as opposed to one out of four) (2,3). As it happens, this patient did have involvement of a single non-sentinel node, but it remains unknown whether, if left alone, this would have resulted in axillary recurrence or affected overall survival in a 70-year-old woman. Some women may decline further axillary surgery

when informed of potential morbidity. Any risk:benefit ratio for detection of disease in non-sentinel nodes must consider subgroups of patients and not individual cases (4).

Related Cases

Screen-detected cancer—*Case Studies 12, 13, 14, 15, 16, and 17*
Breast conservation surgery for impalpable lesions—*Case Studies 14 and 15*

Completion axillary dissection—*Case Studies 10 and 24*

Learning Points

1. Many cancers detected in mammographic screening programs are palpable. In fact, some investigators have argued that screening clinical breast examination (CBE) and screening mammography are equally beneficial in reducing breast cancer mortality. Therefore, screening CBE should remain an integral part of all mammographic screening programs.

2. The potential benefits of axillary surgery are often debated. There are three reasons for considering axillary surgery (sentinel biopsy/axillary clearance): staging, local control, and improved survival. The status of the axillary lymph nodes is an integral part of tumor staging, which can be used to plan adjuvant treatment. Furthermore, axillary clearance reduces the risk of local recurrence (in the axilla) by about 90%. Finally, recent studies indicate that local recurrences may have an adverse effect on survival.

References

1. Benson JR, Querci della Rovere G. Management of the axilla in women with breast cancer. Lancet Oncol 2007; 8:331–348.
2. Cserni G, Gregori D, Merletti F, et al. Non-sentinel node metastases associated with micrometastatic sentinel nodes in breast cancer: metaanalysis of 25 studies. Br J Surg 2004; 91:1245–1252.
3. Rescigno J, Taylor LA, Aziz MS, et al. Predicting negative axillary lymph node dissection in patients with positive sentinel lymph node biopsy: can a subset of patients be spared axillary dissection? Breast Cancer Res Treat 2005; 94:S35.
4. Benson JR, Wishart GC, Forouhi P, et al. The incidence of nodal involvement following completion axillary dissection for sentinel node positive disease. Eur J Cancer 2007; 5:21.

CASE STUDY 14

History

A 51-year-old woman was found to have an opacity in the upper inner quadrant of the right breast on routine screening mammography. She had never previously been recalled from screening and had no family history of breast or ovarian cancer. She reported no discrete lumps in either breast, no areas of tenderness, and no nipple discharge. The patient had four children (eldest 24 years old) and had used the oral contraceptive pill for a cumulative period of two years.

Clinical Findings

Clinical examination was normal, with no palpable discrete lumps or any areas of focal nodularity (E1).

Clinical Assessment

Radiological abnormality detected on routine screening, with no clinical correlate

Investigations

Mammography (Screening)

An ill-defined opacity measuring 10 mm was seen in the upper inner quadrant of the right breast. The mammographic appearances were suspicious for carcinoma (R4) (Fig. 10A, B).

Breast Ultrasound

The opacity seen on mammography corresponded to a 9.2-mm hypoechoic mass lesion with posterior acoustic shadowing (Fig. 11).

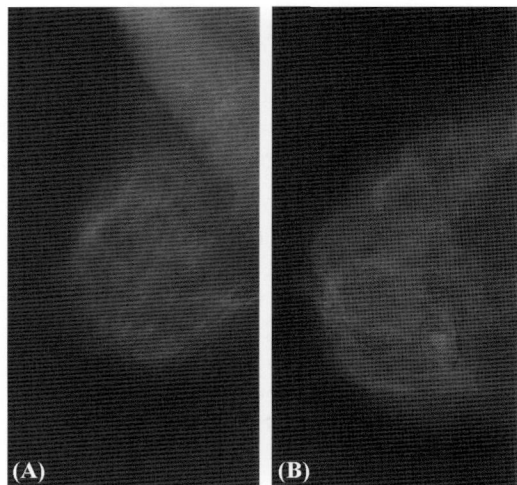

(A)   (B)

Figure 10

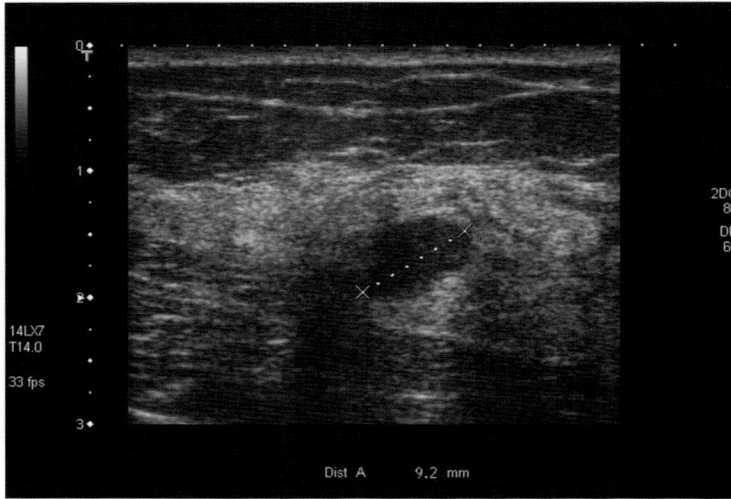

Figure 11

Core Biopsy

Ultrasound-guided core biopsy of the breast mass confirmed an invasive carcinoma (grade III) [Fig. 12A (low power), B (high power)]. The lesion was ER positive and HER2 negative on core biopsy [Fig. 12C (low power), D (high power)].

Diagnosis

Early-stage screen-detected right breast cancer (T1N0)

Multidisciplinary Review 1

It was recommended that the patient be offered a right guide wire–localized wide local excision and sentinel node biopsy.

Treatment and Progress

The patient had a history of hypothyroidism, but was clinically and biochemically euthyroid. She proceeded with the planned surgery three weeks later. The lesion was approached with a curvilinear incision in the medial aspect of the right breast centered over the skin projection of the radiological abnormality (ultrasound skin marker) (Fig. 12E). A specimen radio-graph confirmed that the lesion had been excised (reviewed by radiologist) and was positioned centrally with a good margin of surrounding breast tissue (Fig. 13). Two blue and hot sentinel nodes were removed. The patient made an uneventful recovery and was discharged home the following day.

Definitive Histology

This confirmed an invasive ductal carcinoma (grade III) measuring 13 mm in maximum diameter [Fig. 14A (low power), B (high power)]. There was no in situ component, and the tumor was clear of all margins by >10 mm. None of the three sentinel nodes contained any metastases (0/3 nodes).

Multidisciplinary Review 2

It was recommended that the patient receive radiotherapy to the right breast and systemic adjuvant therapy with tamoxifen for two to three years followed by an early switch to an aromatase inhibitor [NPI: $(0.2 \times 1.3) + 3 + 1 = 4.26$]. Chemotherapy should be discussed with the patient (modest absolute benefit of 2–3% only).

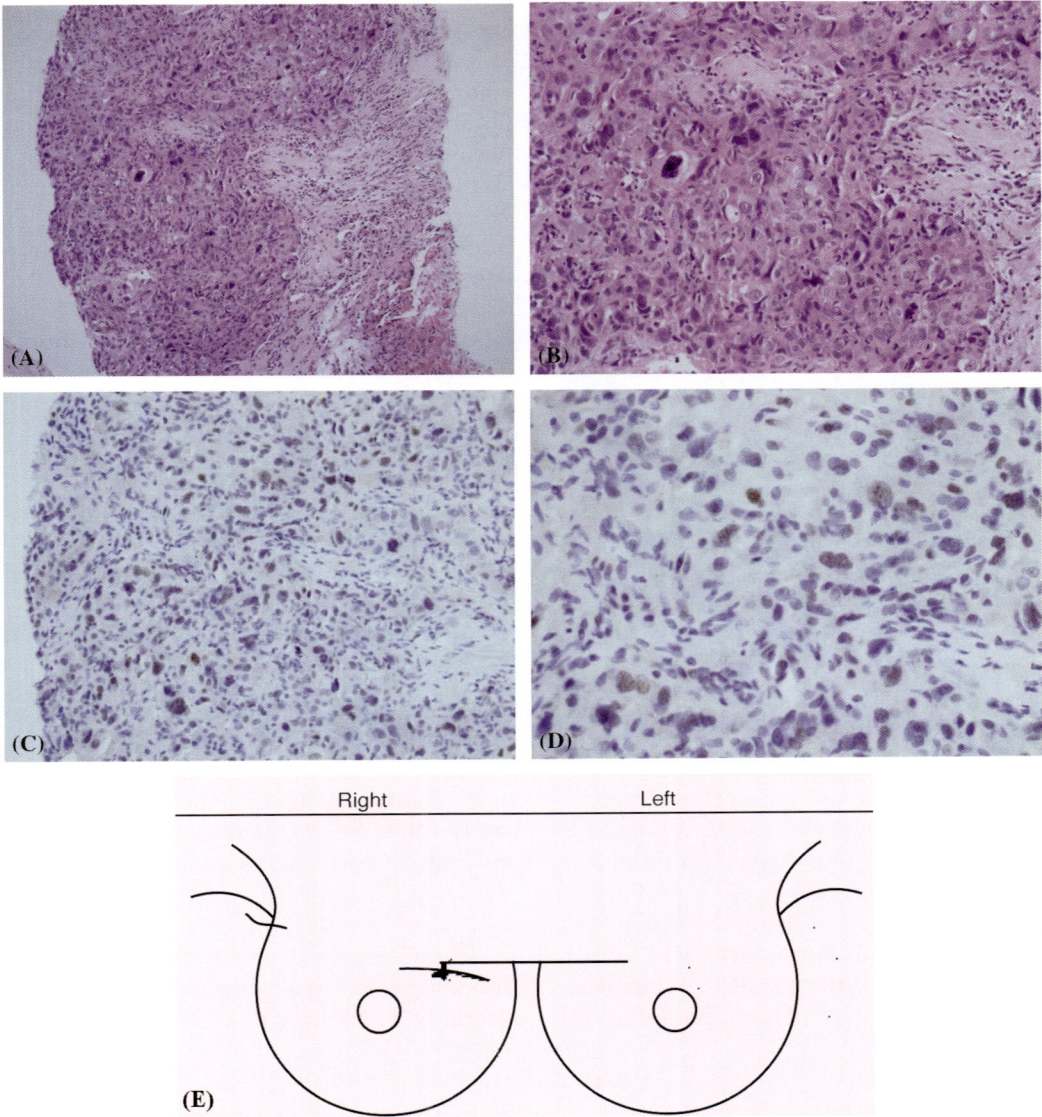

Figure 12

Discussion

This patient had a small invasive carcinoma detected as an opacity on routine screening mammography. Though the histology was a grade III invasive ductal carcinoma, this was otherwise a typical screen-detected breast cancer. Grading of tumors is based on the degree of tubule formation (t), the number of mitoses (m), and the degree of nuclear pleiomorphism (p). Each of these factors is scored by the pathologist, and the overall score determines the grade (this patient scored t3, m3, p3—total score 9). There is an element of subjectivity, and the proportion of tumors graded as I, II, and III varies from one center to another. Non–high grade and special-type tumors are more common in the older screened population (1–4).

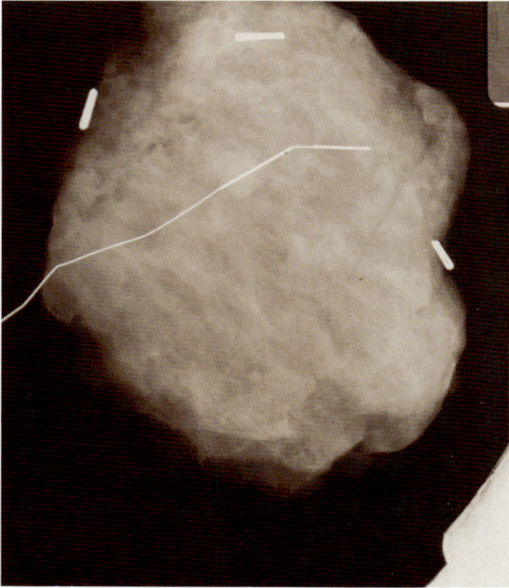

Figure 13

It is helpful to the surgeon if a skin marker is placed by the radiologist in addition to the wire at the time of localization. Sometimes the wire enters the breast at some distance from the radiological abnormality. Under these circumstances, it is preferable to make an incision overlying the lesion and deliver the wire into the surgical field from a more peripheral entry point. To facilitate placement of the skin incision, the radiolog-ists can mark the skin projection of the lesion. The surgeon then aims to excise a column of tissue deep to this, which incorporates the tip of the wire and the adjacent breast tissue (which should contain the lesion). It is imperative to undertake a specimen radiograph that has been appropriately orientated with sutures and ligaclips (the latter are radiopaque). It is conventional to place two sutures superiorly and a single one laterally. The specimen radiograph should be viewed by the radiologist who has performed the localization (5,6). They should comment on

1. the presence of the radiological abnormality (opacity, microcalcification, area of architectural distortion),
2. the position of the tip of the wire in relation to this, and
3. the presence of any clip that has been deployed at the time of core biopsy

In addition, the position of the lesion in relation to the gross specimen should be commented on; if the lesion appears close to one particular margin, then further tissue can be taken before the wound is closed. This will reduce the chance of re-excision at a later stage (7). In this case, the lesion was positioned centrally with an adequate margin of surrounding tissue. This was confirmed on definitive histology, which showed a good clearance of all margins (>10 mm).

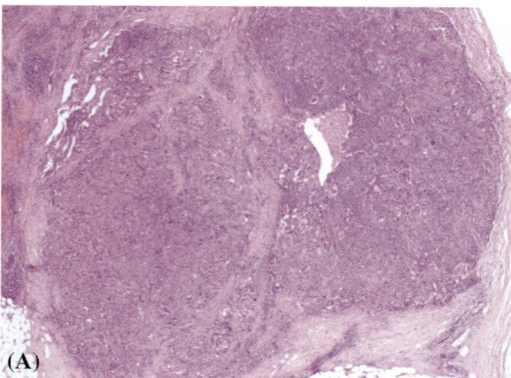

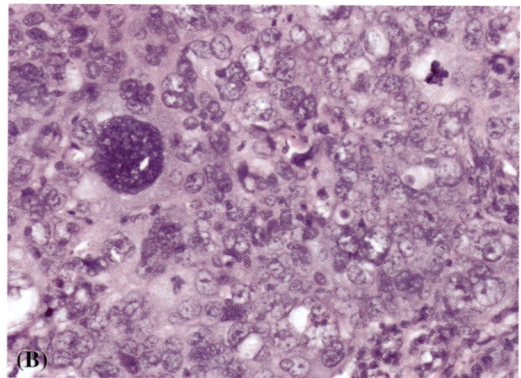

(A)   (B)

Figure 14

Radiotherapy was recommended as adjuvant treatment; there is some evidence that older patients (>55 years) with a non–high grade tumor excised with wide margins might safely avoid radiotherapy (8,9). Such patients have a low risk of local recurrence without irradiation, and the absolute benefits therefrom are small. Nonetheless, radiotherapy will still reduce this risk whatever its relative level (e.g., from 4% to 2% at 10 years). Though this patient had a small, screen-detected node-negative cancer, its high grade pushed up the NPI to 4.25. The patient qualified for systemic adjuvant hormonal therapy with tamoxifen for two to three years, followed by an early switch to an aromatase inhibitor. However, the absolute benefits from chemotherapy were in the range of 3% to 5%, and this was discussed with the patient.

Related Cases

Screen-detected lesions—*Case Studies 13, 15, 16, and 17*

Breast conservation surgery for impalpable lesions—*Case Studies 13 and 15*

Aromatase inhibitors—*Case Studies 1, 4, 9, 10, and 19*

Sentinel lymph node biopsy—*Case Studies 5, 6, 7, 10, 11, 16, 24, and 26*

Learning Points

1. **Mammographic screening reduces breast cancer mortality in postmenopausal women by about 25%, but its benefit in premenopausal women is disputed. However, women should also consider the potential hazards of mammographic screening: lead time (the early detection of cancer may not necessarily result in benefit), false positives (finding lesions on mammography that ultimately prove not to be cancer), overdiagnosis (finding lesions such as DCIS**
that might never pose a threat to life), and the risks of exposure to low dose radiation.
2. After lumpectomy for breast cancer, omission of radiotherapy may increase the risk of local recurrence. A meta-analysis of trials comparing lumpectomy with and without radiotherapy found that omission of radiotherapy was associated with an 8% excess in mortality. However, competing causes of mortality (besides breast cancer) are of greater concern in older patients, so the benefit of radiotherapy is diminished in these patients.

References

1. Anderson TJ, Lamb J, Donnan P, et al. Comparative pathology of breast cancer in a randomised trial of screening. Br J Cancer 1991; 64:108–113.
2. Cole P, Morrison AS. Basic issues in population screening for cancer. J Natl Cancer Inst 1980; 65:1263.
3. Klemi PJ, Joensuu H, Toikkanen J, et al. Aggressiveness of breast cancers found with and without screening. BMJ 1992; 304:467–469.
4. Crisp WJ, Higgs MJ, Cowan WK, et al. Screening for breast cancer detects tumours at an earlier biological stage. Br J Surg 1993; 80:863–865.
5. Hwang ES, Esserman LJ. Management of ductal carcinoma in situ. Surg Clin North Am 1999; 79 (5):1007–1030.
6. Woo CS, Skinner KA, Silverstein MJ. Ductal carcinoma in situ: clinical studies and controversies in treatment. In: Querci della Rovere G, Warren R, Benson JR, eds. Early Breast Cancer. London and New York: Taylor and Francis, 2006:349–374.
7. Mokbel K, Ahmed M, Nash A, et al. Re-excision operations in nonpalpable breast cancer. J Surg Oncol 1995; 58:225–228.
8. Lim M, Bellon J, Gelman R, et al. A prospective study of conservative surgery without radiation therapy in selected patients with stage I breast cancer. Int J Radiat Oncol Biol Phys 2006; 65:1149–1154.
9. Hughes K, Schnaper L, Berry D, et al. Lumpectomy plus tamoxifen with or without irradiation in women 70 years of age or older with early breast cancer. N Eng J Med 2004; 351:971–977.

CASE STUDY 15

History

A 64-year-old woman was recalled from routine screening mammography with bilateral areas of microcalcification. The patient had undergone a core biopsy from the right breast four years previously, which showed benign changes only. She had a weak family history of breast cancer, having a paternal aunt diagnosed with postmenopausal disease. The patient had two children and was 24 years of age at the birth of her first child. She had never used either the oral contraceptive pill or hormone replacement therapy.

Clinical Findings

Clinical examination was normal with no palpable discrete lumps or any areas of focal nodularity (E1).

Clinical Assessment

Bilateral microcalcification detected on routine screening with no clinical correlate

Investigations

Mammography (Screening)

There were localized areas of fine clustered microcalcification in both breasts with no associated soft tissue shadow (opacity) (Fig. 15A–D).

Mammotome Biopsy

Percutaneous biopsy with a vacuum-assisted device (11-gauge needle) revealed high–nuclear grade DCIS with necrosis on the left side (Fig. 16) and fibroadenomatoid changes on the right. Calcium was present within these areas of DCIS and fibroadenomatoid change corresponding to calcium present in the mammotome biopsy specimens (Fig. 17A, B). A clip was deployed at the time of biopsy.

Diagnosis

(1) Localized screen-detected ductal carcinoma in situ left breast (Tis)

(2) Pathologically indeterminate lesion right breast (B3)

Multidisciplinary Review 1

Following multidisciplinary review, it was recommended that the patient undergo a left guide wire–localized wide local excision and a right guide wire–localized diagnostic biopsy.

Treatment and Progress

Wire localization was carried out on the morning of surgery, and the patient was placed early on the list (insulin-dependent diabetic). Once the patient was anesthetized, it was noted that a guide wire was present on the left side only. Localization of the right side had been omitted in error. The patient proceeded with a wide local excision on the left side (Fig. 18); specimen radiography confirmed that the clip was present in the specimen, but calcification was close to the superolateral aspect of the specimen. A cavity shave was therefore taken. An intraoperative ultrasound failed to visualize the area of calcification in the right breast, and no surgical procedure was undertaken on this side.

Definitive Histology

This showed high–nuclear grade DCIS with comedo necrosis extending over an area of 30 mm. In addition, a small focus (6 mm) of invasive ductal carcinoma (grade II; ER positive) was found. All surgical margins were clear of both invasive and in situ disease by >10 mm [Fig. 19A (magnification 5×), B (magnification 10×)].

Multidisciplinary Review 2

In view of the invasive component on the left side, axillary staging was required. It was recommended that a left sentinel lymph node biopsy be undertaken and this be combined with a right guide wire localized biopsy as originally planned.

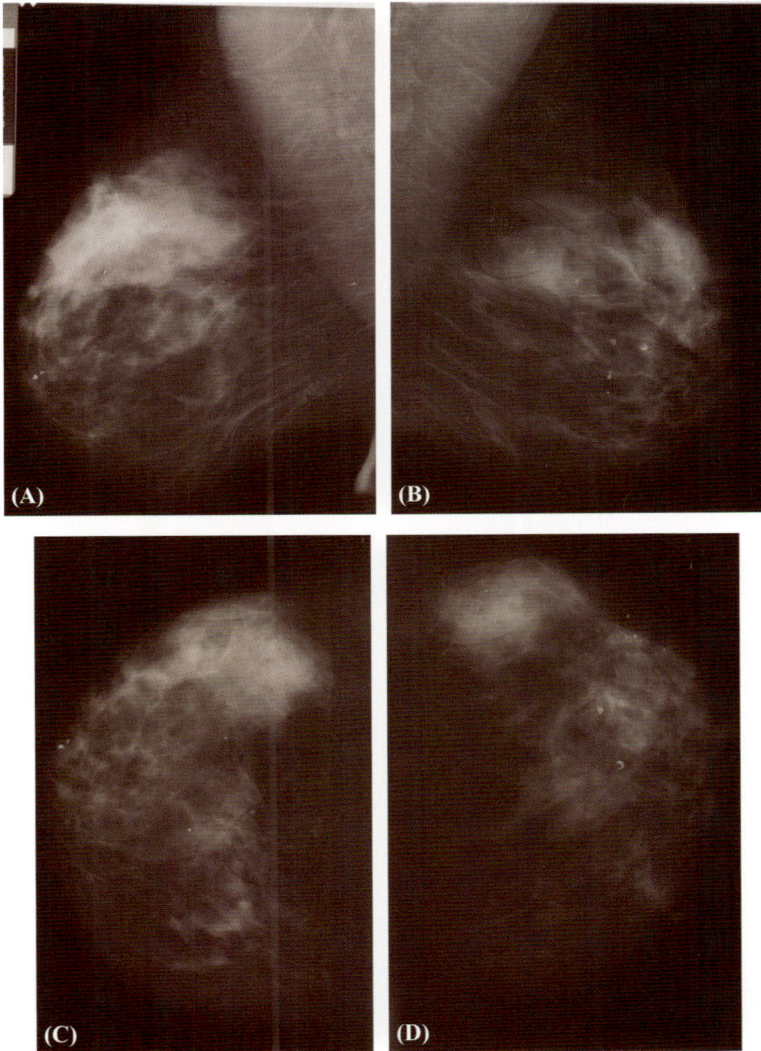

Figure 15

Treatment and Progress

The patient was admitted for further surgery two weeks later (i.e., four weeks from the first surgical procedure). Two hot and blue nodes were identified in the left axilla, and a wire-guided diagnostic biopsy was undertaken from the right breast (Fig. 20). A specimen X ray confirmed the presence of both a clip and calcification (Fig. 21). The patient made an uneventful recovery and was discharged home one day after surgery.

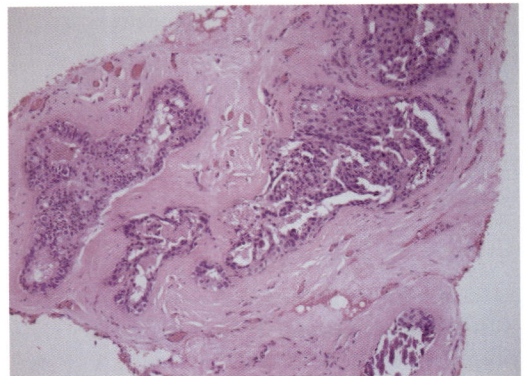

Figure 16

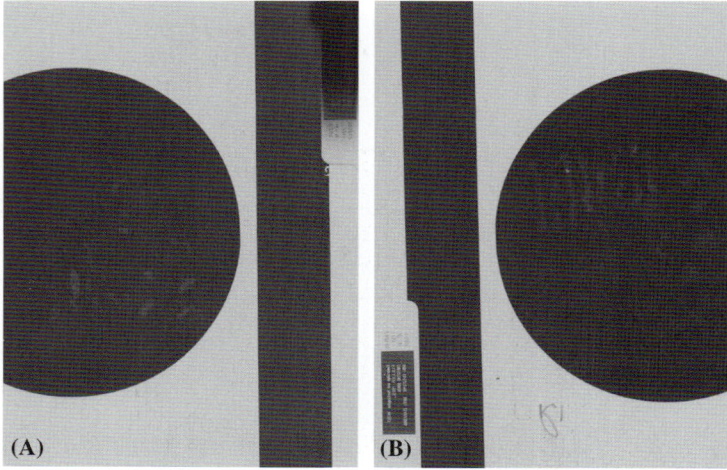

(A)   (B)

Figure 17

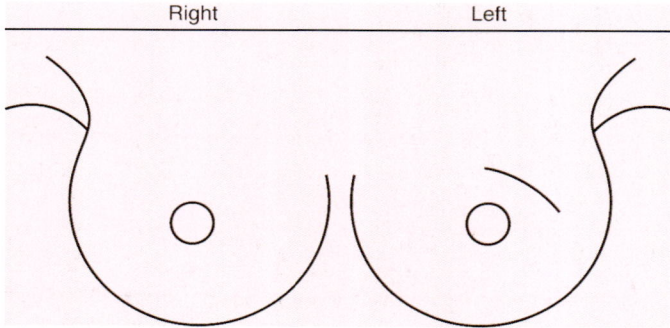

Right   Left

Figure 18

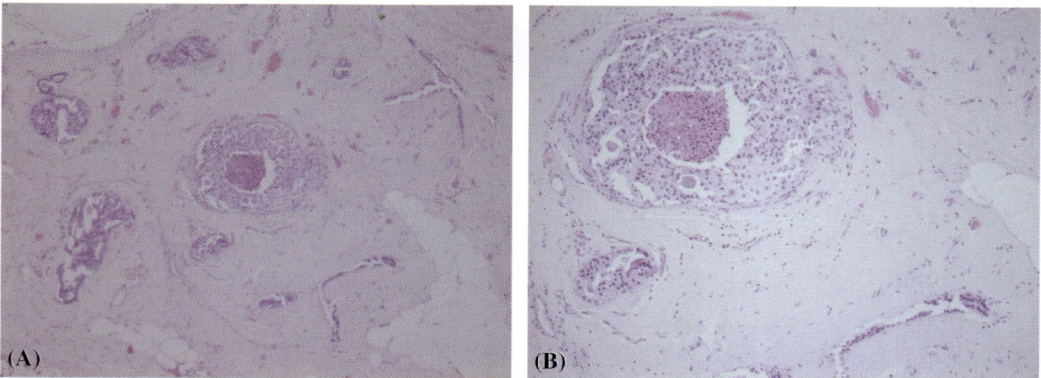

(A)   (B)

Figure 19

Definitive Histology

All four nodes retrieved from the left axilla were free of tumor. Histology of the right breast lesion confirmed the findings of previous core biopsy and showed fibroadenoma- toid hyperplasia with microcalcification [Fig. 22 (magnification 5×)]. There was no evidence of atypia or malignancy, and the mammotome biopsy site was present in the specimen.

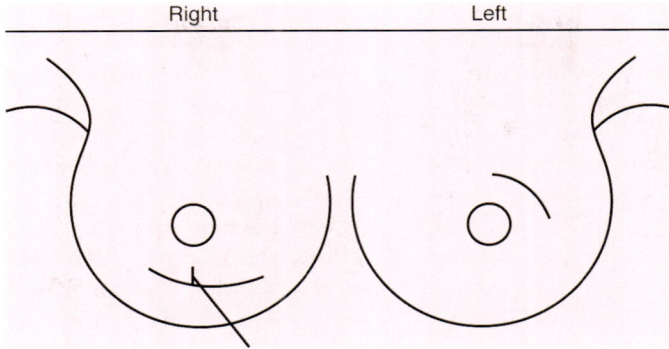

Figure 20

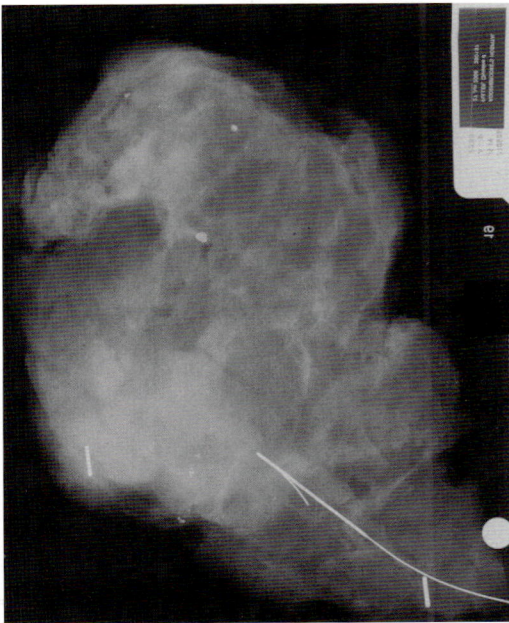

Figure 21

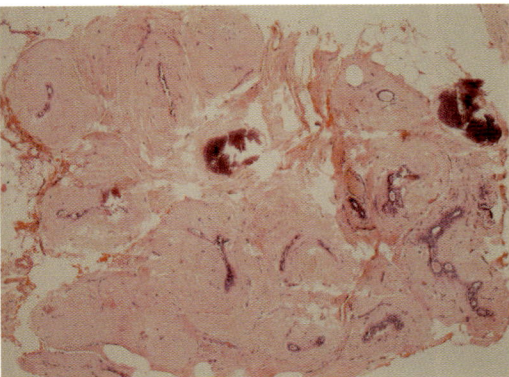

Figure 22

Multidisciplinary Review 3

Further adjuvant therapies included radiotherapy to the left breast and tamoxifen (20 mg daily) for five years (low risk of relapse with an NPI of <4.4).

Treatment and Progress

The patient proceeded with a three-week course of radiotherapy to the left breast (46 Gy in 15 fractions). She was intolerant of tamoxifen, and the option of discontinuing any form of systemic adjuvant hormonal therapy was discussed. However, the patient was keen to receive hormonal treatment (estimated benefit <1%), and she was switched from tamoxifen to the aromatase inhibitor arimidex after eight months.

Discussion

This case demonstrates a failure of communication and organization. Bilateral guide-wire localization should have been undertaken on the day of surgery, but only the left side was localized. By the time this was recognized, the patient was already under general anesthetic and could not return to the breast unit for a further localization. Intraoperative ultrasound can often detect the mammographic abnormality, particularly when there is a focal mass lesion. Calcification alone may not be visualized on ultrasound (as was the case here), and this is one of the main limitations of ultrasound for diagnosis of early breast cancer. Calcium forms an interface, which is opaque to this frequency of sound waves, but higher frequency transducers can detect calcification within small tumors (1). It was perhaps fortuitous that an invasive tumor was found in the left breast on definitive histology, which mandated axillary staging with sentinel lymph node biopsy. This provided an opportunity to perform a right guide wire–localized diagnostic biopsy at the same time. Sentinel node biopsy for localized DCIS (wide excision only) is indicated only when the lesion is palpable or possibly when a focal mass lesion is evident radiologically.

The advantage of a vacuum-assisted biopsy device using an 11-gauge needle (such as a mammotome) is retrieval of a larger volume of tissue than with a conventional core biopsy. The former varies in size from 8 to 14 gauge, while the latter is best undertaken with either a 14- or a 16-gauge needle. These devices are particularly suitable for biopsy of screen-detected areas of microcalcification (2). In the case of a small cluster of microcalcification, this may be completely removed with percutaneous biopsy and a metallic clip must be inserted to mark the biopsy site if subsequent surgery is required. Mammotome biopsy is less likely to underestimate disease; when only DCIS is diagnosed with a vacuum-assisted biopsy, the chance of finding invasive disease at subsequent surgical excision is only 10% (compared with 20% for conventional core biopsy) (3). An unexpected finding of invasion will mandate axillary staging if this has not already been undertaken. Sometimes this can be combined with cavity re-excision or completion mastectomy.

In terms of this patient's in situ disease, the Van Nuys prognostic index (see page 90, case study 16) was [2 (size 30 mm) + 1 (margins > 10 mm) + 3 (high grade with necrosis) + 1 (age 64 years)] = 7.

This patient should receive radiotherapy for DCIS, but also required this as treatment for the invasive component. However, the absolute risk reduction for local recurrence will be very small for a 6-mm tumor. Similarly, the benefits from adjuvant systemic therapy will be modest (approximately 1%). In the presence of troublesome side effects from tamoxifen, it would be reasonable to withhold any hormonal treatment (rather than switching to an aromatase inhibitor).

Hot flushes and night sweats can adversely impact on a woman's quality of life and are often exacerbated by tamoxifen (or aromatase inhibitors) if preexistent. Simple remedies like vitamin B6 may help, but more severe and persistent symptoms usually require more specific treatment with agents such as clonidine or propanolol. The antidepressant agent venlafaxine has been extensively trialed, and studies have shown a 40% to 60% reduction in incidence of hot flushes at a dosage of either 37.5 or 75 mg daily (4). Similarly, the selective serotonin reuptake inhibitor fluoxetine has shown promising results in pilot studies for management of persistently troublesome hot flushes and night sweats (5). These can be justifications for switching from tamoxifen to an aromatase inhibitor as adjuvant therapy.

Related Cases

Screen-detected lesions—*Case Studies 13, 14, 16, and 17*

Breast conservation surgery for impalpable lesions—*Case Studies 13 and 14*

Adjuvant hormonal therapy—*Case Studies 1, 4, 9, 10, and 19*

Sentinel lymph node biopsy—*Case Studies 5, 6, 7, 10, 11, 16, 24, and 26*

Learning Points

1. In the United States, approximately 11% of all women who undergo screening mammograms are recalled. Approximately 0.3% of these women are found to have either DCIS or invasive cancer, so the false-positive rate for screening mammography in the United States is about 10.7%. The false-positive rate is much higher in the United States than in Europe, owing to the heightened medicolegal environment.
2. False-positive mammograms are one of the major drawbacks of breast cancer screening. False positives may result in unnecessary anxiety and psychological distress.

3. In general, cancers detected on mammograms have a better prognosis than those detected clinically. This is partly attributable to lead time bias (screening advances the time of diagnosis, so the interval of time from diagnosis to death is automatically extended). However, the better prognosis of screen-detected cancers is also partly attributable to length bias (slow-growing, indolent tumors are more likely to be detected by screening, while the faster-growing tumors are more likely to be detected in the intervals between screening sessions). Yet, the benefit of mammography screening is best discerned through randomized prospective trials, which seem to indicate that mammography screening reduces breast cancer mortality by about 25% in postmenopausal women.

References

1. Cheung YC, Wan YL, Chen SC, et al. Sonographic evaluation of mammographically detected microcalcifications without a mass prior to stereotactic core needle biopsy. J Clin Ultrasound 2002; 30:323–331.
2. Jackman RJ, Burbank F, Parker SH, et al. Atypical ductal hyperplasia diagnosed at stereotactic breast biopsy: improved reliability with 14 gauge, directional, vacuum-assisted biopsy. Radiology 1997; 204:485–488.
3. Jackman RJ, Nowels KW, Rodriguez-Soto J, et al. Stereotactic, automated, large-core needle biopsy of nonpalpable breast lesions: false-negative and histologic underestimation rates after long term follow up. Radiology 1999; 210:799–805.
4. Loprinzi CL, Sloan JA, Perez EA, et al. Phase III evaluation of fluoxetine for treatment of hot flashes. J Clin Oncol 2002; 20:1578–1583.
5. Loprinzi CL, Kugler JW, Sloan JA, et al. Venlafaxine in management of hot flashes in survivors of breast cancer: a randomized controlled trial. Lancet 2000; 356:2059–2063.

Incidental Breast Cancer

3

Part I: Mastectomy

CASE STUDY 16

History

A 47-year-old woman presented with a three-week history of a lump in the left breast, which was slightly tender but not associated with any nipple discharge. The lump had not changed in size over this time period.

Clinical Findings

Examination revealed an area of focal nodularity in the upper outer quadrant of the left breast, but no discrete or dominant lump. There was no axillary lymphadenopathy (E2) (Fig. 1).

Clinical Assessment

The presentation was suggestive of benign breast disease (fibrocystic changes) with no clinically suspicious features.

Investigations

Mammography

The mammographic appearances of the left breast were normal, but multiple clusters of coarse granular microcalcification were seen in the upper outer quadrant of the contralateral breast (Fig. 2A–D). The calcification extended over an area of 23 mm and there was a low index of suspicion for malignancy (R3/4).

Breast Ultrasound

Several small cysts were present in the upper outer quadrant of the left breast corresponding to the area of palpable nodularity. The sonographic interpretation of both breasts

was benign and consistent with fibrocystic changes (R2).

Mammotome Biopsy

Stereotactic core biopsy of the microcalcification in the right breast revealed high nuclear grade DCIS (ductal carcinoma in situ) with comedo necrosis [Fig. 3A (magnification 10×), B (magnification 20×)]. There were associated foci of lobular neoplasia (atypical lobular hyperplasia/lobular carcinoma in situ) (Fig. 3C). Calcium was present in the biopsy specimen.

Diagnosis

Incidental noninvasive cancer of the right breast cancer (Tis).

Multidisciplinary Review 1

Following multidisciplinary review, it was recommended the patient undergo a right guidewire-localized wide local excision of the DCIS, which appeared localized to the upper outer quadrant of the right breast radiologically.

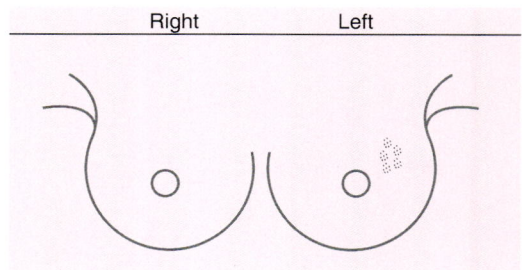

Figure 1

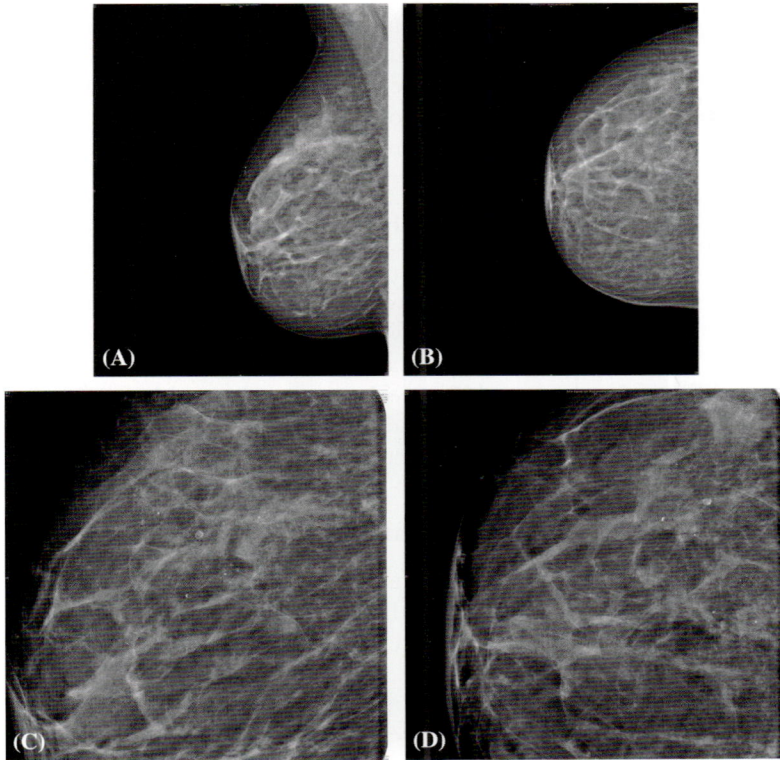

Figure 2

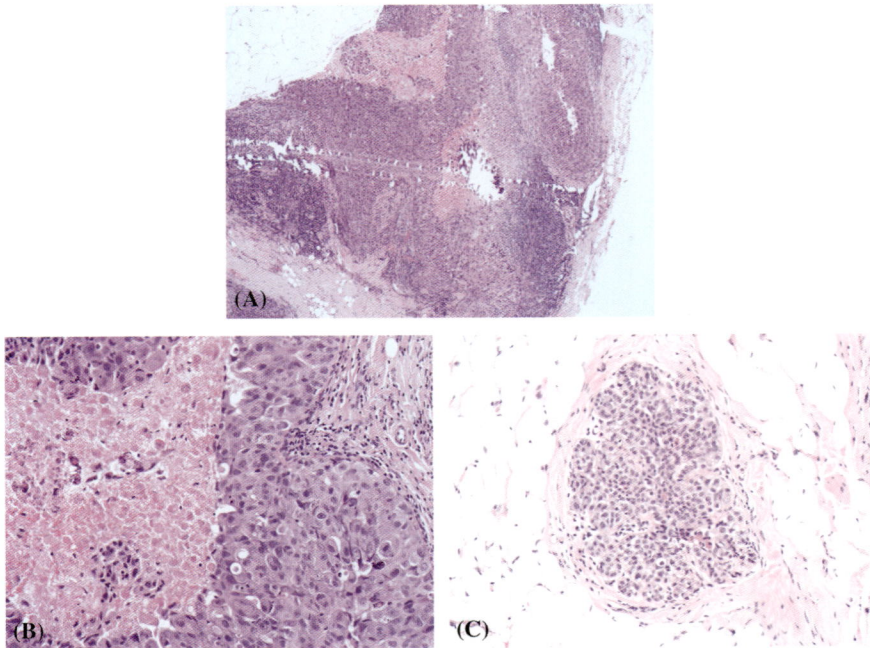

Figure 3

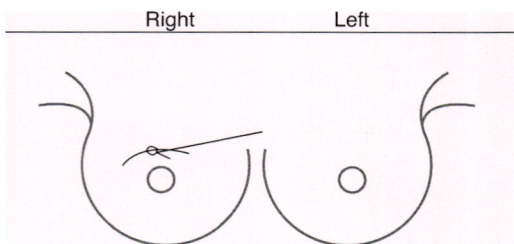

Figure 4

Treatment and Progress

The patient proceeded to surgery four weeks later (holiday during interim) as a day case (Fig. 4). A guidewire was inserted on the morning of surgery and a specimen radiograph confirmed that all calcification had been removed together with a satisfactory margin of surrounding breast tissue. The patient made an uneventful recovery and was discharged home on the same day.

Definitive Histology

This revealed extensive ductal [Fig. 5A (low power); B (high power)] and lobular (Fig. 5C) carcinoma in situ extending over an area of at least 52 mm (Fig. 5A–C). Tumor extended to the lateral and inferior margins (Fig. 5D) and there was columnar cell change with atypia at the superior margin. The medial margin was clear of tumor (>5 mm).

Multidisciplinary Review 2

In view of the extent of the lesion (>50 mm) together with involvement of several margins, it was recommended the patient undergo a right completion mastectomy together with a sentinel lymph node biopsy. She would be offered immediate breast reconstruction.

Treatment and Progress

Immediate breast reconstruction was discussed with the patient, but she was rather undecided on this issue. After further consideration, the patient expressed a wish to pursue immediate breast reconstruction and was referred to the plastic surgeons for discussion of reconstructive options. A right sentinel lymph node biopsy was undertaken in advance of definitive surgery and revealed no evidence of nodal metastases. The patient

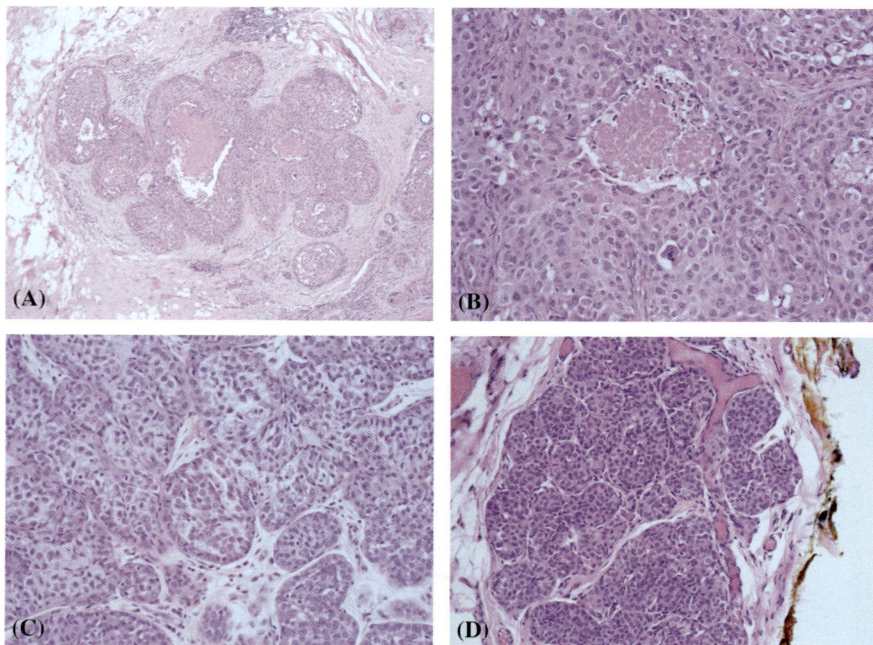

Figure 5

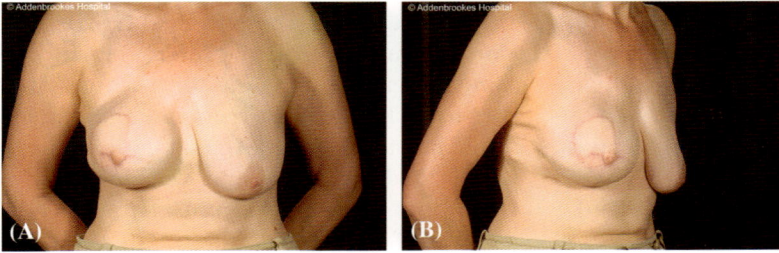

Figure 6

proceeded to a right simple mastectomy (no further axillary surgery indicated) and immediate breast reconstruction with a latissimus dorsi (LD) flap and implant. A skin-sparing technique was employed and the scar from the previous wide local excision was not disturbed. This allowed for preservation of much of the skin envelope and provided optimal cosmetic results (Fig. 6A, B). The patient made an excellent postoperative recovery and was discharged home on the seventh postoperative day. The time interval between the original diagnosis and definitive surgery was four months.

Definitive Histology

This showed extensive residual LCIS around the surgical cavity and within a random section taken from the upper outer quadrant. There was no residual DCIS or invasive disease (Fig. 7).

Multidisciplinary Review 3

Having undergone mastectomy for DCIS/LCIS with no evidence of invasive disease

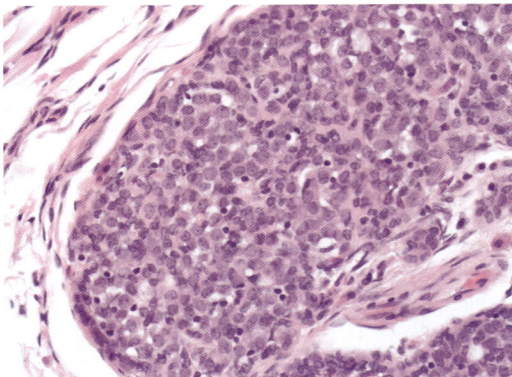

Figure 7

(sentinel node biopsy negative), the patient required no further treatment. There was no indication for either radiotherapy or tamoxifen as adjuvant systemic hormonal therapy in the context of in situ disease treated by mastectomy. The patient had an excellent prognosis and was entered into the patient-led follow-up program. She would receive contralateral mammography at two and four years posttreatment.

Discussion

This patient presented with a symptomatic breast lump and was found to have incidental calcification in the contralateral breast. This had rather coarse features and the initial index of radiological suspicion was low, though sufficiently high to warrant biopsy. The calcification was associated with high nuclear grade DCIS in the core biopsy specimens. Calcification is commonly seen with comedo necrosis, where dystrophic calcification occurs within necrotic material in the center of the ducts. The initial radiological estimate of the size of this DCIS was 23 mm. This was deemed suitable for breast-conserving surgery with wide local excision. Until relatively recently, the majority of DCIS was managed with mastectomy. With the introduction of screening programs, diagnosis of DCIS has increased form about 7% of all breast cancers in 1985 to approximately 20% to 25% of current new diagnoses (1). Moreover, most of these screen-detected cases of DCIS are relatively localized areas involving a single quadrant of the breast. It is difficult to justify mastectomy for such cases and breast conservation surgery has been increasingly used for treatment of these small areas of DCIS over the past two decades. When breast-conserving surgery is undertaken for DCIS, the primary tumor must be excised with clear histological margins as a minimum. The use of radiotherapy after wide local excision for DCIS remains controversial, but the majority of high nuclear grade lesions receive this (2–5). The crucial issue with breast-conserving surgery for localized DCIS is the risk of recurrence. In most published series, approximately half of all local recurrences for DCIS were invasive disease—herein lies the importance of local control and the dilemma it sometimes presents (2,3,6). Clinicians must be confident that the risk of local recurrence is at an acceptable level (<10% at 5–10 years) when anything less than mastectomy is offered for surgical treatment of DCIS.

The risk of local recurrence is related to three principle factors:

1. Size of the lesion
2. Margin width
3. Grade of the lesion

These are each statistically independent predictors of local tumor recurrence and have been quantified in an attempt to make them clinically useful. The Van Nuys Prognostic Index (VNPI) (7) and its recent modification (which incorporates age) (8) has been popularized in recent years. The scoring system for the VNPI is shown in Table 1. The recommendations for treatment based on the VNPI are as follows:

4, 5, 6—excision only
7, 8, 9—excision plus radiotherapy
10, 11, 12—mastectomy

Although radiotherapy significantly decreases the risk of local recurrence by about 50% when compared with excision alone, it may represent over treatment for some patients undergoing breast-conserving surgery. The blanket recommendation by American authorities (4) that radiotherapy is indicated for all patients with high-grade DCIS does not take account of the heterogeneity of DCIS or variation in absolute benefits from radiotherapy between different subsets. Radiotherapy not only has significant side effects but also changes the texture of the breast and renders subsequent mammography more difficult to interpret. Moreover, the breast cannot receive further irradiation should an ipsilateral invasive breast cancer develop at a later date.

Following initial wide local excision, this patient had a VNPI of:
[3 (size 52 mm) + 3 (margins < 1 mm) + 3 (high grade with necrosis) + 2 (age 48 years)] = 11

Therefore, completion mastectomy was appropriate based on the above treatment recommendations. From a surgical point of view, mastectomy is usually indicated for a lesion >40 mm in size. However, it may be possible to excise more extensive DCIS in a large breast with satisfactory margins of clearance (particularly using some of the newer oncoplastic techniques such as therapeutic mammoplasty). If the calculated VNPI is below 10, then the estimated risk of recurrence would be sufficiently low to accept breast conservation (with radiotherapy).

This patient opted for immediate breast reconstruction and underwent sentinel lymph node biopsy in advance of definitive surgery. Final histology revealed no evidence of invasive disease and no further treatment was indicated. Despite having a scar in the upper

Table 1   The Modified University of Southern California/Van Nuys Prognostic (USC/VNPI) Scoring System

	Score		
	1	*2*	*3*
Size	<15 mm	16–40 mm	>41 mm
Margins	>10 mm	1–9 mm	<1 mm
Pathology	Non-high grade without necrosis	Non-high grade with necrosis	High-grade with or without necrosis
Age	≥61 yr	40–60 yr	≤39 yr

Source: Adapted from Ref. 9

outer quadrant of the right breast from initial wide local excision, the patient was very happy with the cosmetic result. A two-stage procedure necessarily incurs additional scarring and whenever possible the need for mastectomy should be anticipated at the outset. This will avoid a second surgical procedure and confine scarring to the periareolar region (skin-sparing mastectomy).

Related Cases

DCIS—*Case Studies 12, 13, 17, and 18*

Immediate breast reconstruction—*Case Studies 3, 17, 18, and 37*

Learning Points

1. Following mastectomy for DCIS, some oncologists might offer a patient tamoxifen (20 mg/day for 5 years) to reduce the risk of contralateral breast cancer. Yet, in general, tamoxifen is not indicated after total mastectomy for DCIS.
2. If breast-conserving surgery is attempted in a patient with a diffuse area of DCIS, then two wires might be placed to localize two ends of the lesion, thereby providing guideposts for wide excision of the entire lesion.
3. The LD muscle alone generally does not provide sufficient tissue bulk, so reconstruction with an LD flap usually requires placement of an implant. In contrast, the transverse rectus abdominis muscle (TRAM) flap provides sufficient tissue bulk and an implant is not required. Yet, the TRAM flap procedure is technically more challenging, and it is associated with a greater risk of morbidity. An extended autologous LD flap provides additional bulk without the need for an implant but can be associated with increased donor site morbidity.

References

1. Bland KI, Menck HR, Scott-Conner CE, et al. The National Cancer Data Base 10 year survey of breast carcinoma treatment at hospitals in the United States. Cancer 1998; 83:1262–1273.
2. Solin L, Kurtz J, Fourquet A, et al. Fifteen results of breast conserving surgery and definitive breast irradiation for treatment of ductal carcinoma-in-situ of the breast. J Clin Oncol 1996; 14: 754–763.
3. Fisher B, Dignam J, Wolmark N, et al. Lumpectomy and radiation therapy for the treatment of intra-ductal breast cancer: findings from the National Surgical Adjuvant Breast and Bowel Project B-17. J Clin Oncol 1998; 16:441–452.
4. Fisher B, Land S, Mamounas E, et al. Prevention of invasive breast cancer in women with ductal carcinoma in situ: an update of the National Surgical Adjuvant Breast and Bowel Project experience. Semin Oncol 2001; 28:400–418.
5. Julien J, Bijker N, Fentiman I, et al. Radiotherapy in breast conserving treatment for ductal carcinoma-in-situ: first results of EORTC randomized phase III trial 10853. Lancet 2000; 355:528–533.
6. Silverstein M, Barth A, Poller D, et al. Ten year results comparing mastectomy to excision and radiotherapy for ductal carcinoma in situ of the breast. Eur J Cancer 1995; 31:1425–1427.
7. Silverstein MJ, Lagios MD, Craig PH, et al. A prognostic index for ductal carcinoma in situ of the breast. Cancer 1996; 77:2267–2274.
8. Silverstein MJ. USC/Van Nuys Prognostic Index. In: Silverstein MJ, ed. Ductal Carcinoma In Situ of the Breast. 2nd ed. Philadelphia: Lippincott, Williams and Wilkins, 2002.
9. Woo CS, Skinner KA, Silverstein MJ. Ductal carcinoma in situ: clinical studies and controversies in treatment. In: Querci della Rovere G, Warren R, Benson JR, eds. Early Breast Cancer. New York/London: Taylor and Francis, 2005; 365.

CASE STUDY 17

History

A 45-year-old woman presented with a 12-month history of left breast pain. This had no clear relationship to the menstrual cycle and was not associated with any breast lumps or nipple discharge. The patient had no previous breast problems and no family history of breast or ovarian cancer. She had two children (eldest 16 years of age) and had used the oral contraceptive pill for a cumulative period of 10 years.

Clinical Examination

Examination of both breasts was normal with no areas of nodularity and no dominant

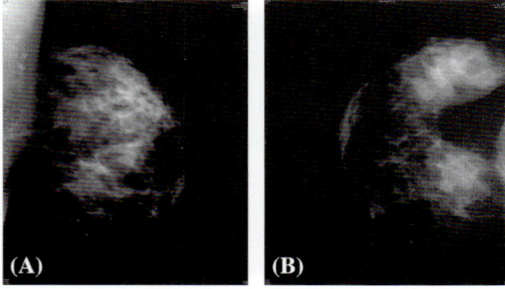

Figure 8

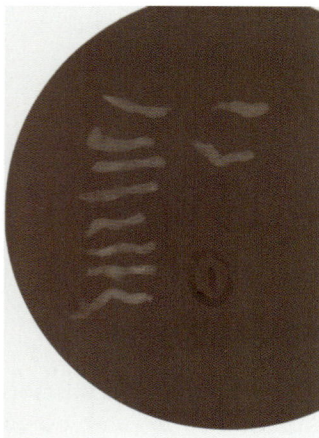

Figure 10

lumps palpable. There was no axillary lymphadenopathy (E1).

Clinical Assessment

The patient was considered to have noncyclical breast pain most likely attributed to a degree of fibrocystic change. She was reassured and provided with information on evening primrose oil (gamolenic acid 160–320 mg daily).

Investigations

Mammography

Mammographic interpretation of the left breast was normal, but two separate areas of linear and branching fine microcalcification were seen in the upper outer quadrant of the right breast (Fig. 8A, B).

Breast Ultrasound

No mass lesion was evident sonographically and these areas of suspicious microcalcification were not seen on ultrasound examination of the breasts.

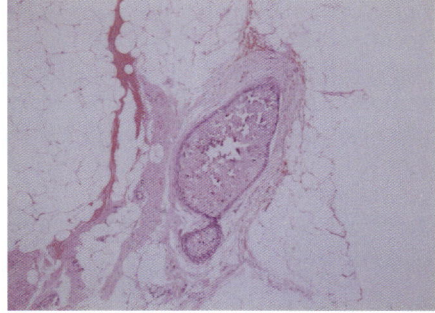

Figure 9

Mammotome Biopsy

Percutaneous biopsy was undertaken using an 11-gauge needle with a vacuum-assisted device. Specimen X ray confirmed that calcium was present in the biopsy material (Fig. 9) and histopathological examination showed high nuclear grade DCIS with comedo necrosis. Biopsies were taken from both areas in the right breast and displayed similar features (Fig. 10).

Diagnosis

Extensive multifocal ductal carcinoma in situ of the right breast cancer (Tis).

Multidisciplinary Review 1

Following multidisciplinary discussion and careful review of the mammograms, it was recommended the patient undergo a right simple mastectomy. The areas of microcalcification were separated by several centimeters and represented multicentric disease. Because of the possibility of a small focus of invasive carcinoma being found on definitive histology (approximately 20%) sentinel lymph node biopsy was advised. The patient was suitable for a skin-sparing mastectomy (periareolar incision) and would be offered immediate breast reconstruction.

Treatment and Progress

It was very difficult for the patient to come to terms with the prospect of a right mastectomy; she had presented with left breast pain and was found incidentally to have areas of suspicious microcalcification in the contralateral breast, which had no clinical correlate. The patient accepted the need for

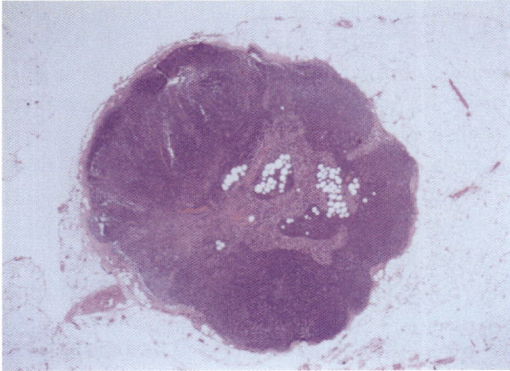

Figure 11

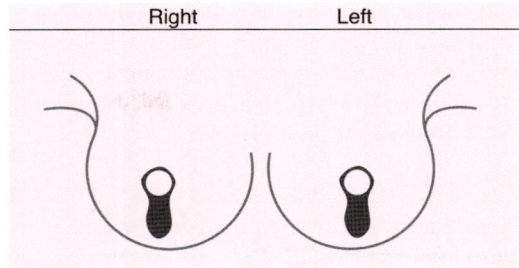

Figure 12

mastectomy and was referred to the plastic surgeons for discussion of reconstructive options. A right sentinel lymph node biopsy was carried out in advance of definitive surgery and revealed no evidence of regional metastases in any of the five nodes retrieved (Fig. 11).

The patient proceeded to a right skin-sparing mastectomy (no further axillary surgery) and immediate breast reconstruction with a free TRAM flap. A contralateral breast reduction was performed at the same time to achieve symmetrization. The incision chosen for the skin-sparing mastectomy was modified in accordance with the contralateral procedure and extirpation of breast tissue was incorporated into a vertical-type mammoplasty incision, which permitted a similar pattern of scarring in the two breasts and maximized the chance of achieving symme-

try of shape and volume (Fig. 12) and (Fig. 13A–C). The patient made an uneventful recovery and in particular experienced no problems with the healing of the abdominal wound.

Definitive Histology

This revealed extensive high nuclear grade DCIS involving much of the breast tissue (Fig. 14A). The two main foci of disease measured 30 mm and 40 mm and in addition there was a small focus of invasive carcinoma (grade II, ER positive) measuring 6 mm in maximum extent [Fig. 14B (low power), C (high power)].

Multidisciplinary Review 2

In the absence of any invasive component, no further treatment for extensive DCIS treated with mastectomy would be indicated. In the presence of a 6 mm focus of grade II,

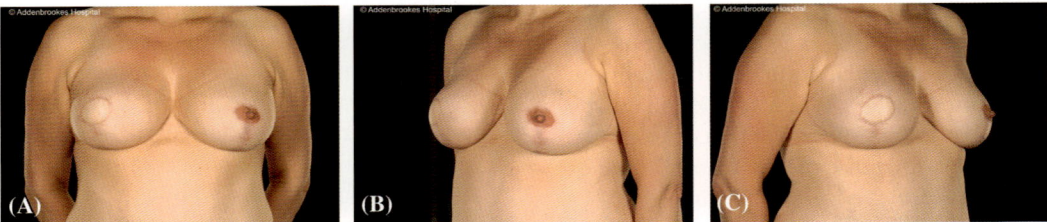

Figure 13

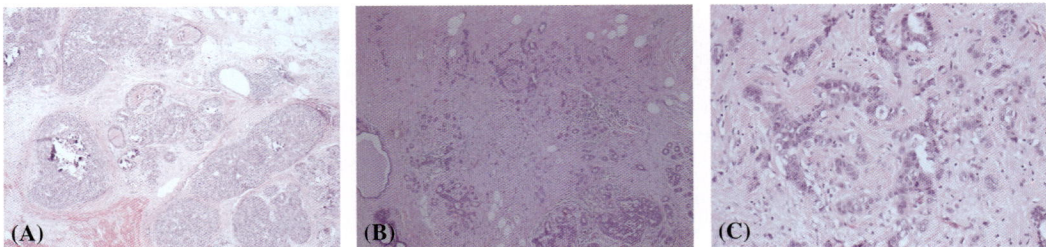

Figure 14

ER-positive node-negative invasive ductal carcinoma, adjuvant systemic hormonal therapy with five years tamoxifen is appropriate (without an early switch to an aromatase inhibitor).

Discussion

This relatively young woman was found incidentally to have multifocal high nuclear grade DCIS (with comedo necrosis) of the right breast. Two areas of suspicious microcalcification were present in separate quadrants of the breast, which mandated mastectomy. Definitive surgery, including immediate breast reconstruction, could be confidently planned on the basis of the preoperative investigations, which provided histological evidence of multifocality. There is up to a 20% chance of finding invasive disease when mastectomy is undertaken for extensive high nuclear grade DCIS, though this is reduced by use of a vacuum-assisted device with a larger bore needle (11 gauge). Sentinel node biopsy is now routinely performed in such circumstances and is best undertaken in advance of mastectomy and immediate breast reconstruction; should there be metastases within the sentinel node, then completion axillary lymph node dissection can be done at the same time as mastectomy. The latter is usually undertaken with a periareolar incision that minimizes scarring and yields excellent cosmetic results. In this particular case, a modified skin incision was employed that mirrored the vertical mammoplasty-type incision used to reduce the contralateral breast (Fig. 13) (1). This type of incision provides excellent access to the axillary contents and a counter incision in the axilla is unnecessary. When autologous tissue is transferred, the nipple-areolar complex can be replaced with a disc of skin from the donor site (in this case the lower abdomen).

Final histology revealed two areas of DCIS within the right breast measuring 30 mm and 40 mm (aggregate size 70 mm). In addition, a small 6-mm focus of invasive carcinoma was found. This was hormonally sensitive and tamoxifen was prescribed for five years as adjuvant systemic hormonal treatment (low risk of relapse).

This patient had problems coming to terms with the need for mastectomy; it is important to emphasize to these women that their long-term prognosis is excellent following mastectomy for extensive DCIS, albeit with a small invasive component (at least 90% 10-year survival). In a series of patients from Memorial Sloan-Kettering Cancer Center with node-negative and node-positive tumors less than or equal to 2 cm (T1N0 and T1N1), comparison of observed to expected survival at a median follow-up of 18 years revealed that 89% of patients with node-negative tumors less than or equal to 1 cm were estimated to be cured (2). Many of these patients will have achieved a "personal" cure and are likely to eventually succumb from non–breast cancer related causes. This patient was discharged into a patient-led follow-up program and will have contralateral mammography at two and four years and thereafter enter the NHS Breast Screening Programme.

Related Cases

DCIS—*Case Studies 12, 13, 16, and 18*

Immediate breast reconstruction—*Case Studies 3, 17, 18, and 37*

Adjuvant hormonal therapy for "minimal" breast cancer—*Case Studies 9 and 18*

Learning Points

1. This patient presented with mastalgia and no palpable breast masses. Many clinicians would not have obtained a mammogram in such an instance, unless the patient was due for an annual screening mammogram. Patients with mastalgia are often managed with evening primrose oil, dietary modification (caffeine restriction), and reassurance. If the mastalgia persists and is severe, a short course of tamoxifen therapy might be considered.

2. In patients with multicentric DCIS, the risk of invasive cancer is about 20% and a sentinel node biopsy should be obtained prior to mastectomy. If the sentinel node biopsy had not been obtained, and the invasive cancer was discovered incidentally after the mastectomy, then a level I and II axillary dissection might be required (sentinel node biopsy would no longer be feasible after mastectomy).

References

1. Lejour M. Vertical mammoplasty without infra-mammary scar and with liposuction. Perspect Plast Surg 1990; 4:67.

2. Rosen PP, Groshen S, Saigo P, et al. A long-term follow up study of survival in stage I (T1N0M0) and stage II (T1N1M1) breast carcinoma. J Clin Oncol 1989; 7:355–366.

CASE STUDY 18

History

A 42-year-old woman presented with a two-week history of a non-tender lump in the right breast. This had not changed in size and there was no associated nipple discharge. There were no previous breast problems and the patient did not report having particularly "lumpy" breasts. The patient's maternal grandmother and great aunt had developed breast cancer postmenopausally. The patient had two children both of whom were breast-fed and was aged 28 years when giving birth to her eldest child. The oral contraceptive pill had been used for a cumulative period of 15 years, including 7 years usage prior to the patient's first pregnancy. She had a relatively early menarche at the age of 10 years.

Clinical Findings

Examination revealed large pendulous breasts with an area of focal nodularity in the upper inner quadrant and a smooth round tender lump immediately inferior to the right nipple areolar complex measuring 0.5 cm in maximum diameter (E2). There was no axillary lymphadenopathy (Fig. 15).

Clinical Assessment

The clinical impression was of benign breast disease involving localized fibroadenotic change and duct ectasia with possible peri-ductal cyst formation. There were no clini-cally suspicious features.

Investigations

Mammography

This showed an area of pleiomorphic micro-calcification in the superior aspect of the right breast extending over at least 40 mm. There was a vague mass lesion associated with microcalcification and the appearances were highly suspicious for DCIS (Fig. 16A–C).

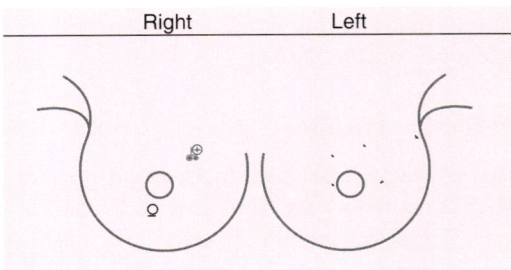

(A)

(B)   (C)

Figure 16

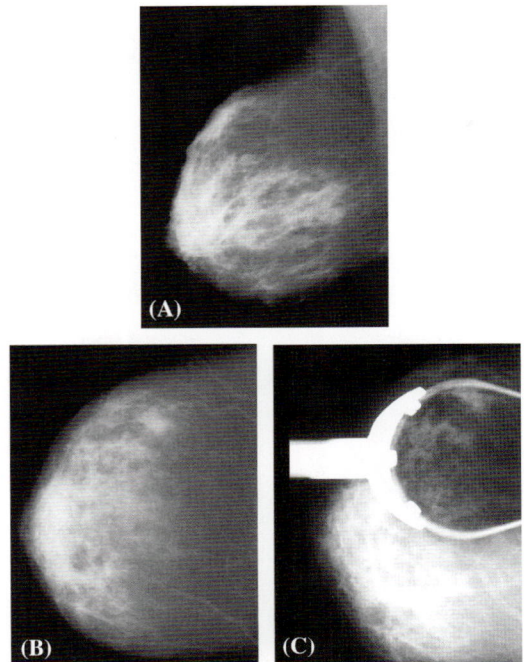

Right   Left

Figure 15

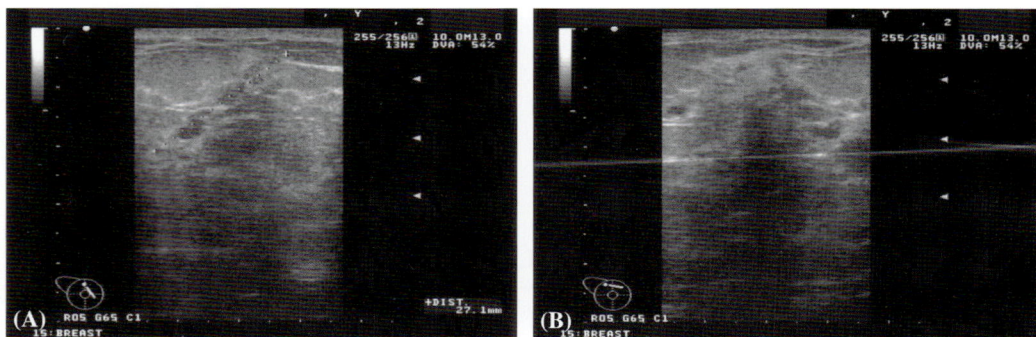

Figure 17

Breast Ultrasound

The sonographic correlate of the microcalcification was an extensive area of altered echogenicity between 11 and 12 o'clock. In addition, a more well-defined mass lesion was seen in the lateral aspect of the right breast (Fig. 17A, B).

Core Biopsy

Stereotactic core biopsy of the microcalcification revealed low and intermediate nuclear grade DCIS with no evidence of invasion [Fig. 18A (low power), B (high power)]. Calcium was present within the biopsy specimens. Ultrasound-guided core biopsy of the lesion in the lateral aspect of the breast revealed fat and normal breast tissue only.

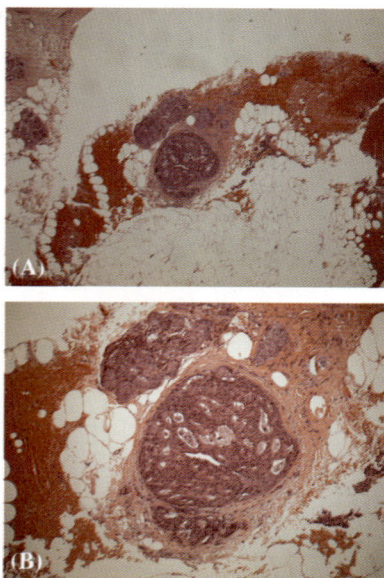

Figure 18

Diagnosis

Extensive noninvasive right breast cancer (Tis)

Multidisciplinary Review 1

The microcalcification involved an area of at least 40 mm and it was possible the DCIS extended beyond the zone of microcalcification. Following multidisciplinary review, it was recommended the patient undergo a right simple mastectomy and be offered immediate breast reconstruction. It was felt that MRI examination of the breasts would not influence the patient's management and was therefore not performed preoperatively.

Treatment and Progress

Reconstructive options were discussed with the plastic surgeons; the patient's large body habitus precluded reconstruction with a TRAM flap and therefore she proceeded to a right simple mastectomy and immediate breast reconstruction with an LD flap and implant. A skin-sparing technique was employed using a periareolar incision. The nipple-areolar complex was replaced with a disc of skin from the dorsal donor site. The patient made an uneventful recovery with no infective complications.

Definitive Histology

This revealed extensive high nuclear grade DCIS of comedo, cribriform, and micropapillary types [Fig. 19A (magnification 5×), B (magnification 20×)]. The DCIS measured up to 130 mm and was present within 1 mm of several

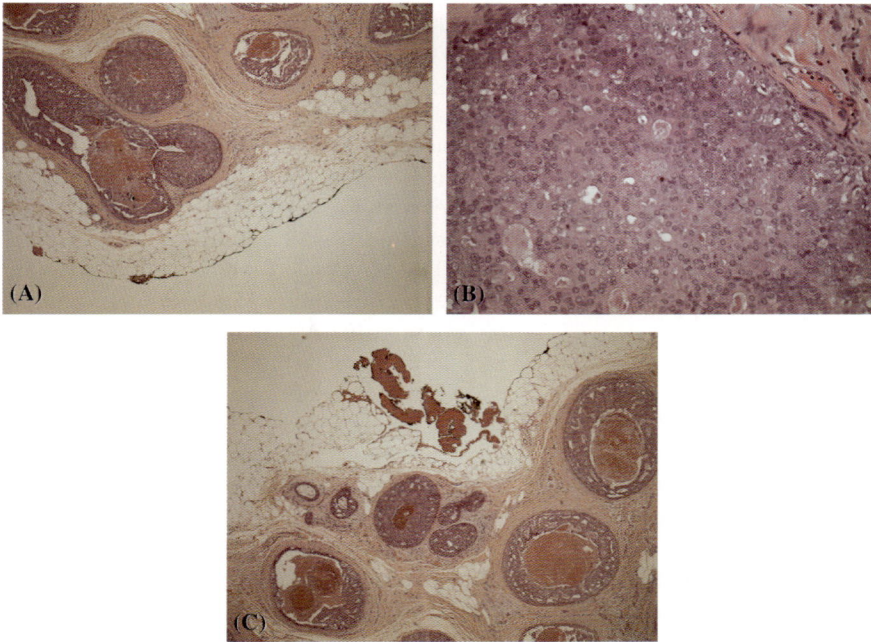

Figure 19

resection margins. Two small foci of invasion were found measuring 2 mm and 6 mm (both grade I) [Fig. 19C (magnification 5×)]. An inferior flap shave showed extensive DCIS while a superior flap shave was free of any tumor.

Multidisciplinary Review 2

In view of the total extent of DCIS and its proximity to several resection margins, chest wall radiotherapy was recommended. The two foci of grade I invasive ductal carcinoma had an aggregate diameter of 8 mm and it was considered inappropriate to undertake a delayed axillary lymph node dissection due to the low probability (<5%) of nodal involvement. Similarly, the absolute benefits from adjuvant hormonal therapy (tamoxifen) were <2% and systemic therapy was withheld.

Treatment and Progress

The patient proceeded to chest wall radiotherapy with a total dose of 50 Gy given in 25 fractions over five weeks. She developed

acute radiation sequelae with marked erythema of the breast but no skin breakdown. The patient was prescribed flamazine cream for topical usage. Over the next 18 months, she developed progressive hardening and discomfort of the reconstructed breast. Examination confirmed a degree of capsule formation with prominent telangiectasia over the region of the right inframammary fold. Despite the presence of a significant degree of contracture, this was not of particular concern to the patient who declined any offer of capsulectomy and implant exchange. She was further reviewed 12 months later when capsular contracture had worsened; at this stage the patient was prepared to undergo further surgery to reduce the hardness and heaviness of the breast (Fig. 20).

Discussion

At the time this patient underwent surgery, sentinel lymph node biopsy was not routinely offered to all patients undergoing mastectomy for extensive high nuclear grade DCIS. There is up to a 20% chance of finding invasion in these circumstances, which

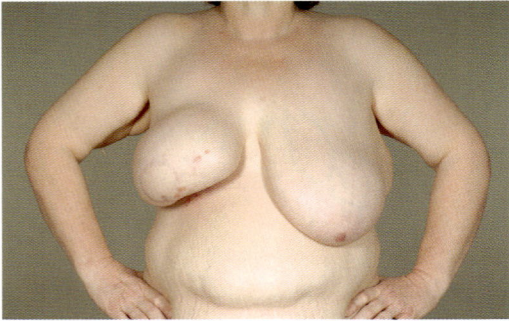

Figure 20

either mandates subsequent axillary staging (with axillary lymph node dissection) or, as in this case, no axillary surgery with observation only (1). This patient had two foci of grade I invasive ductal carcinoma with a combined diameter of 8 mm. The incidence of nodal involvement for grade I invasive ductal carcinomas or special type cancers measuring less than 1 cm is very low (<5%) (2). It would have been difficult to justify a delayed axillary lymph node dissection in this patient who had undergone immediate breast reconstruction with transposition of a LD flap. Sentinel node biopsy or guided axillary sampling cannot be carried out once all the breast tissue has been removed. This patient is highly unlikely to have any adverse clinical consequences in terms of regional recurrence or longer-term survival from failure to undertake any form of axillary staging (3). Many clinicians intuitively feel that with the advent of sentinel node biopsy, all patients with invasive disease (whatever the size) should at least undergo this procedure. Axillary staging can almost certainly be omitted for some tubular cancers <1 cm (any age group) and probably safely omitted in some older women with small, ER-positive, non-high-grade tumors. The latter group would be treated with adjuvant hormonal therapy irrespective of nodal status. Rates of axillary relapse at five years follow-up have been reported to be only 3% after omission of axillary surgery in a group of patients with mainly T1c clinically node-negative tumors (4). Despite the detection of invasive disease on final histology, this

patient had an excellent prognosis and her absolute benefit from adjuvant systemic treatment would be <2%. Some clinicians may have prescribed five years of tamoxifen as adjuvant hormonal therapy with the proportional benefits being similar for pre- and postmenopausal women.

This patient had relatively large breasts and a TRAM flap would have provided better volume replacement. However, the patient was obese with a BMI in excess of 35 and considered to be a high risk for these major tissue-transfer techniques. An extra large implant was ordered for this patient and the breast became very hard and heavy following capsular contracture. There is some evidence that contracture is more likely after irradiation of very large implants. The decision to give radiotherapy to the chest wall was carefully considered in this patient. She had very extensive DCIS (>100 mm) extending close to several margins of the resected specimen.

Related Cases

DCIS—*Case Studies 12, 13, 16, and 17*

Immediate breast reconstruction—*Case Studies 3, 17, and 37*

Omission of completion axillary dissection—*Case Studies 10 and 24*

Capsular contracture—*Case Study 3*

Adjuvant hormonal therapy for "minimal" breast cancer—*Case Studies 9 and 17*

Learning Points

1. In this particular case, some oncologists might have opted to place this patient on tamoxifen to reduce the risk of contralateral breast cancer. Additionally, in this patient's case, the axilla might have been appropriately treated with either surgery or radiotherapy (either will reduce the risk of axillary recurrence by about 90%). However, this patient's risk of nodal metastasis was very low, so omission of axillary treatment was a reasonable choice.

2. Some plastic surgeons recommend a two-stage reconstruction option for patients

undergoing mastectomy for DCIS or invasive cancer. In the first stage, an expander prosthesis is placed immediately after the mastectomy. A few months later (once the final histology is available and the patient has completed any radiotherapy or chemotherapy), the second stage procedure is completed (tissue reconstruction or placing a permanent implant). One advantage of this option is that there is less risk of damage to the tissue reconstruction from radiotherapy.

References

1. Dowlatshahi K, Fan, Bloom KJ, et al. Occult metastases in sentinel lymph nodes of patients with early stage breast carcinoma: a preliminary study. Cancer 1999; 86:990–996.
2. Querci della Rovere G, Bonomi R, Ashley S, et al. Axillary staging in women with small invasive breast tumors. Eur J Surg Oncol 2006; 32: 733–737.
3. Benson JR, Querci della Rovere G. Management of the axilla in women with breast cancer. Lancet Oncol 2007; 8:331–348.
4. Greco M, Agresti R, Cascinella N, et al. Breast cancer patients treated without axillary surgery. Ann Surg 2000; 232(1):1–7.

Part II: Breast-Conservation Surgery

CASE STUDY 19

History

A 76-year-old woman presented with a three-week history of a lump in the left breast, which had developed a few weeks after the patient sustained bruising of the left breast from a fall (since settled). There was minimal pain but no nipple discharge and the patient had undergone regular screening mammograms up to the age of 64 years. She had no family history of breast or ovarian cancer and was nulliparous. She had used HRT (hormone replacement therapy) for a total period of 10 years in the past but never been prescribed the oral contraceptive pill.

Clinical Findings

Examination revealed a slightly irregular and ill-defined lump in the medial aspect of the left breast, corresponding to the site of previous bruising. No discrete lump was palpable in the right breast and there was no axillary lymphadenopathy (E3) (Fig. 21).

Clinical Assessment

The lump in the left breast was clinically indeterminate, but would be consistent with a diagnosis of fat necrosis (suggested from the history).

Investigations

Mammography

An asymmetric density was seen in the lower inner quadrant of the left breast, corresponding to the palpable abnormality. There was no discrete mass lesion on mammography in the left breast. However, in the upper outer quadrant of the contralateral (nonpresenting) side was a spiculate mass lesion measuring 22 mm in diameter. This had the appearances of a carcinoma (R5) (Fig. 22A, B).

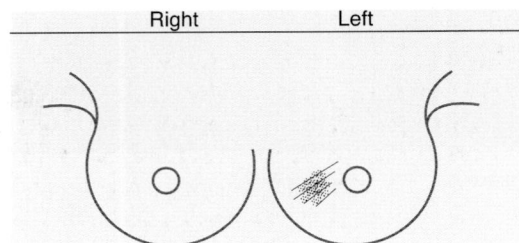

Figure 21

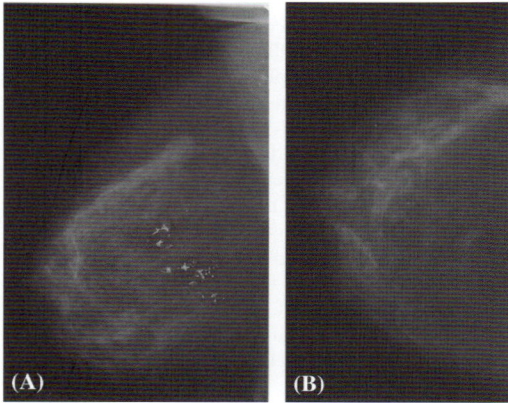

(A)   (B)

Figure 22

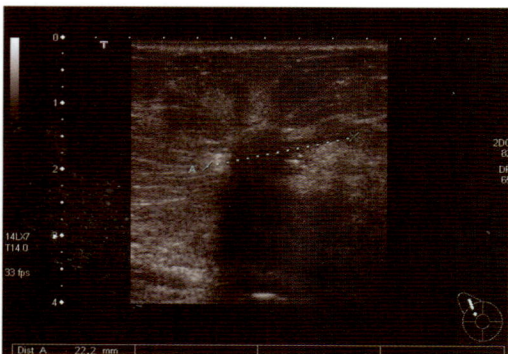

Figure 24

Breast Ultrasound

There was evidence of fat necrosis in the lower inner quadrant of the left breast on ultrasound examination. Moreover, the sonographic correlate of the spiculate mass lesion in the upper outer quadrant of the right breast was a heterogeneous, ill-defined hypoechoic mass with posterior acoustic attenuation. This corresponded in size with the mammographic estimate (22 mm) and was sonographically a carcinoma (U5) (Fig. 23).

Core Biopsy

Ultrasound-guided 16-gauge core biopsy of the right breast mass confirmed the radiological impression of malignancy and showed

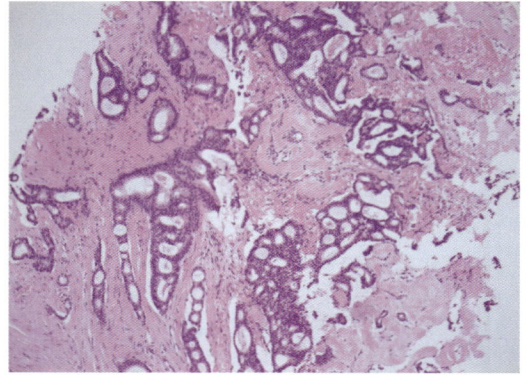

Figure 23

an invasive ductal carcinoma (grade I, ER-positive[a], HER2 negative) (Fig. 24). No biopsy was taken on the left side.

Diagnosis

1. Incidental early-stage impalpable right breast cancer (T2N0)
2. Fat necrosis left breast

Multidisciplinary Review 1

Following multidisciplinary review, it was recommended the patient be offered a right guidewire-localized wide local excision and sentinel lymph node biopsy. It was confirmed upon reexamination that the right breast lump was impalpable, though there was a suggestion of subtle skin tethering.

Treatment and Progress

The patient proceeded to surgery within three weeks and a quadrantic style resection was performed using a single radial incision and excising a narrow ellipse of skin overlying the tumor (Fig. 25). The sentinel node biopsy was carried out through the lateral one-third of the incision and yielded two blue and "warm" nodes (one nonsentinel node was also removed). A specimen radiograph confirmed that the lesion had been removed with an adequate margin of tissue (radiologically) (Fig. 26).

[a] Allred score 8/8

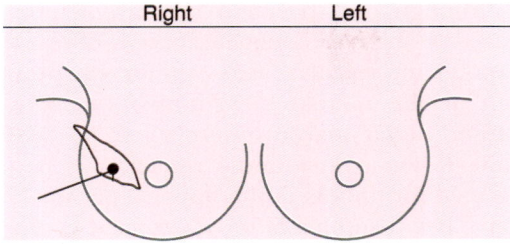

Figure 25

The patient made an uneventful recovery and was discharged home on the second rather than first postoperative day for social reasons (husband disabled).

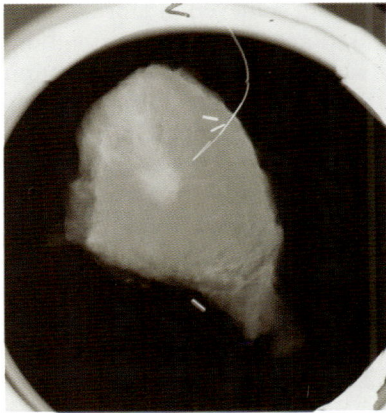

Figure 26

Definitive Histology

This revealed an invasive ductal carcinoma (grade I) measuring 24 mm in maximum diameter (Fig. 27A). There were multiple intratumoral foci of intermediate nuclear grade DCIS, but these did not extend beyond the invasive component. Perineural invasion was noted, but no lymphovascular invasion was seen. The lateral, superior, and inferior resection margins were clear of tumor by >10 mm, but tumor was present at the medial margin (Fig. 27B). There was no evidence of metastases in either of the two sentinel nodes or the single nonsentinel node.

Multidisciplinary Review 2

The patient required re-excision of the medial margin and if satisfactory clearance

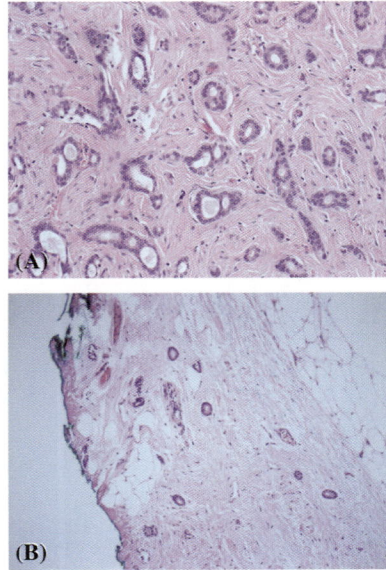

Figure 27

of the tumor achieved, this would be followed by radiotherapy to the right breast and tamoxifen as adjuvant systemic hormonal therapy (low risk of relapse).

Treatment and Progress

The patient underwent re-excision of the medial cavity margin almost four weeks after the original surgery (further surgery delayed at request of patient). There was no further tumor in the re-excision specimen and the patient proceeded to radiotherapy planning shortly after completion of surgery. Final cosmetic results following surgery and radiotherapy were satisfactory with minor loss of volume in the lateral aspect of the right breast (Fig. 28A, B).

Discussion

This patient was found to have an incidental, impalpable cancer in the right breast when she presented symptomatically with a lump in the left breast. The history was very suggestive of fat necrosis; the patient had sustained trauma to the left breast, which had caused bruising. This was followed two to three weeks later by the appearance of a lump at the site of bruising. Fat necrosis can mimic a carcinoma both clinically and

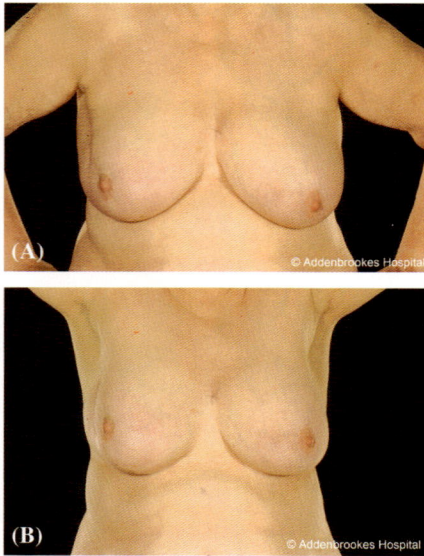

Figure 28

Though the specimen radiograph app-eared to show an adequate margin of tissue around the spiculate mass, tumor was pres-ent at the medial margin histologically. Other radial margins were clear by >10 mm. When a quadrantic resection is per-formed for tumors in the upper outer quad-rant, less tissue tends to be resected at the medial and lateral margins and proportion-ately more tissue superiorly and inferiorly. The opposite applies to a curvilinear incision.

Approximately 25% of patients undergo-ing breast-conserving surgery require re-excision to either attain negative margins or a wider margin of clearance, with negative margins being achieved in more than 90% of cases (3). Rates of re-excision tend to be higher when a 5 mm margin is stipulated rather than 2 to 3 mm. Residual tumor is identified in approximately 50% of cases with positive or unknown margins. When there is an extensive in situ component, the chance of residual disease is up to 70% (4–8). Patients should be warned of the pos-sibility of re-excision when consenting to breast-conserving surgery. This patient had a low risk of distant relapse with an NPI of $(0.2 \times 2.4) + 1 + 1 = 2.48$ (24 mm, grade I, node negative). Tamoxifen only for five years was the recommended adjuvant hor-monal treatment.

Related Cases

Re-excision after breast conservation sur-gery—*Case Studies 7, 11, and 16*

Adjuvant hormonal therapy—*Case Studies 1, 2, 4, 9, 10, and 15*

mammographically (1,2). However, the ultrasound features are characteristic and when the history is consistent with fat necro-sis, no core biopsy is necessary. Often patients cannot recollect any history of trauma, and if there is doubt about the nature of a lump on clinical and radiological criteria, then core biopsy should be under-taken. The carcinoma in the right breast measured 22 mm and was located in the extreme lateral aspect of the breast. It was suitable for breast-conserving surgery, but required localization prior to excision.

The breast excision and sentinel node biopsy were undertaken through a single radial incision rather than two separate inci-sions (curvilinear breast, transverse axilla). This is an ideal incision for a more periph-erally sited tumor in the upper outer quad-rant of the breast. When a formal axillary dissection is undertaken, it allows the breast lesion to be removed in continuity with the axillary contents. This en bloc dissection incorporates the intervening breast tissue containing the lymphatics coursing toward the axillary nodes. The lower axilla can easily be accessed through the lateral one-third of the incision for sentinel node biopsy.

Learning Points

1. A diagnostic mammogram should be obtained whenever a patient presents with a suspicious breast mass. The mam-mogram may not only help establish a diagnosis, but may also discern occult lesions in the ipsilateral or contralateral breast, which could prove useful in plan-ning local therapy. In this instance, the palpable lesion proved to be benign, but

the mammogram led to the discovery of an occult cancer in the contralateral breast.

2. Approximately 77% of all breast cancers are ER positive. However, ER-positive tumors are more common in the elderly than in younger women. Breast cancers with better prognostic features (ER positive, HER2 negative, low grade, node negative) are more common in elderly patients.

3. Population-based statistics indicate that breast cancer mortality rates in the industrialized countries have declined by about 25% since 1990. However, this decline in mortality rates has largely affected women below the age of 70 with ER-positive tumors.

References

1. Bilgen IG, Ustun EE, Memis A. Fat necrosis of the breast: clinical, mammographic and sonographic features. Eur J Radiol 2001; 39:92–99.

2. Harrison RL, Britton P, Warren R, et al. Can we be sure about a radiological diagnosis of fat necrosis of the breast? Clin Radiol 2000; 55:119–123.

3. Kearney TJ, Morrow M. Effect of re-excision on the success of breast conserving surgery. Ann Surg Oncol 1995; 2:303–307.

4. Schnitt SJ, Abner A, Gelman R, et al. The relationship between microscopic margins of resection and the risk of local recurrence in patients with breast cancer treated with breast conserving surgery and radiation therapy. Cancer 1994; 74:1746–1751.

5. Gage I, Schnitt SJ, Nixon AJ, et al. Pathological margin involvement and the risk of recurrence in patients treated with breast conserving therapy. Cancer 1996; 78:1921–1928.

6. Singletary SE. Surgical margins in patients with early stage breast cancer treated with breast conservation therapy. Am J Surg 2002; 184:383–393.

7. Taghian A, Mohiuddin M, Jagsi R, et al. Current perceptions regarding surgical margin status after breast conserving therapy: results of a survey. Ann Surg 2005; 241:629–639.

8. Morrow M, Harris JR. Practice guidelines for breast conserving therapy in the management of invasive breast cancer. J Am Coll Surg 2007; 205:362–376.

Ipsilateral Breast Tumor Recurrence

4

History

A 58-year-old practice nurse presented with a lump in the right breast. She had undergone breast conservation surgery with wide local excision and axillary sampling for an invasive lobular carcinoma of the right breast 18 years earlier. Radiotherapy was administered to the right breast, but the patient received no form of adjuvant systemic hormonal therapy (not standard of care at the time). She was otherwise well and reported no weight loss, cough, or unusual back pain. There was no family history of breast cancer, and the patient had two children. She had received regular mammography within the NHS Breast Screening Programme and never been recalled.

Clinical Findings

On examination there was a firm, irregular mass lying immediately superior to the previous scar in the superior aspect of the right breast. This measured approximately 2 cm in maximum diameter, and there was some associated skin tethering and indrawing of the right nipple. The patient claimed the latter signs were longstanding, but the lump in the right breast was new. There were telangiectatic changes of the skin consistent with previous radiotherapy but neither axillary nor supraclavicular lymphadenopathy. Moreover, the lung fields were clear, there was no spinal tenderness, and no hepar was palpable (E4).

Clinical Assessment

Clinically suspicious lump in the ipsilateral breast almost two decades after conservation surgery for an invasive carcinoma of the right breast.

Investigations

Mammography

An area of increased density was seen in the central zone of the right breast corresponding to the site of previous surgery. This appeared to have increased since mammography was last undertaken (Fig. 1A, B).

Breast Ultrasound

The sonographic correlate of this density was a 25-mm hypoechoic lesion with the radiological features of a carcinoma (U5) (Fig. 2).

Core Biopsy

Ultrasound-guided core biopsy of the breast mass confirmed an invasive lobular carcinoma

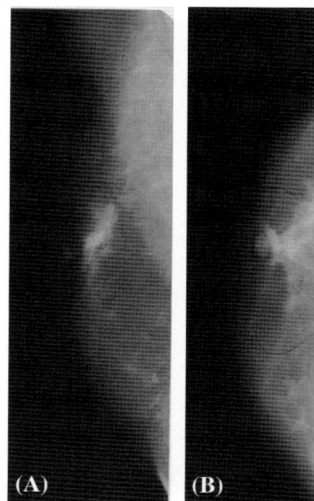

Figure 1

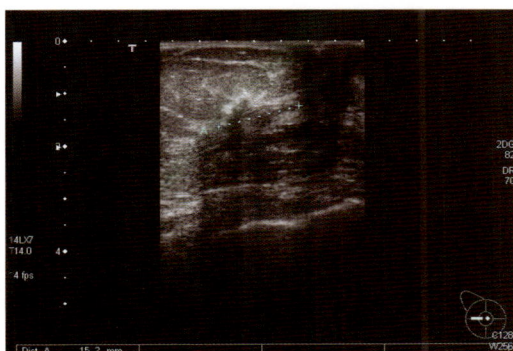

Figure 2

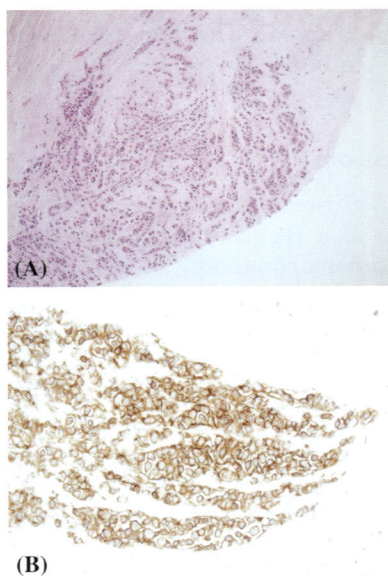

(A)

(B)

Figure 3

(grade II) (Fig. 3A), which was strongly ER (estrogen receptor) positive (Allred score 8/8) and also HER2 positive (Fig. 3B).

Diagnosis

Probable recurrent (rather than de novo) right breast cancer.

Multidisciplinary Review 1

It was recommended that the patient undergo a right completion mastectomy and be offered immediate breast reconstruction. The location of the tumor in relation to the previous scar together with its lobular phenotype supported a diagnosis of recurrent rather than de novo breast cancer. However, it was noted that almost 20 years had elapsed since the time of the patient's original presentation. The risk of ipsilateral breast cancer recurrence persists for up to 15 to 20 years (see below). In view of this tumor most likely representing recurrence, staging investigations were requested, including CT imaging of the chest, abdomen, and pelvis. These revealed no evidence of distant metastatic disease, though abnormalities of bone texture were noted in the lumbar spine and pelvis with evidence of sclerosis. After careful scrutiny by more than one radiologist, these changes were considered consistent with Paget's disease of bone rather than metastatic tumor. Indeed, it transpired that the patient had undergone a bone biopsy 10 years earlier, which corroborated this diagnosis. Some post-radiotherapy changes were noted in the lung fields, but no evidence of secondary pulmonary deposits was found.

The patient reported that the axillary sampling procedure had retrieved 10 nodes at the time of primary surgical treatment 18 years earlier. It was proposed to remove any further nodes at operation, which lay below the level of the axillary vein or were palpable.

Treatment and Progress

The patient expressed an initial interest in immediate breast reconstruction and was reviewed by the plastic surgeon. After further consideration, the patient declined any immediate reconstructive procedure and underwent a right completion mastectomy within only six weeks of tissue diagnosis (core biopsy) (Fig. 4). There was some delay in definitive surgery because of a plastic surgery consultation and reduction of surgical activity over the festive season. At the time of surgery, the mastectomy flaps were very thin, and a wide skin excision was performed to encompass the skin overlying the tumor, the previous scar, and areas of skin damaged by radiotherapy (telangiectatic). Some residual axillary tissue was removed in continuity with the breast.

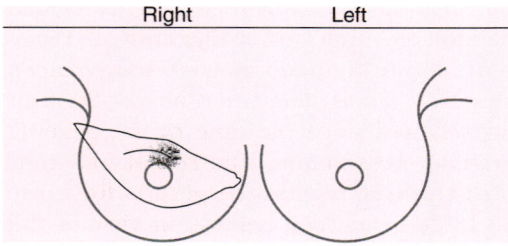

Figure 4

Definitive Histology

This revealed a grade III invasive lobular carcinoma measuring 30 mm in maximum diameter [Fig. 5 (magnification 20×)]. The tumor extended into the dermis of the nipple, though there was no evidence of Paget's disease. There was no associated DCIS (ductal carcinoma in situ), but LCIS (lobular carcinoma in situ) was present. A total of seven nodes were identified within the axillary tissue. None of these contained metastases, and there was no lymphovascular invasion.

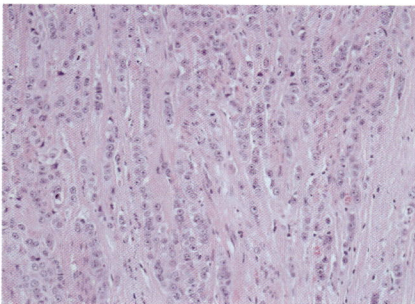

Figure 5

Multidisciplinary Review 2

The final histology confirmed an invasive lobular carcinoma similar to the patient's original breast cancer diagnosed almost 20 years previously. The lesion was hormone sensitive and HER2 receptor positive with evidence of neither lymphovascular invasion nor nodal disease. It was recommended the patient receive a course of anthracycline-based chemotherapy combined with a taxane [FEC (5-fluorouracil, epirubicin, cyclophosphamide)/taxotere] together with Herceptin. She had previously received radiotherapy to the breast and was ineligible for chest wall radiotherapy.

Treatment and Progress

The patient proceeded to four cycles of FEC (5-fluorouracil, epirubicin, and cyclophosphamide) followed by four cycles of docetaxel with concomitant Herceptin (see Appendix III). She tolerated FEC well, though she developed grade I nausea, vomiting, and stomatitis with grade II lethargy. After the first cycle of docetaxel, she experienced moderately severe symptoms of sensory changes (grade III) together with alopecia, arthralgia, myalgia, and lethargy (grade II). The dosage of taxane was therefore reduced, but the patient received the first cycle of Herceptin in the presence of a satisfactory left ventricular ejection fraction [normal MUGA (Multigated Acquisition) scan].

Discussion

Ipsilateral breast tumor recurrence (IBTR) persists at a regular rate beyond five years, with patients continuing to be exposed to a risk of 1% to 3% per annum. There is long-standing controversy over the significance of IBTR following conservation surgery and whether rates of local recurrence affect overall survival. Of particular concern is the relationship to distant relapse and whether local recurrence within the conserved breast acts as a source of distant metastases or is a marker of risk for development of distant disease and de facto poor prognosis. Several studies have confirmed that local recurrence confers an increased risk of distant relapse, varying from 2.72- to 4.62-fold, implying that local recurrence and distant metastases are linked.

The most recent overview by the Early Breast Cancer Trialists Collaborative Group (EBCTCG) in 2005 revealed that moderate differences in rates of local recurrence at five years can impact on breast cancer mortality after more prolonged follow-up of 15 years (1). This suggests that local recurrence has a determinant role with patients developing disseminated disease as a direct consequence of failure to remove residual but viable cancer cells at the time of primary treatment. By implication, inadequate locoregional treatment may ultimately compromise longer-term survival.

It can be difficult to distinguish between a true local recurrence within the conserved breast and a new primary. The site of recurrence and morphology can be helpful—a lesion occurring within the same quadrant and of the same morphology as the original tumor is likely to be a true local recurrence. However, most cancers are invasive ductal carcinomas of no special type (IDC-NST), and therefore, histological type is not a useful discriminator unless the tumor types are different. There is usually no progression of grade between in situ, invasive, locally recurrent, and metastatic phases (2). Flow cytometric analyses of DNA ploidy in primary and matching recurrent lesions reveals concordance in more than 70% of cases (3).

An analysis of 82 cases of local recurrence in 990 patients undergoing breast conservation surgery concluded that 47 (59%) were true local recurrences and 33 (41%) new primaries (4). The latter were classified on the basis of (i) relapse at a different site from the original tumor, (ii) histology consistent with a new primary, and (iii) differences in ploidy between original tumor (aneuploid) and recurrence (diploid). True local recurrences are associated with a shorter time to relapse and poorer five-year survival compared with a new primary lesion (36% versus 89%). Immunohistochemical profiling may assist in differentiating a true recurrence from a new primary; p53 is generally not useful, but MIBI can be helpful together with a panel of markers including ER, PgR (progesterone receptor), EGFR (epidermal growth factor receptor), HER2, and CK (creatinine kinase). Microsatellite instability and LOH (loss of heterozygosity) confer a distinctive chromosomal pattern, which is shared by a true recurrence and the original tumor (but not a new primary) (5). Comparative genomic hybridization (CGH) has also been employed to show a genetic link between the original tumor and a true recurrence (6).

It remains unclear where new primary tumors come from and whether radiotherapy to the breast induces malignant epithelial changes. Furthermore, some cases of IBTR represent neither a true recurrence nor a new primary but persistence of disease within the breast at the site of surgery. There is some uncertainty over differential prognosis between a true local recurrence and a new primary, and some believe that the distinction is irrelevant in terms of the type of treatment; local recurrence occurring within two years has a greater chance of being associated with distant disease.

Two factors emerge as principle determinants of true local recurrence within the ipsilateral breast: (i) margin status (7–12) and (ii) the presence or absence of an extensive intraduct component (EIC) (13,14). Other factors have been implicated in determining risk of local relapse, but correlations are in general much weaker than for margin status and EIC. Amongst these, lymphatic invasion (15) and young age (35 years) (11) have been shown to be primary predictors for increased risk of local recurrence. Consistent associations have been found for larger tumor size (>2 cm) and higher histological grade but not for tumor subtype or nodal status. These findings are consistent with the notion that local recurrence develops from regrowth of residual cancer cells in peri-tumoral tissue. Increased rates of local recurrence associated with positive margins and EIC suggest that incomplete removal of tumor may contribute to local recurrence. Rates of local recurrence are more than threefold greater for tumorectomy compared with quadrantectomy in which a larger volume of tissue is excised. Furthermore, true recurrences occur within the index quadrant and are of the same histological type and grade as the primary tumor. In the NSABP B-06 (National Surgical Adjuvant Breast and Bowel Project B-06) trial, the annual local recurrence rate was 8.5% in the first three years of follow-up and 4.6% in years 4 to 9 for patients undergoing WLE (wide local excision) only compared with a constant rate of 1.4% for patients receiving adjuvant RT (radiotherapy). Moreover, within the NSABP B-06 trial, 39.2% of patients undergoing WLE only had developed local recurrence at 20 years follow-up compared with only 14.3% for those receiving radiotherapy post-lumpectomy (16). Despite great variation in incidence of IBTR, this does not translate into survival differences, and it was concluded that no causal relationship existed between IBTR and distant disease (17). IBTR was found to be the strongest predictor for distant disease and was considered to be a marker for increased risk but not a cause of distant metastases (3.41-fold increased risk, 95% CI 2.70–4.30). Early local recurrence was associated with a shorter disease-free interval, and IBTR was better correlated with distant disease than with tumor size, which has been reported to be highly predictive for development of distant metastases (17). IBTR is an independent predictor of distant disease and a marker of risk, but not an instigator of distant metastases. Though locoregional treatment in the form of surgery or radiotherapy may prevent or reduce chance of expression of the marker, such therapy does not alter the intrinsic risk of developing distant disease.

The meta-analysis by the EBCTCG showed an overall survival benefit at 15 years from local radiation treatment to either the breast following breast conservation surgery or the chest wall after mastectomy (1). For treatment comparisons where the difference in local recurrence rates at five years was less than 10%, survival was unaffected. Amongst the 25,000 women in whom differences in local relapse were substantial (>10%), there were moderate reductions in breast cancer–specific and overall mortality. The absolute reduction in local recurrence at five years was 19%, and the absolute reduction in breast cancer mortality at 15 years was 5.0%. This represents one life saved for every four locoregional recurrences prevented by radiotherapy at five years. It is unclear precisely what the proportional contributions of local versus regional reductions were as absolute nodal recurrence rates were very low.

This important meta-analysis based on individual patient data from 42,000 women in 78 randomized treatment comparisons provides conclusive evidence that differences in locoregional treatments, which substantially improve rates of local control, will impact on longer-term survival of breast cancer patients.

It must therefore be conceded that up to one quarter of local recurrences are a deter-

minant and not simply a marker of risk for distant metastases and death.

It is clear that IBTR does reflect biology of a tumor and is a manifestation of risk for distant relapse (Fisherian paradigm). Though clinical trials should provide conclusive evidence on whether surgery affects local or distant relapse, there are now relatively fewer relapse events. If rates of local recurrence can be minimized in the first five years, this will eventually impact on overall survival (Halstedian paradigm).

When both surgical resection (wide local excision/quadrantectomy) and radiotherapy have already been employed as treatment for the primary tumor, recurrence in the breast should be treated by mastectomy. This yields a 10-year disease-free survival of 50% to 60%, and rates of complications for salvage mastectomy are comparable to those for primary mastectomy despite surgery within an irradiated field (18,19). In cases where the axilla has not been previously treated, a formal axillary dissection should be carried out at the time of salvage mastectomy. Rates of subsequent local recurrence are higher in patients treated with an additional conservation procedure. Nonetheless, further breast conservation surgery can be used selectively and should be restricted to local recurrences which are isolated mobile lesions ≤2 cm in diameter occurring in an originally node-negative patient. Larger recurrences can be managed initially with induction chemotherapy either to render them operable or to permit further breast conservation surgery.

More treatment options should be available for local recurrence after BCT (breast conservation therapy). In most breast units, completion mastectomy is the only treatment for IBTR. Alternative options include reconserving the breast and possibly further SLN (sentinel lymph node) biopsy, though prior disruption of lymphatic pathways may increase false negative rates for "second time round" sentinel node biopsy (20). It may be feasible to consider re-irradiation with brachytherapy where a booster dose has not been employed at the time of primary treatment.

It remains unclear who should receive systemic treatment at the time of IBTR, but overtreatment should be avoided (40–50% of patients). Local treatment alone is potentially curative in the absence of distant metastases, and recurrent tumor nodules must be excised with clear margins. It is suggested that systemic treatment should be considered for the following:

1. Patients whose original disease was node positive
2. Evidence of lymphovascular invasion at the time of IBTR
3. High nuclear grade
4. Short time interval to local recurrence (IBTR)

The efficacy of chemotherapy after IBTR is unknown; the BIG 1-02 (Breast International Group 1-02) trial is an international collaboration, which will randomize patients to chemotherapy (investigator's choice) or observation (20). Patients with a recurrence of HER2-positive disease in the breast should receive Herceptin. HER2 status should be reassessed at the time of IBTR as 10% to 12% can change from being HER2 negative to HER2 positive upon recurrence. There is currently no evidence that treatment with chemotherapy at the time of IBTR will prolong survival and many patients treated with taxanes at the time of IBTR will eventually develop distant metastases (21).

Estrogen receptor and progesterone receptor status should be measured at the time of IBTR and if the result is positive for hormone receptors, then endocrine therapy should either be changed or introduced. Tamoxifen can prevent further local recurrence but does not improve overall survival in this setting.

Related Cases

Mastectomy without reconstruction—*Case Studies 1, 2, and 22*

Aromatase inhibitors—*Case Studies 1, 4, 9, 10, and 19*

Adjuvant chemotherapy—*Case Studies 2, 3, 6, 8, 11, and 37*

Herceptin—*Case Studies 8, 11, and 26*

Locally recurrent disease—*Case Study 26*

Learning Points

1. Approximately 15% of all patients who undergo breast-conservative surgery and radiotherapy for early breast cancer will experience an IBTR within 10 years. The risk of IBTR is diminished if clear margins are obtained around the tumor.
2. There are several factors that increase the risk of IBTR. The omission of radiotherapy after conservative surgery results in a 30% to 40% risk of IBTR. Also, the presence of lymphatic invasion or positive axillary lymph nodes increases the risk of IBTR. There is now evidence that IBTR increases mortality risk.
3. If a patient develops IBTR after breast-conserving surgery and radiotherapy, then additional radiotherapy cannot be administered. A salvage mastectomy is therefore warranted in such instances.

References

1. Early Breast Cancer Trialists Collaborative Group. Effects of radiotherapy and of differences in the extent of surgery for early breast cancer on local recurrence and 15 year survival: an overview of the randomized trials. Lancet 2005; 366:2087–2106.
2. Millis R, Barnes D, Lampejo OT, et al. Tumour grade does not change between primary and recurrent mammary carcinoma. Eur J Cancer 1998; 34:548–553.
3. Tsutsui S, Ohno S, Murakami S, et al. Flow cytometric analysis of DNA ploidy in primary, metastatic and recurrent breast cancers. Oncol Rep 2002; 9:793–799.
4. Haffty B, Carter D, Flynn SD. Local recurrence versus new primary: clinical analysis of 82 breast relapses and potential applications for genetic fingerprinting. Int J Radiat Oncol Biol Phys 1993; 27:575–583.
5. Regitnig P, Moser R, Thalhammer M, et al. Microsatellite analysis of breast carcinoma and corresponding local recurrences. J Pathol 2002; 198: 190–197.
6. Waldman FM, DeVries S, Chew KL, et al. Chromosomal alterations in ductal carcinomas in situ and their in situ recurrences. J Natl Cancer Inst 2000; 92:313–320.
7. Singletary SE. Surgical margins in patients with early stage breast cancer treated with breast conservation therapy. Am J Surg 2002; 184:383–393.
8. van Dongen JA, Bartelink H, Fentimen I, et al. Factors influencing local relapse and survival and results of salvage treatment after breast conserving treatment in operable breast cancer. EORTC trial

10801. Breast conservation compared with mastectomy in TNM stage I and II breast cancer. Eur J Cancer 1992; 28A:808–815.

9. Smitt MC, Nowels K, Carlson RW, et al. Predictors of re-excision findings and recurrence after breast conservation. Int J Radiat Oncol Biol Phys 2003; 57:979–985.

10. Fisher ER, Costantino J, Fisher B, et al. Pathologic findings from the National Surgical Adjuvant Breast and Bowel Project (NSABP) Protocol B-17. Cancer 1995; 75:1310–1319.

11. Kurtz JM, Jacquemir J, Amalric R, et al. Risk factors for breast recurrence in premenopausal and postmenopausal patients with ductal cancers treated by conservation therapy. Cancer 1990; 65:1867–1878.

12. Smitt MC, Nowels KW, Zdeblick MJ, et al. The importance of the lumpectomy surgical margin status in long term results of breast conservation. Cancer 1995; 76:259–267.

13. Vicini FA, Recht A, Abner A, et al. Recurrence in the breast following conservative surgery and radiation therapy for early-stage breast cancer. J Natl Cancer Inst Monogr 2002; 11:33–39.

14. Veronesi U, Volterrani F, Luini A, et al. Quadrantectomy versus lumpectomy for small size breast cancer. Eur J Cancer 1990; 26:671–673.

15. Borger JH. The impact of surgical and pathological findings on radiotherapy of early breast cancer. Radiother Oncol 1991; 22:230–236.

16. Fisher B, Anderson S, Bryant J, et al. Twenty-year follow up of a randomized trial comparing total mastectomy, lumpectomy and lumpectomy plus irradiation for the treatment of invasive breast cancer. N Engl J Med 2002; 347:1233–1241.

17. Fisher B, Anderson S, Fisher ER, et al. Significance of ipsilateral breast tumour recurrence after lumpectomy. Lancet 1991; 338:327–331.

18. Osborne MP, Simmons RM. Salvage mastectomy for recurrence after breast conservation surgery. World J Surg 1994; 18:93–97.

19. Osteen RT. Risk factors and management of local recurrence following breast conservation surgery. World J Surg 1994; 18:76–80.

20. Hansen N. Sentinel Node Biopsy for Local Recurrence After Breast Conserving Surgery. Miami Breast Cancer Conference, Orlando, FL, 2008.

21. International Breast Cancer Study Group, National Surgical Adjuvant Breast and Bowel Project (NSABP). Adjuvant chemotherapy in treating women who have undergone resection for relapsed breast cancer. Clinical Trials.gov 2002; http://clinicaltrials.gov/ct/show/NCT00074152.

Diagnostic Excision Biopsy

5

History

A 45-year-old woman presented with a one-week history of asymmetrical lumpiness of the left breast. She had not noticed any particular lump in the left breast, but thought this felt more "lumpy." There was no tenderness or associated nipple discharge and the patient had not experienced a period since the onset of these breast symptoms. She had no previous breast problems and no family history of breast or ovarian cancer. She had two children and gave birth to her eldest child at the age of 28 years. The oral contraceptive pill had been used for a cumulative period of eight years.

Clinical Findings

Examination revealed a firm area of prominent focal nodularity in the upper outer quadrant of the left breast, but no discrete or dominant lump was palpable. There was no axillary lymphadenopathy (E3) (Fig. 1).

Clinical Assessment

The clinical findings were considered to be slightly suspicious, but likely benign.

Investigations

Mammography

A discrete mass lesion was seen in the upper outer quadrant of the left breast. In close proximity to this was a small cluster of fine granular microcalcification (Fig. 2A, B). The mammographic appearances were indeterminate (R3/4).

Breast Ultrasound

A cyst measuring 31 mm in maximum diameter was found in the upper outer quadrant of the left breast. This was aspirated to dryness with no residual lump. Material was not sent for routine cytology (Fig. 3).

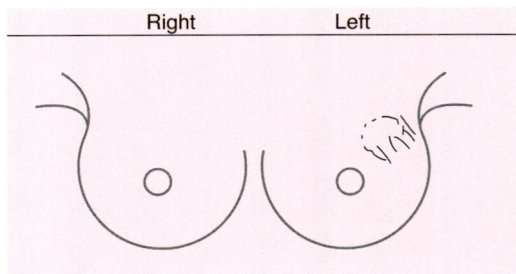

Figure 1

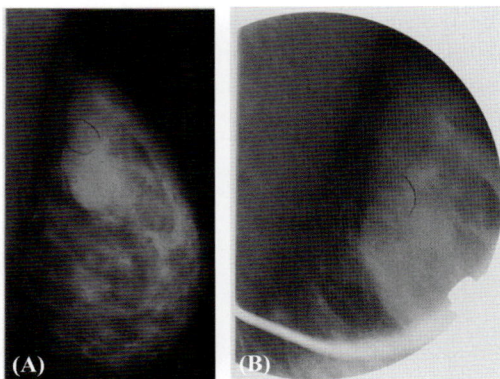

Figure 2

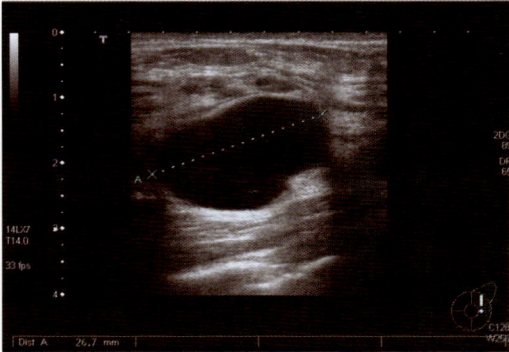

Figure 3

Mammotome Biopsy

The patient returned at a later date for a mammotome biopsy (11-gauge needle) of the area of microcalcification in the upper outer quadrant of the left breast. Calcium was present in the specimen radiograph (Fig. 4A), and histology showed extensive fibrocystic change with apocrine metaplasia and columnar cell change. The latter exhibited focal areas of mild nuclear atypia and architectural atypia but no in situ or invasive malignancy. Luminal calcification was present (B3) (Fig. 4B, C).

Diagnosis

Uncertain; premalignant changes in left breast.

Multidisciplinary Review 1

The biopsy was classified as B3 on the basis of nuclear and architectural atypia and a left guidewire localized diagnostic excision biopsy was therefore recommended.

Treatment and Progress

The patient proceeded to surgery as a day case within two weeks of mammotome biopsy (Fig. 5). An intraoperative specimen radiograph confirmed that the microcalcification had been removed (Fig. 6). A hematoma was present from the mammotome biopsy and this helped guide the surgical excision. A medial cavity shave was taken.

Definitive Histology

Both the main specimen and the medial cavity shave were examined in their entirety. Sections showed similar features to the mammotome biopsy—fibrocystic change with areas of apocrine metaplasia and columnar cell change with mild nuclear, but no architectural atypia. These areas of atypia occurred around the site of the previous biopsy and the majority of columnar cell change showed no atypia (Fig. 7A). A single focus of atypical lobular hyperplasia was seen (Fig. 7B).

Multidisciplinary Review 2

On account of the single focus of atypical lobular hyperplasia, it was recommended that the patient undergo enhanced radiological surveillance with annual mammography until the age of 50 years followed by entry into the NHS Breast Screening Programme (3 yearly mammographies) with interim imaging at 18 months.

Discussion

Mammographic abnormalities with a Breast Imaging Reporting and Data System (BIRADS) classification of 4 or 5 require some

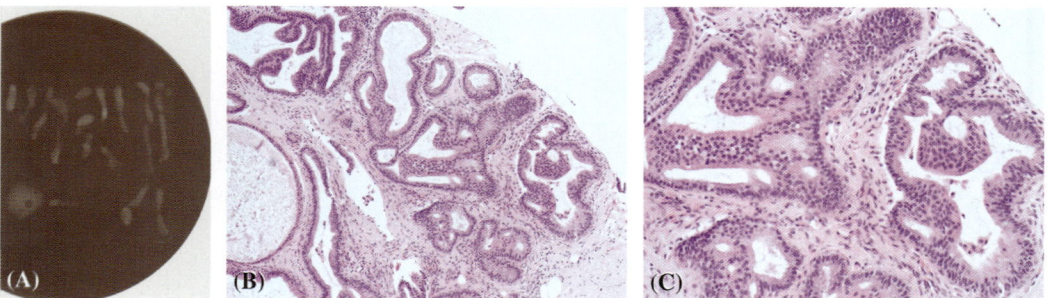

(A)   (B)   (C)

Figure 4

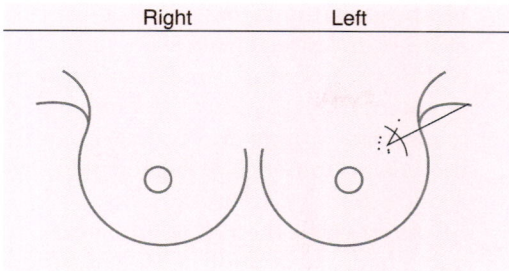

Right   Left

Figure 5

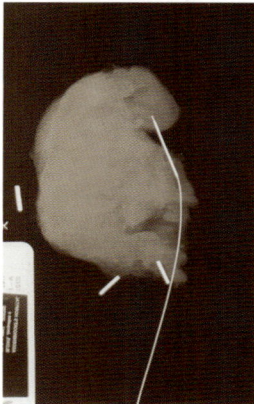

Figure 6

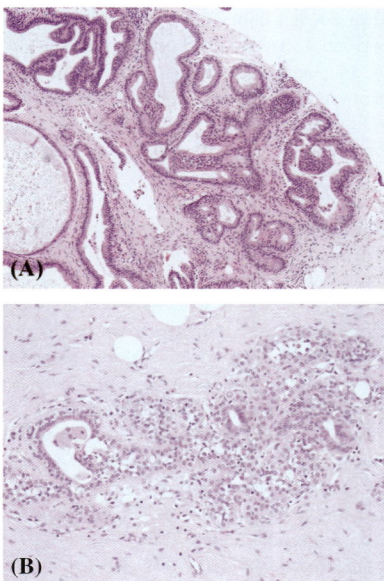

(A)

(B)

Figure 7

form of tissue diagnosis (1). Those lesions with a BIRADS score of 3 may subsequently warrant biopsy if shown to progress on short-term follow-up imaging. Before the introduction of image-guided biopsy techniques, all tissue acquisition involved open excision biopsy. For impalpable, screen-detected lesions, wire localization was necessary (2). Percutaneous needle biopsy techniques can now provide a definitive diagnosis for the majority of benign and malignant conditions (3,4). Wide bore needle core biopsy is preferred to fine needle aspiration cytology and yields solid cores of tissue that maintain tissue architecture and permit distinction between invasive and noninvasive carcinoma (5). Mass lesions can be biopsied using ultrasound or stereotactic guidance, whereas microcalcification usually mandates stereotactic methods (6). The standard core biopsy needle is either 14 or 16 gauge (7), but larger volumes of tissue can be obtained from vacuum-assisted core biopsy devices using a range of needle sizes, most often an 11-gauge needle (8). These latter devices reduce the chance of "underdiagnosis" and increase the chance of obtaining a definitive preoperative cancer diagnosis, which allows appropriate planning of breast cancer surgery (9,10).

A B2 core biopsy result indicates benign changes only, which may include epithelial hyperplasia of the usual type. Any core biopsy results classified as B3 implies a lesion of uncertain malignant potential such as the following:

1. Atypical ductal hyperplasia with moderate degrees of atypia
2. Lobular neoplasia [atypical lobular hyperplasia, lobular carcinoma in situ (LCIS)]
3. Papillary lesions
4. Columnar cell change with atypia
5. Phylloides tumor

For all such cases, diagnostic excision biopsy is necessary (+/− wire localization). In addition to the above histological diagnoses, surgical excision is also warranted for a radial scar or when there is lack of concordance between the clinical, radiological, and core biopsy findings. A radial scar (otherwise termed a complex sclerosing lesion) may be associated with a tubular carcinoma in up to 20% of cases (11). A radial scar is not a premalignant lesion, but when atypical hyperplasia coexists, the relative risk for developing cancer is increased sixfold. As radial scars can be difficult to distinguish from a carcinoma radiologically, all must be excised. When atypical ductal hyperplasia is diagnosed on conventional core biopsy, DCIS (ductal carcinoma-in-situ) will be found on excision biopsy in 40% to 50% of cases (12). This figure is much reduced for mammotome biopsy where the larger volume of tissue retrieved is more likely to contain DCIS (12). Though the term lobular neoplasia is used to embrace both atypical lobular hyperplasia and LCIS, these two lesions should be distinguished histologically as they possess different risk factors for subsequent development of malignancy. Both are considered to be markers of risk rather than precursor lesions of breast cancer. The absolute risk for development of invasive cancer is 8% and 10% at 15 years for atypical lobular hyperplasia and 25% to 30% at 15 to 20 years for LCIS (13,14). Patients with a diagnosis of lobular neoplasia on excision biopsy require mammographic surveillance with annual mammography until the age of 50 years and thereafter interim mammography at 18 months within the NHS Breast Screening Programme (normally triennial screens).

Columnar cell change involves dilatation of the terminal duct lobular unit with preservation of two cell layers. Cytological atypia is usually low grade and is an indication for excision biopsy. Some authorities recommend careful mammographic surveillance for patients with columnar cell change and atypia on excision biopsy. However, the risk of developing an invasive breast cancer appears to be very low.

Related Cases

Diagnostic excision biopsy—*Case Study 15*

Learning Points

1. If atypia is found on core biopsy of a mammography abnormality, then a needle-localized excisional biopsy is generally recommended because up to 50% of these patients may harbor occult DCIS or invasive cancer.

2. Although frequent surveillance (with mammography) is often recommended for women with atypia on breast biopsy, there is no evidence to suggest that this reduces breast cancer mortality.

3. Atypia increases the risk of breast cancer, and chemoprevention with tamoxifen (20 mg/day for 5 years) substantially reduces that risk. In clinical trials, tamoxifen has been shown to reduce the risk of developing breast cancer by about 50%, but this has not translated to a reduction in breast cancer mortality.

References

1. American College of Radiology. Breast Imaging Reporting and Data System (BIRADS). 2nd ed. Reston, VA: American College of Radiology, 1995.

2. Gallagher WJ, Cardenosa G, Rubens JR, et al. Minimal-volume excision of non-palpable breast lesions. AJR Am J Roentgenol 1989; 153:957–961.

3. Dronkers DJ. Stereotactic core biopsy of breast lesions. Radiology 1992; 183:631–634.

4. Britton PD, McCann J. Needle biopsy in the NHS Breast Screening Programme: how much and how accurate? Breast 1999; 8:5–11.

5. Britton PD, Flower CDR, Freeman AH, et al. Changing to core biopsy in an NHS breast screening unit. Clin Radiol 1997; 52:764–767.

6. Helbich TH, Matzek W, Fuchsjager MH. Stereotactic and ultrasound-guided breast biopsy. Eur Radiol 2004; 14:383–393.

7. Liberman L, Dershaw DD, Rosen PP, et al. Stereotaxic 14-gauge breast biopsy: how many core biopsy specimens are needed? Radiology 1994; 192:793–795.

8. Parker SH, Burbank F, Jackman RJ, et al. Percutaneous large-core breast biopsy: a multiinstitutional study. Radiology 1994; 193:359–364.

9. Burbank F. Stereotactic breast biopsy of atypical ductal hyperplasia and ductal carcinoma in situ lesions: improved accuracy with directional, vaccum-assisted biopsy. Radiology 1997; 202:843–846.

10. Jackman RJ, Nowels KW, Rodriguez-Soto J, et al. Sterotactic, automated, large-core needle biopsy of nonpalpable breast lesions: false-negative and histologic underestimation rates after long term follow up. Radiology 1999; 210:799–805.

11. Linell F. Precursor lesions of breast carcinoma. Jackman RJ, Nowels KW, Rodriguez-Soto J, et al. Sterotactic, automated, large-core needle biopsy of nonpalpable breast lesions: false-negative and histologic underestimation rates after long term follow up. Breast 1993; 203:202–205.

12. Jackman RJ, Burbank, Parker SH, et al. Atypical ductal hyperplasia diagnosed at stereotactic breast

biopsy: improved reliability with 14 gauge, directional, vaccum-assisted biopsy. Radiology 1997; 204:485–488.

13. Rosen PP. Lobular carcinoma in situ and atypical lobular hyperplasia. In: Rosen's Breast Pathology. Philadelphia: Lippincott Williams and Williams, 2001:527–538.

14. Page DL, Steel CM, Dixon JM. Carcinoma in situ and patients at high risk of breast cancer. Br Med J 1995; 310:39–42.

Bilateral Breast Cancer

6

History

A 52-year-old woman presented with a six-month history of hardening and change in consistency of the left breast. She had noticed this while "comfort feeding" her child and over the preceding six weeks had been aware of several red nodules overlying the left breast (which she described as "mosquito bites"). Furthermore, there had been a progressive change in shape of the left breast, though no discrete lump or nipple discharge was reported. There were no previous breast problems except for an episode of mastitis in the past. The patient's maternal grandmother had developed breast cancer in her 70s, and she had four children all of whom were breast-fed (first child at age 34 years). The patient was perimenopausal and had never used any form of exogenous hormonal preparation.

Clinical Findings

Examination revealed gross changes in the left breast; the whole of the breast had undergone generalized contracture and a large mass was palpable in the central portion of the left breast measuring at least 7 cm in maximum diameter. This was associated with nipple retraction and skin dimpling. In addition, there were multiple cutaneous deposits overlying the left breast and extending toward the inframammary fold. Several clinically suspicious, but mobile, nodes were palpable in the left axilla (E5) (Fig. 1).

Clinical Assessment

Large clinical carcinoma of the left breast, which was locally advanced rather than inflammatory (no erythema).

Investigations

Mammography

Bilateral mammography revealed a spiculate mass in the upper inner quadrant of the left breast measuring 27 mm in maximum dimension (R5) (Fig. 2A, B). Diffuse thickening of the skin was noted, and on the right side, architectural distortion was apparent in the inner half of the breast on the cranio-caudal view (R4) (Fig. 2C, D).

Breast Ultrasound

The sonographic correlate of the spiculate mass in the left breast was a 26-mm hypoechoic, poorly defined lesion with posterior acoustic shadowing (U5) (Fig. 3A). A further suspicious area measuring 15 mm was seen in the upper outer quadrant (Fig. 3B). Finally, a hypoechoic lesion measuring 20 mm was seen in the upper inner quadrant of the right breast (U5) (Fig. 3C).

Core Biopsy

Image-guided core biopsy (14-gauge needle) of both lesions in the upper outer and inner

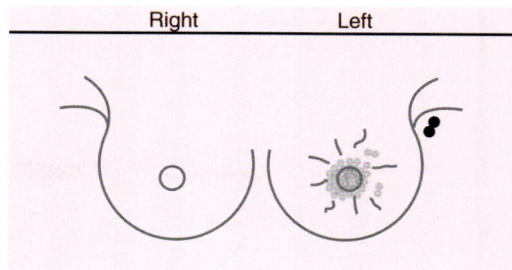

Figure 1

116

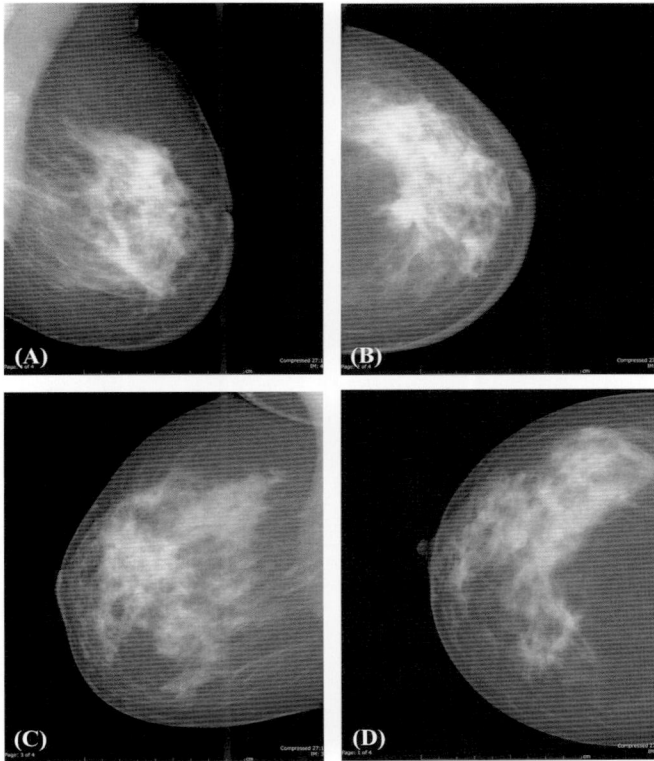

Figure 2

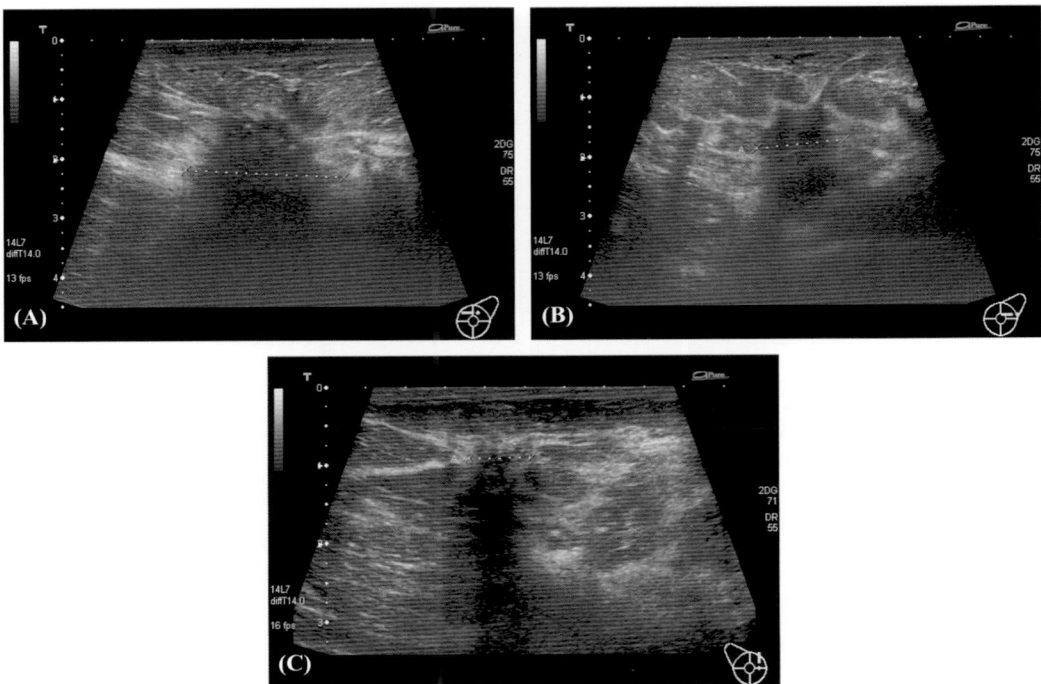

Figure 3

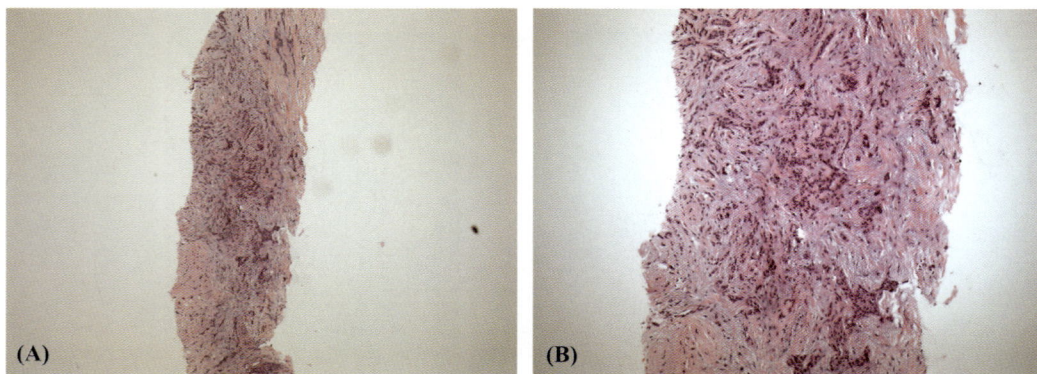

Figure 4

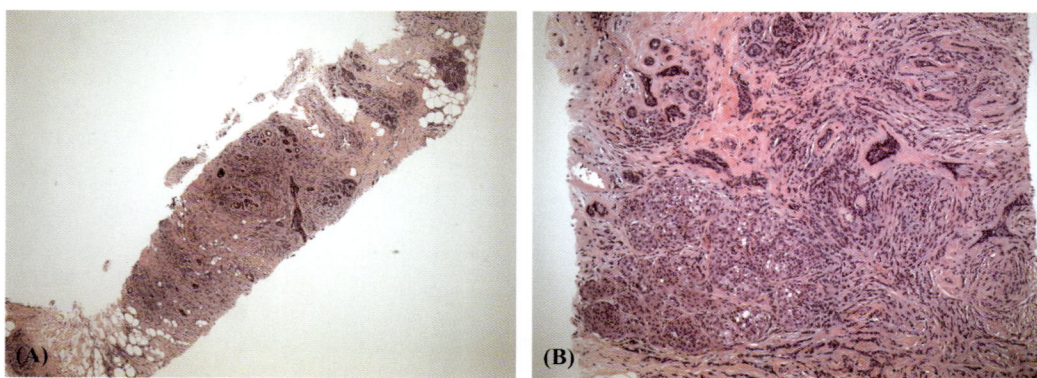

Figure 5

quadrants of the left breast revealed invasive ductal carcinoma (grade II, ER positive) [Fig. 4A (low power), B (high power)]. Core biopsy of a single tumor focus in the upper inner quadrant of the right breast revealed an invasive lobular carcinoma (grade II, ER positive) [Fig. 5A (low power), B (high power)]. HER2 testing was not routinely performed on core biopsy specimens at the time of diagnosis.

Diagnosis

Bilateral breast cancer; locally advanced and multifocal with possible inflammatory component on the left side (T4N1); early-stage breast cancer on the right side (T2N0).

Multidisciplinary Review 1

Following multidisciplinary discussion, it was recommended that the patient undergo neo-adjuvant chemotherapy and subsequent

bilateral modified radical mastectomy (without immediate breast reconstruction). The patient would likely require radiotherapy to the left chest wall (and possibly supraclavicular fossa) and hormonal therapy after completion of chemotherapy. Staging investigations were requested to exclude distant disease.

Further Investigations

1. Isotope bone scan—no evidence of bony metastases
2. CT scan (chest, abdomen, pelvis)—no evidence of pulmonary or hepatic metastases
3. HER2 status—negative

Treatment and Progress

The patient underwent four cycles of combination chemotherapy with epirubicin and

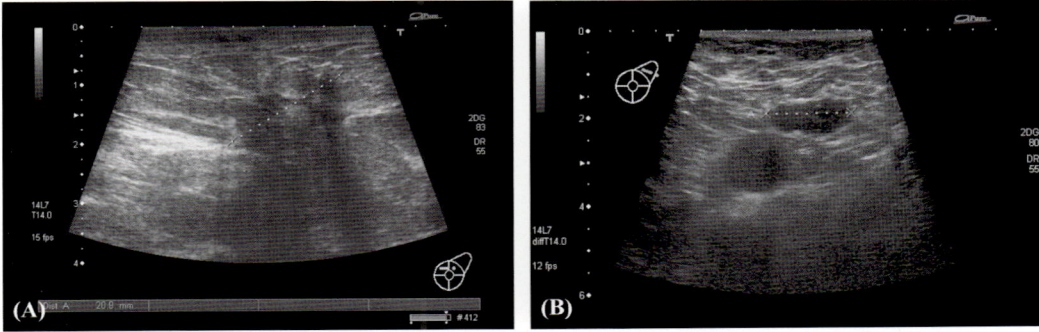

Figure 6

cyclophosphamide followed by four cycles of a taxane (EC/docetaxel—see Appendix III). This was tolerated well with minimal side effects [mild nausea, constipation (grade I)], and repeat imaging with ultrasound after three cycles of EC showed a good tumor response in both breasts. On the left side the larger lesion in the upper inner quadrant had reduced in size to 21.4 mm (from 26 mm) (Fig. 6A) and the smaller one in the upper outer quadrant to 12.5 mm (from 15 mm). The enlarged nodes in the left axilla had also shrunk in size significantly from initial measurements of 25 mm, 17 mm, and 14 mm to 19 mm, 10.5 mm, and 7 mm, respectively (Fig. 6B). An area of poorly defined shadowing corresponded to the lesion in the right breast that no longer had a distinct radiological correlate.

After completion of the seventh cycle of chemotherapy (EC × 4 cycles, docetaxol × 3 cycles), no further reduction in tumor dimensions was evident on the left side. The tumor in the right breast was invisible at this stage. The patient proceeded to surgery six weeks after completion of the eighth and final cycle of chemotherapy (Fig. 7):

1. Left—modified radical mastectomy with level III axillary lymph node dissection[a]
2. Right—modified radical mastectomy with level II axillary lymph node dissection

On the left side a very wide skin excision was performed to encompass areas of skin previously involved clinically. Primary closure was achieved and both mastectomy wounds healed well with only moderate seroma formation (requiring aspiration) (Fig. 8).

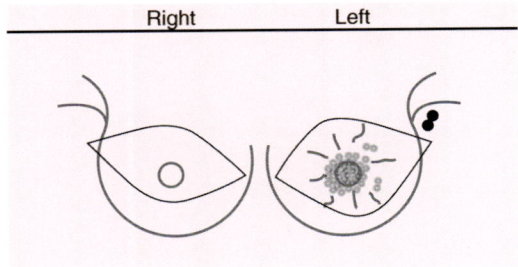

Figure 7

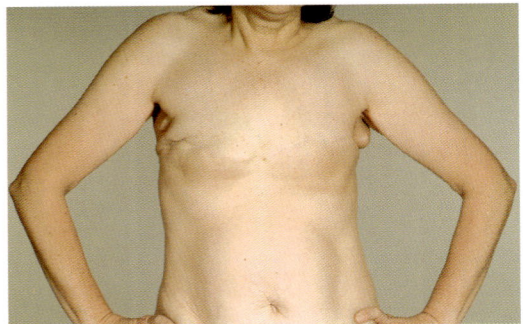

Figure 8

[a]Intraoperative evidence of gross disease at level II.

Definitive Histology

1. Left: An invasive ductal carcinoma (grade II) measuring 55 mm in maximum extent and clear of all resection margins [Fig. 9A (magnification 10×), B (magnification 20×)]. Nine out of 14 lymph nodes contained metastatic tumor [Fig. 9C (magnification 10×)] and there was extensive lymphovascular invasion [Fig. 9D (magnification 10×)].
2. Right: An invasive lobular carcinoma (grade II) measuring 40 mm in maximum extent. All resection margins were clear of tumor and only 1 out of 13 lymph nodes contained metastatic tumor (despite extensive lymphovascular invasion) [Fig. 10A (low power), B (high power)].

Multidisciplinary Review 2

Following further discussion, it was recommended that the patient receive bilateral chest wall radiotherapy together with irradiation of the left supraclavicular fossa (40 Gy

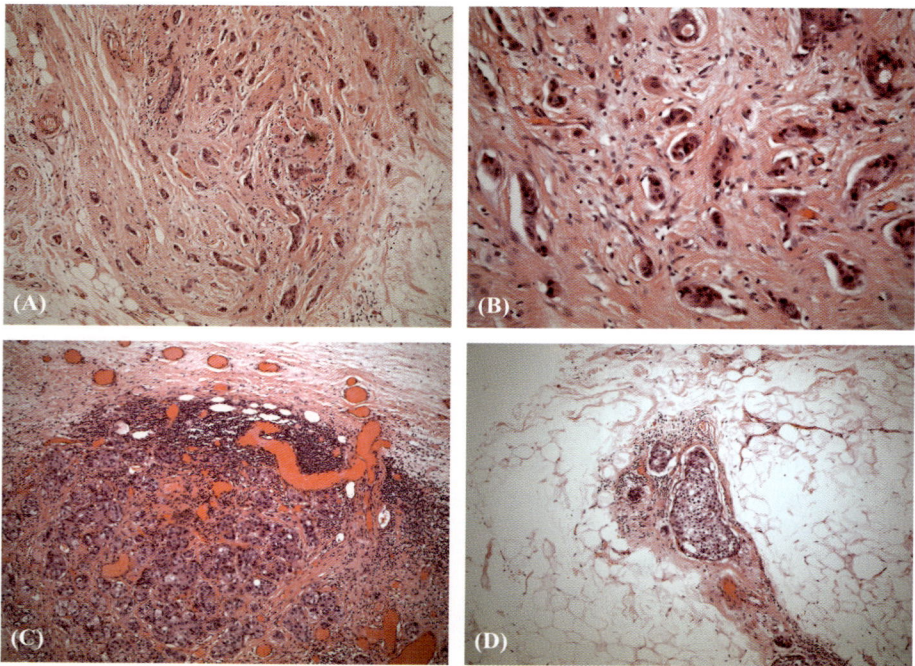

Figure 9

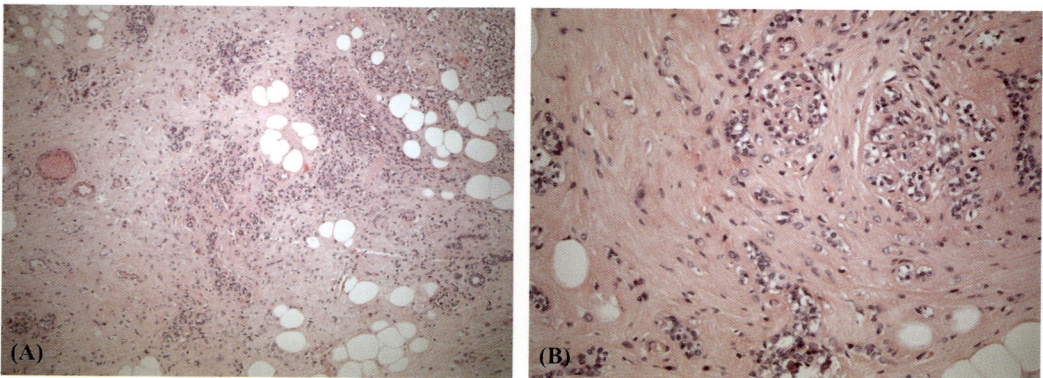

Figure 10

in 15 fractions to the right and left chest walls and a similar dose to the supraclavicular fossa). The decision to irradiate the right chest wall was based on final pathological tumor size and nodal status. Involvement of ≥4 nodes on the left side reinforced the previous anticipation of left supraclavicular fossa irradiation. The patient was not eligible for Herceptin (HER2 negative), but should receive an aromatase inhibitor as a component of adjuvant hormonal therapy (high risk of locoregional relapse).

Discussion

Despite being at the lower age range for the NHS Breast Screening Programme, this patient presented with a large, locally advanced cancer of the left breast and was found to have an incidental contralateral breast cancer. She had a weak family history of breast cancer and though she had four children (all breast-fed) she bore her first child at the relatively late age of 34 years. It is perhaps surprising that she had not become concerned about the lesion in her left breast at an earlier stage. Though several cutaneous nodules were evident, there was no erythema or edema of the breast and the tumor was therefore considered to be locally advanced rather than inflammatory. The clinical distinction between a locally advanced and inflammatory carcinoma can be difficult, and these may not represent distinct clinicopathological entities, but an advanced breast cancer continuum with a poor prognosis and high risk of locoregional relapse (1). Nonetheless, the patient was advised against immediate breast reconstruction because of the high risk of locoregional relapse (clinically node-positive disease). The left-sided tumor was not only locally advanced but also multifocal and mandated mastectomy following induction chemotherapy. The right-sided tumor was unifocal and <3 cm in maximum diameter. However, in view of the lobular phenotype and the synchronous left-sided tumor, bilateral mastectomy was recommended. The patient accepted this decision and had a very positive outlook to her management plan. The left-sided tumor was successfully downstaged

clinically, which facilitated surgical extirpation. Though the residual tumor size was 55 mm, this was clear of all resection margins. The right-sided tumor had been underestimated in size on ultrasound with a final size of 40 mm. This justified the decision to perform a mastectomy on that side. There was bilateral nodal involvement and therefore axillary dissection was also indicated on the right side (clinically node negative). Bilateral axillary dissection can be associated with significant morbidity and sentinel node biopsy should be offered wherever appropriate. Bilateral arm lymphedema can be very disabling for patients and restrict daily activities.

There was a clear indication for irradiation of the left chest wall and supraclavicular fossa based on the extent of nodal involvement (≥4 nodes) (2). The decision to irradiate the right chest wall was based on the tumor size, extensive lymphovascular invasion, and the presence of one to three positive nodes. The latter is not an absolute indication for inclusion of a supraclavicular field, and the American Society of Clinical Oncology guidelines (2) conclude that there is insufficient evidence to make a recommendation on this issue, which is currently being investigated in the SUPREMO trial (3).

The patient was not eligible for Herceptin (HER2 negative), but both tumors were ER positive. Arimidex (upfront) was prescribed as adjuvant hormonal therapy as the patient was considered to be at high risk for locoregional relapse. The optimum strategy for incorporation of aromatase inhibitors into standard adjuvant endocrine schedules remains unclear. Benefits in terms of disease-free and overall survival must be balanced against longer-term risks (bone health, cognitive function) and costs. The evidence available at the present time favors an early switch policy for the majority of patients with hormone receptor–positive postmenopausal breast cancer. The absolute benefits of an aromatase inhibitor for the average patient are very small in the first 36 months and some argue that the additional benefit of an aromatase inhibitor in the first two to three years is difficult to justify. Fewer than 5% of patients have early relapse in the first two to three years while receiving tamoxifen as adjuvant therapy. However, an upfront aromatase inhibitor might be indicated in those patients (such as in this case) at higher risk of relapse for whom the amplitude of the hazard peak for recurrence is proportionately greater in magnitude (4,5). Though interim results of the BIG 1-98 study reveal greater benefit from aromatase inhibitors for node-positive patients (6), the converse is true for the ATAC study (7). Moreover, patients with higher-grade tumors derive no additional benefit from upfront aromatase inhibitors and there is no conclusive evidence for HER2 status being predictive of response to aromatase inhibitors.

Related Cases

Bilateral breast cancer—*Case Studies 23, 24, and 32*

Mastectomy without reconstruction—*Case Studies 1, 2, and 20*

Aromatase inhibitors—*Case Studies 1, 4, 9, 10, and 19*

Taxane-based neoadjuvant chemotherapy—*Case Studies 25, 26, 27, 28, and 29*

Postmastectomy radiotherapy—*Case Studies 2, 3, 26, and 28*

Learning Points

1. Approximately 1.2% of all breast cancer patients present with synchronous bilateral disease. This underscores the need for a bilateral diagnostic mammogram in the evaluation of all women with primary breast cancer. Recently, some investigators have argued for the use of breast MRI in the evaluation of women with primary breast cancer, which increases the detection of bilateral synchronous cancers.

2. Preoperative chemotherapy is also referred to as "induction," "neoadjuvant," or "primary systemic" chemotherapy. It is widely utilized in women with locally advanced or inflammatory breast cancer and reduces the tumor burden in these women, thereby facilitating mastectomy.

3. Many surgeons advise against immediate breast reconstruction for women with locally advanced or inflammatory breast cancer, because the risk of locoregional recurrence is relatively high.

References

1. Gluck S. Inflammatory breast cancer. Miami Breast Cancer Conference, Orlando, Florida, 2008.
2. Recht A, Edge SB, Solin SJ, et al. Post-mastectomy radiotherapy: clinical practice guidelines of the American Society of Clinical Oncology. J Clin Oncol 2001; 19:1539–1569.
3. NHS Scotland. Selective use of postoperativeradio-therapy after mastectomy. Available at: www.supremo-trial.com. Accessed November 17, 2008.
4. Howell A. ATAC trial update. Lancet 2005; 365:1225–1226 (letter).
5. Benson JR, Ravisekar O. Aromatase inhibitors in the treatment of breast cancer. Curr Cancer Treat Rev 2007; 3:67–79.
6. Coates AS, Keshaviah A, Thurlimann B, et al. Five years of letrozole compared with tamoxifen as initial adjuvant therapy for postmenopausal women with endocrine-responsive early breast cancer: update of study BIG 1-98. J Clin Oncol 2007; 25:486–492.
7. ATAC Trialists Group. Effect of anastrozole and tamoxifen as adjuvant treatment for early stage breast cancer: 100 month analysis of the ATAC trial. Lancet Oncol 2008; 9:45–53.

CASE STUDY 23

History

A 37-year-old professional woman presented with a four-week history of a painless lump in the right breast, which had slightly decreased in size. There was no associated nipple discharge and the patient had no previous breast problems. Her maternal grandmother had developed breast cancer in her 40s and her paternal grandmother had the disease at the age of 79 years. The patient was nulliparous and had used the oral contraceptive pill for a cumulative period of 15 years.

Clinical Findings

On examination there was an area of focal nodularity in the upper outer quadrant of the right breast with the impression of a more dominant lump. There was no skin tethering or axillary lymphadenopathy (E3) (Fig. 11).

Clinical Assessment

The history of a lump, which had decreased in size, was suggestive of a benign breast condition, although clinical examination was suspicious of malignancy.

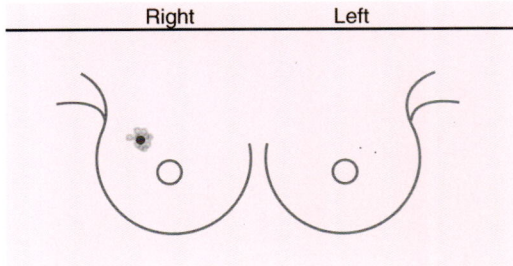

Figure 11

Investigations

Mammography

Two clusters of fine microcalcification were seen in the right breast, one of which coincided with the clinical abnormality (Fig. 12A, B).

Breast Ultrasound

Ultrasound revealed an area of altered texture in the upper outer quadrant of the right breast measuring approximately 3 cm (U4) (Fig. 13).

Core Biopsy

Ultrasound-guided core biopsy (14-gauge needle) of the right breast mass confirmed an invasive carcinoma with mucinous features (grade II, ER positive, HER2 negative). No in situ component was seen on core biopsy [Fig. 14A (low power), B (high power)].

Diagnosis

Early-stage right breast cancer (T2N0)

Multidisciplinary Review 1

Neither mammography nor ultrasound provided clear information on the dimensions of the tumor in the right breast (approximately

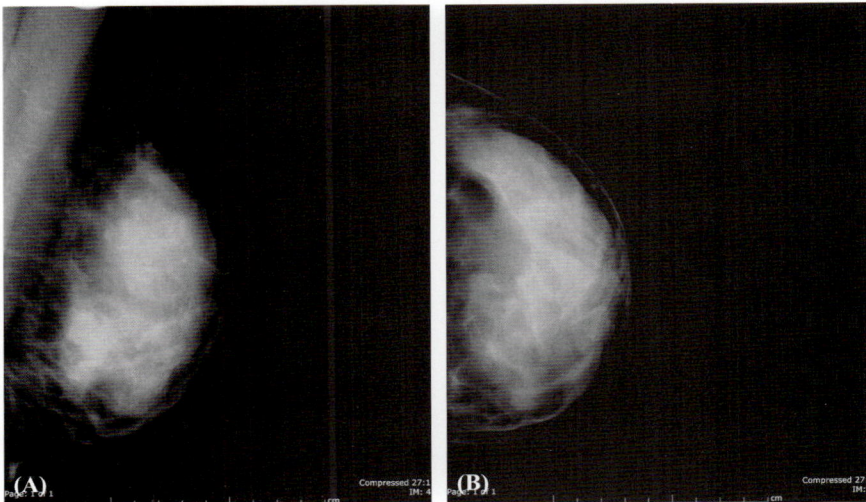

Figure 12

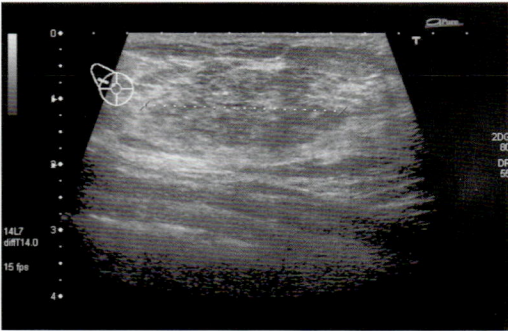

Figure 13

3 cm). MRI examination of the breasts was recommended to clarify the extent of the lesion, which was otherwise borderline conservable. In the event that the lesion exceeded 3 cm in maximum size, then either a right-modified radical mastectomy (+/- immediate reconstruction) or possibly neoadjuvant chemotherapy would be indicated.

Further Investigations

MRI Examination

This upstaged the right breast tumor to a maximum diameter of 4.1 cm (Fig. 15). Furthermore, two lesions with high intensity signals were evident in the left breast (Fig. 16). The larger of these measured 7 mm and lay in the upper outer quadrant of the left breast. The smaller lesion (4.5 mm) lay relatively close to the nipple-areolar complex.

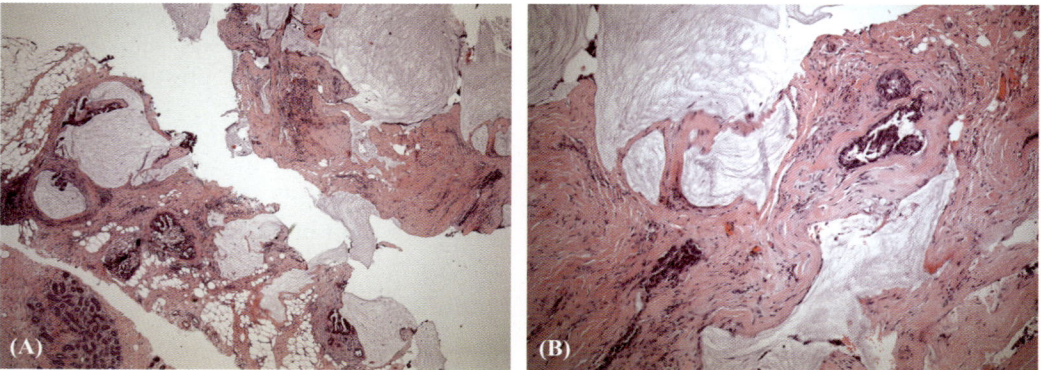

Figure 14

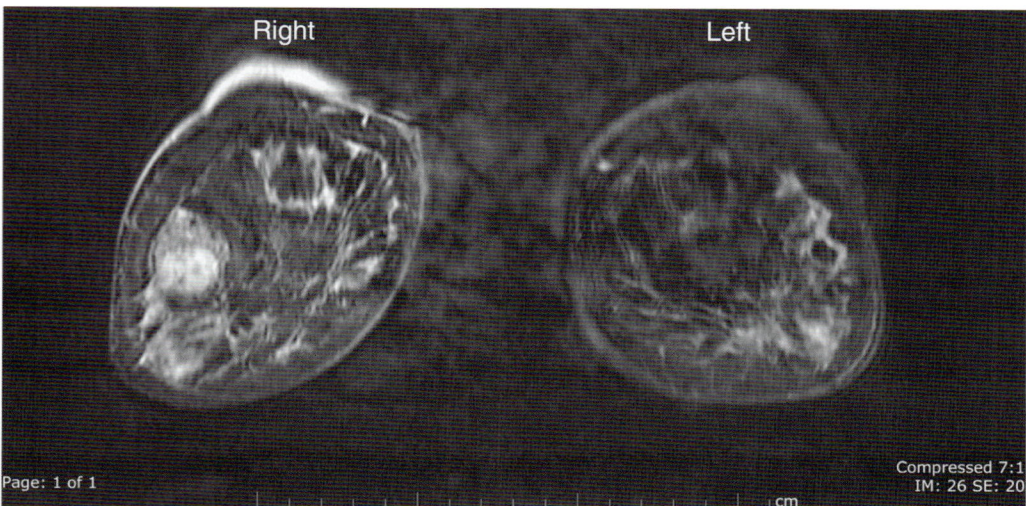

Figure 15

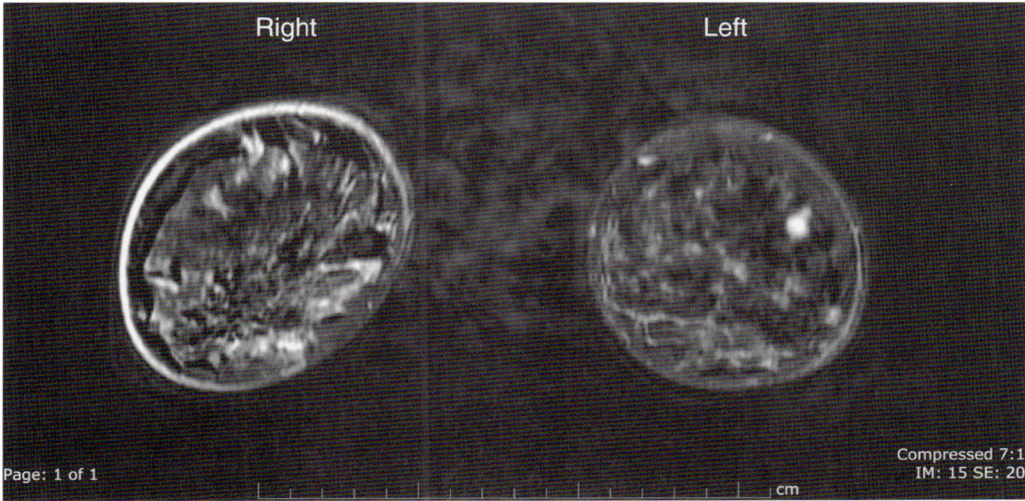

Figure 16

Core Biopsy

Ultrasound-guided core biopsy (14-gauge needle) of the 7-mm lesion revealed an invasive carcinoma (grade II, ER positive, HER2 negative) [Fig. 17A, B (low power), C (high power)] while biopsy of the smaller lesion yielded benign tissue only.

Multidisciplinary Review 2

The patient had confirmed bilateral breast cancer with a large, unifocal tumor on the right and a probable multicentric tumor on the left (though not proven histologically). Treatment options included bilateral mastectomy with an axillary clearance on the

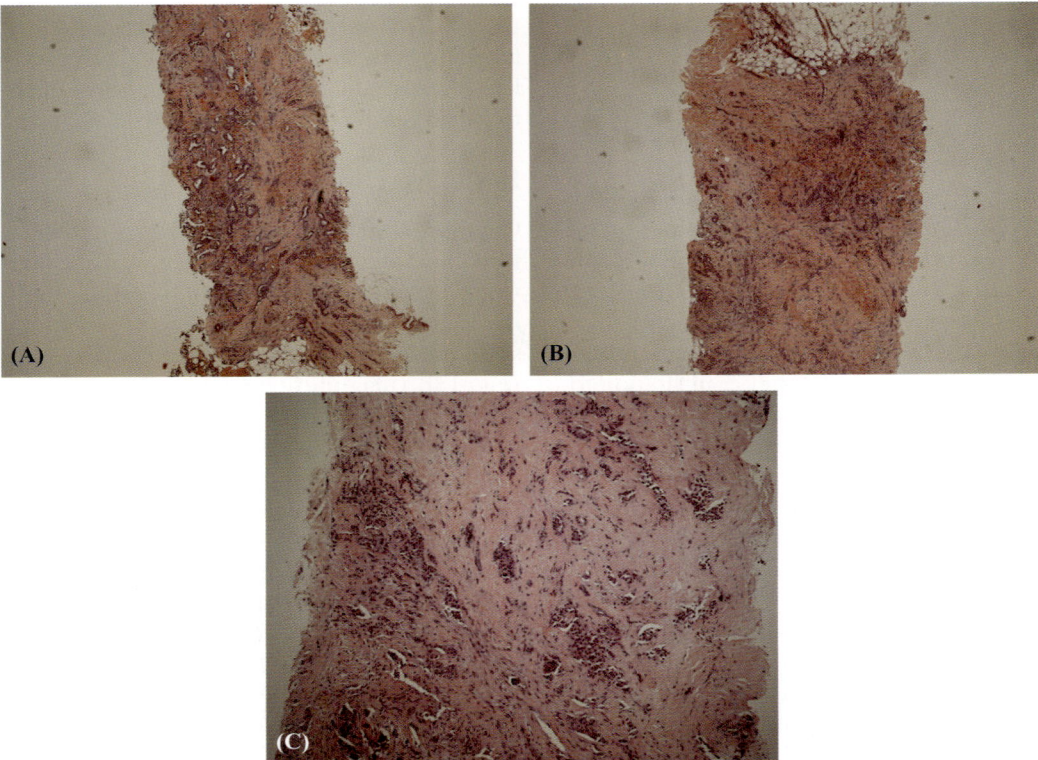

Figure 17

right (tumor >4 cm) and some form of axillary sampling on the left (aggregate tumor size 11.4 mm). Alternatively, neoadjuvant chemotherapy could be offered that may permit breast conservation on the right side after downstaging. It was noted that the patient was relatively young with a family history of breast cancer that would favor complete mastectomy rather than wide local excision on the right whatever the response to chemotherapy may be. Staging investigations with CT scan of chest/abdomen/pelvis and bone scan were requested.

Treatment and Progress

The patient was very keen to avoid mastectomy if at all possible and preferred to embark on neoadjuvant chemotherapy with the possibility of breast preservation (on the right). Moreover, she wished to explore ovarian protection with an LHRH (luteinizing hormone releasing hormone) analogue (Zoladex) as she had not yet borne any children. Staging investigations revealed no evidence of distant metastatic disease and the patient was commenced on a regimen of four cycles epirubicin/cyclophosphamide followed by four cycles of docetaxel (see Appendix III). She tolerated chemotherapy well with mild (grade II) nausea, fatigue, and indigestion. An ultrasound performed after the third cycle chemotherapy showed a partial tumor response on the right side. The biopsy proven lesion in the upper outer quadrant of left breast could no longer be seen on ultrasound, but the smaller 4-mm lesion (not biopsy proven cancer) was still present.

Following the seventh cycle of chemotherapy, the patient had a further consultation to discuss surgical management. Though the right breast cancer had reduced to a size that permitted conservation, there were two potential tumors in the contralateral breast. One of these had disappeared radiologically in response to chemotherapy.

It was recommended that the patient undergo bilateral mastectomy (with or without immediate reconstruction) with an axillary clearance on the right side and an axillary sampling on the left side. The patient was in agreement and did not wish to undergo treatment for either recurrent or de novo treatment in the future. She requested immediate breast reconstruction and was referred to the plastic surgeons for discussion of reconstructive options. The patient had size 36C cup breasts and was of slim build; she had inadequate infraumbilical abdominal tissue for a bilateral "split" TRAM (transverse rectus abdominus myocutaneous flap) and was therefore suitable for either a bilateral procedure with implant only or latissimus dorsi myocutaneous flap with an implant. The patient expressed a desire to have a "good and normal" result as possible and therefore opted for the latter. She was informed that this was a major surgical intervention and could be associated with much postoperative pain and discomfort (from bilateral donor sites on the back).

The patient proceeded with surgery six weeks after completion of chemotherapy. Bilateral skin-sparing mastectomies were carried out with the nipple-areolar complex replaced by a disc of skin from the back (skin island paddle on myocutaneous flap). A formal level II axillary lymph node dissection was performed on the right and a BDANS (blue dye-assisted node sampling). McGhan style 150 implants were used for reconstruction in conjunction with 2 latissimus dorsi flaps. The patient made an excellent postoperative recovery and was well enough to attend her brother's wedding two weeks later.

Definitive Histology

Chemotherapy changes relating to neoadjuvant therapy were evident on the right side (Fig. 18A) with an area of residual high nuclear grade DCIS (ductal carcinoma in situ) measuring 22 m in maximum extent [Fig. 18B (magnification 10×), C, D (magnification 20×)]. There was no residual invasive disease and no lymphovascular space invasion, but lakes of mucin were seen (Fig. 18E). None of the 15 lymph nodes on the right side contained metastatic carcinoma, and there was no suggestion of downstaging secondary to chemotherapy. On the left side there was no evidence of any residual invasive or in situ disease, and the lymph nodes sampled were free of tumor. The tumors from both breasts were ER positive and HER2 negative on core biopsy.

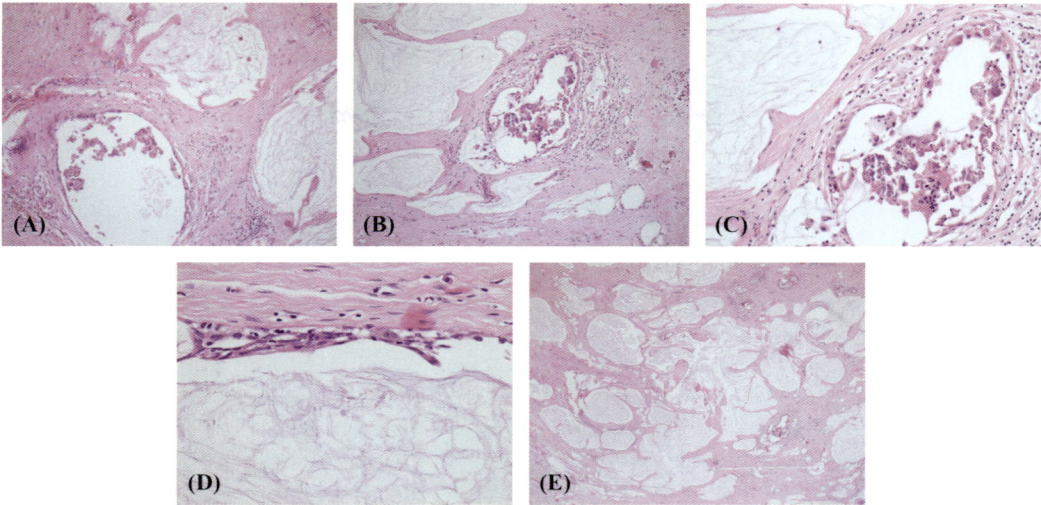

Figure 18

Multidisciplinary Review 3

It was recommended that the patient continue with the LHRH analogue Zoladex for a total period of three years followed by tamoxifen for five years. The patient wished to conceive in the future and laparoscopic oophorectomy was declined. Moreover, there was no indication for chest wall radiotherapy in the absence of any evidence of extensive nodal involvement at the outset or following chemotherapy (HER2 negative).

Treatment and Progress

There was a minor degree of capsular contracture on clinical review at six months. Otherwise there was an excellent cosmetic result (Fig. 19). However, there was discussion of possible implant exchange on the right side at the time of nipple reconstruction.

Discussion

This young patient with bilateral synchronous tumors had several risk factors for breast cancer, including family history, nulliparity, and prolonged usage of the oral contraceptive pill prior to any pregnancy (1). The patient presented with unilateral symptoms on the right side, and the mammographic and ultrasound abnormalities were confined to the ipsilateral side. The left-sided lesions were detected on MRI examination, which was undertaken

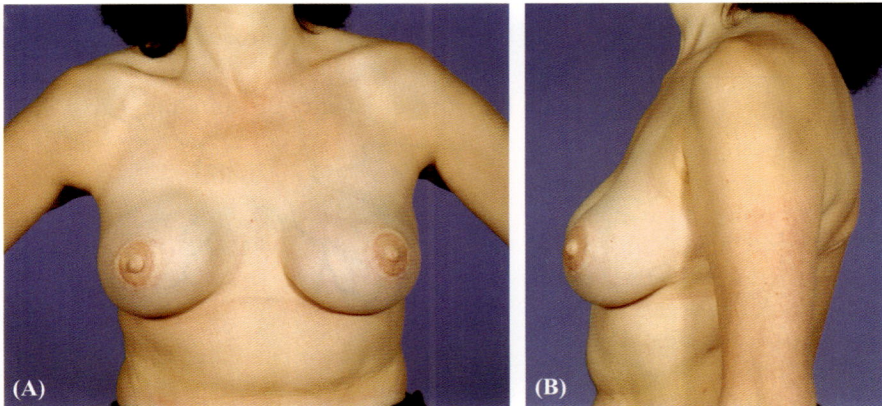

Figure 19

primarily to clarify the extent of the tumor in the right breast that had ill-defined margins on routine imaging (2). However, for those patients deemed to be at higher risk for development of breast cancer, MRI examination has an important role in screening the contralateral breast (3). Bilateral breast cancer has an incidence of approximately 4%, and one-third of tumors are synchronous and two-thirds metachronous (4, 5). Younger women (<50 years) have been reported to have a 10- to 14-fold higher risk of developing contralateral cancers than the general population. Had this patient not undergone MRI examination for investigation of the ipsilateral tumor, it is likely that these small impalpable left-sided tumors would have presented clinically at a future date as metachronous cancer (alternatively they could have been detected radiologically on routine follow-up mammography to the contralateral breast). This increased risk of bilaterality strengthens the argument for undertaking MRI examination in all younger women presenting with unilateral breast cancer.

This patient could have been managed with primary surgery at the outset. This would have necessarily involved bilateral mastectomy on the basis of tumor size on the right and multifocality on the left. Neoadjuvant chemotherapy offered the potential for downstaging the right-sided tumor to permit breast conservation (6,7). Surgical evaluation after the seventh cycle of chemotherapy suggested that this was technically feasible. However, in view of the patient's relatively young age, family history of breast cancer, and the need for contralateral mastectomy, a right-sided mastectomy was recommended.

The patient was of slim build, and immediate reconstruction could have been done with an implant-only technique. When carried out as a simultaneous bilateral procedure, subpectoral placement of implants can create a good cosmetic result with symmetrical breasts, matched for size and shape (8). However, the patient wished to have the best chance of a "normal-looking breast" and opted for autologous tissue transfer. There was inadequate infraumbilical tissue for a split TRAM flap and therefore bilateral latissimus dorsi flaps were raised and used in conjunction with implants as the reconstructive method of choice. There was also a possibility that radiotherapy to the right chest wall might be required.

Facilities for radioisotope usage were not available; sentinel lymph node biopsy with dual localization was not possible. On the basis of the original tumor size on the right side, a level II axillary dissection was performed. Both tumors visualized in the left breast on MRI were small (7 mm and 4.5 mm). The chance of nodal involvement on this side was low and a blue dye–assisted node sampling was carried out.

Definitive histology revealed a complete pathological response bilaterally in respect of invasive carcinoma. Often there is residual DCIS as this is less responsive to induction chemotherapy (lower rate of cell cycling) (9). Furthermore, there was no suggestion that any of the axillary nodes on the right side had previously been involved by tumor and subsequently downstaged by chemotherapy. The patient elected to have ovarian suppression with an LHRH analogue, which would potentially allow restoration of ovarian function in the future. This case illustrates the increasing problem of professional women developing breast cancer prior to conception. Childbearing is deferred due to career commitments, and women are faced with a diagnosis of breast cancer while nulliparous or possibly during pregnancy.

Related Cases

Bilateral breast cancer—*Case Studies 22, 24, and 32*

Immediate breast reconstruction—*Case Studies 3, 16, 17, 18, and 37*

Blue dye–assisted node sampling—*Case Study 8*

Neoadjuvant chemotherapy—*Case Studies 27–29*

Ovarian suppression—*Case Studies 8 and 27*

Learning Points

1. Breast MRI has been increasingly utilized in the evaluation of women with primary breast cancer. In about 3% of all women

with primary breast cancer, MRI will detect lesions in the contralateral breast that are not evident on mammography. The wider use of breast MRI may therefore increase bilateral mastectomy rates.

2. There is mounting evidence to suggest that the anthracylines (epirubicin and doxorubicin) are primarily effective in patients with HER2-positive tumors. Thus, its use in women with HER2-negative tumors may diminish in the years ahead.

3. Important information on primary tumor characteristics might be lost following preoperative chemotherapy. For instance, node-positive tumors might convert to node-negative status. This could potentially result in under treatment (e.g., postmastectomy radiotherapy might be withheld in patients with extensive nodal involvement who convert to node-negative status after preoperative chemotherapy).

References

1. Sellers TA, Grabrick DM. The epidemiology of breast cancer. In: Jatoi I, ed. Manual of Breast Diseases. Philadelphia: Lippincott Wilkins & Williams, 2002:149–175.
2. Kumar NA, Schnall MD. MR imaging: its current and potential utility in the diagnosis and management of breast cancer. Magn Reson Imaging Clin N Am 2000; 8:715–728.
3. Lehman CD, Gatsonis C, Kuhl CK, et al. MRI evaluation of the contralateral breast in women with recently diagnosed breast cancer. N Engl J Med 2007; 356:1295–1303.
4. Wanebo HJ, Senofsky GM, Fechner RE, et al. Bilateral breast cancer: risk reduction of contralateral biopsy. Ann Surg 1985; 201:667–677.
5. Robbins GF, Berg JW. Bilateral primary breast cancers: a prospective clinicopathological study. Cancer 1964; 17:1501–1527.
6. Makris A, Powles TJ, Ashley SE, et al. A reduction in the requirements for mastectomy in a randomized trial of neoadjuvant chemoendocrine therapy in primary breast cancer. Ann Oncol 1998; 9:1179–1184.
7. Bonadonna G, Veronesi U, Brambilla C, et al. Primary chemotherapy to avoid mastectomy in tumours with diameters of three centimeters or more. J Natl Cancer Inst 1990; 82:1539–1545.
8. Nava M, Bonavita M, Arioli N, et al. Breast reconstruction with subpectoral prosthesis or tissue expanders. In: Querci della Rovere G, Benson JR, Breach N, Nava M, eds. Oncoplastic and Reconstructive Surgery of the Breast. London: Martin Dunitz, 2004 (ISBN 1 84184 351 2).
9. Fisher B, Brown A, Mamounas E, et al. Effect of preoperative chemotherapy on loco-regional disease in women with operable breast cancer: findings from the National Surgical Adjuvant Breast and Bowel Project B-18. J Clin Oncol 1997; 15:2483–2493.

CASE STUDY 24

History

An 81-year-old woman presented with a four-week history of a lump in the right breast. She had noticed some dimpling of the skin overlying the lump, but no indrawing of the nipple or discharge therefrom. There was no family history of breast or ovarian cancer, and the patient had no previous breast problems. She had never used any form of exogenous hormones.

Clinical Findings

Examination revealed a hard irregular mass in the upper outer quadrant of the right breast lying well away from the nipple-areolar complex. There was tethering of the overlying skin, but the mass was mobile on the chest wall. There was no axillary lymphadenopathy (E4) (Fig. 20).

Clinical Assessment

The lesion in the right breast was highly suspicious for malignancy.

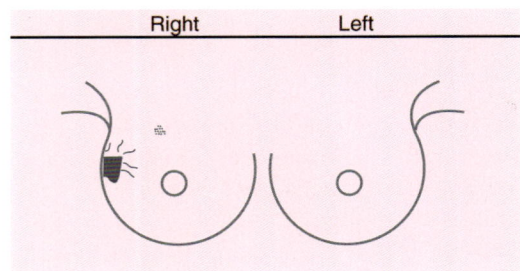

Figure 20

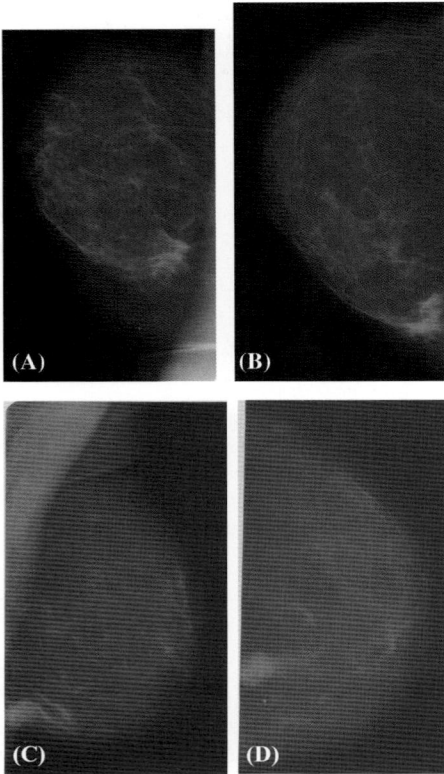

Figure 21

Investigations

Mammography

An asymmetric density was apparent in the upper outer quadrant of the right breast. This measured 25 mm in maximum extent and had the features of a carcinoma (R5) (Fig. 21A, B). A further radiologically

suspicious lesion was seen in the lower inner quadrant of the left breast measuring 20 mm in maximum diameter (R5) (Fig. 21C, D).

Breast Ultrasound

The sonographic correlate of the right breast lesion was a 27-mm ill-defined heterogenous mass with a hypoechoic pattern and posterior attenuation (U5) (Fig. 22A). A 19-mm mass was seen in the left breast with similar ultrasound features (U5) (Fig. 22B).

Core Biopsy

Ultrasound-guided core biopsy of the right breast mass showed an invasive lobular carcinoma (grade II) (Fig. 23A) while the left-sided lesion was an invasive ductal carcinoma (grade II). Both lesions were ER positive and HER2 negative on core biopsy (Fig. 23B).

Diagnosis

Bilateral breast cancers: right (T2N0), left (T1N0).

Multidisciplinary Review 1

Both breast cancers were potentially suitable for breast-conserving surgery with bilateral wide local excision and sentinel lymph node biopsy. In view of the left breast cancer being of the lobular phenotype and associated with skin tethering, it was recommended that MRI imaging of the breasts be undertaken prior to surgery. On review of

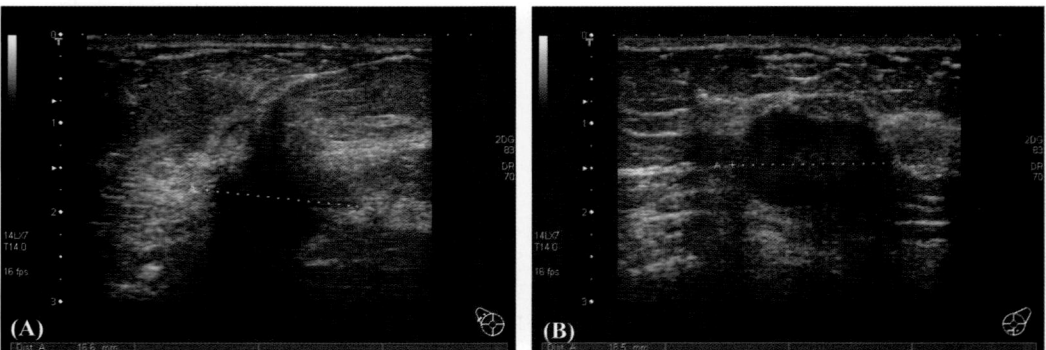

Figure 22

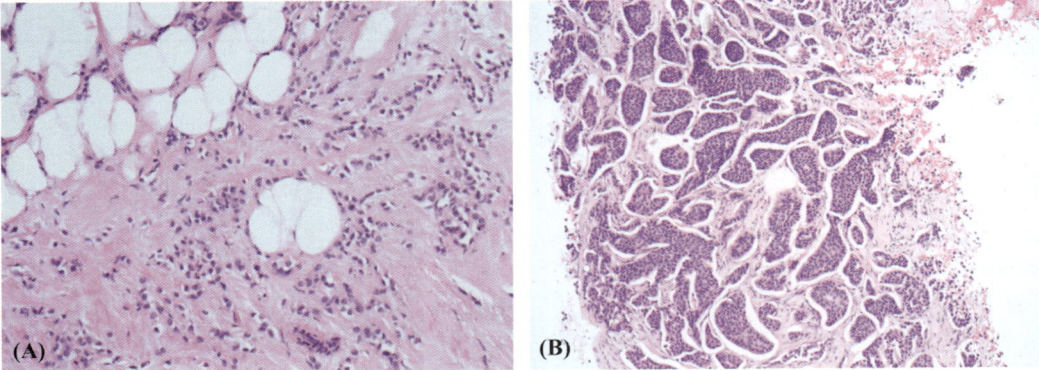

Figure 23

the mammogram, there was a suggestion of a further opacity in the right breast lying several centimeters from the main index lesion. MRI examination of the breasts was requested to clarify the extent of the right-sided breast cancer and to further elucidate the nature of the second opacity on the right side, close to the index lesion. Bilateral axillary ultrasound and possible core biopsy was also recommended preoperatively.

Investigations

MRI Breasts

MRI examination revealed multifocal tumors of both breasts; on the right side there were two enhancing lesions lying in separate quadrants measuring 22.7 mm and 7.3 mm (Fig. 24A). These showed time-intensity curves with malignant-type enhancement (Fig. 24B); on the left side a further lesion was seen

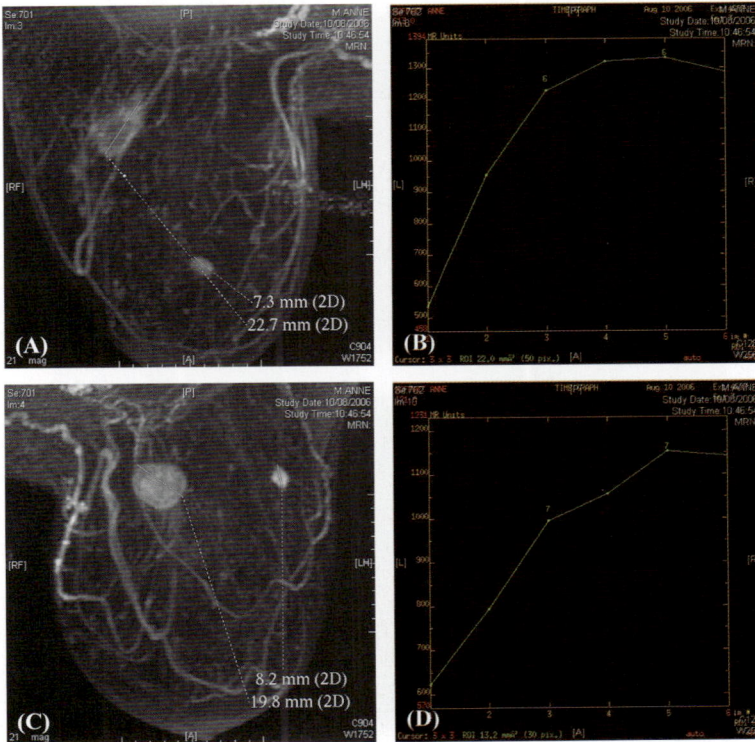

Figure 24

lateral to the main tumor in the superior aspect of the breast (Fig. 24C). This also displayed a malignant enhancement curve (Fig. 24D).

Axillary Ultrasound

Bilateral axillary ultrasound and core biopsy of axillary nodes revealed no evidence of malignancy.

Multidisciplinary Review 2

The MRI had confirmed that both right and left tumors were multifocal and therefore bilateral mastectomy and sentinel lymph node biopsy were mandated.

Treatment and Progress

The patient was keen to proceed with surgery as soon as possible and was issued with an operation date some eight days later. At the time of surgery, sentinel lymph node biopsy was carried out through the lateral end of the mastectomy incision, and there were no suspicious nodes on intraoperative digital examination. A wide skin ellipse was

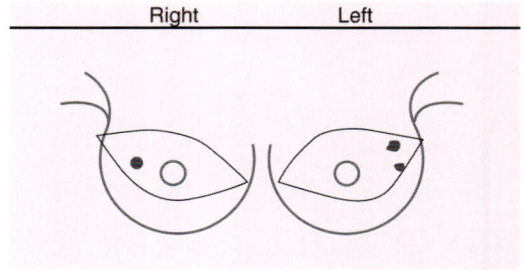

Figure 25

performed on the right side to encompass the area of skin tethering (Fig. 25).

The patient made an excellent postoperative recovery and was discharged home with a single drain each side on the third postoperative day. There was extensive bruising of the chest wall, but no discrete hematoma. The patient developed bilateral seromas that were aspirated in the clinic.

Definitive Histology

Right: An invasive lobular carcinoma (grade II) with the main index lesion measuring 23 mm in maximum diameter (concordant with radiological estimate) [Fig. 26A (low

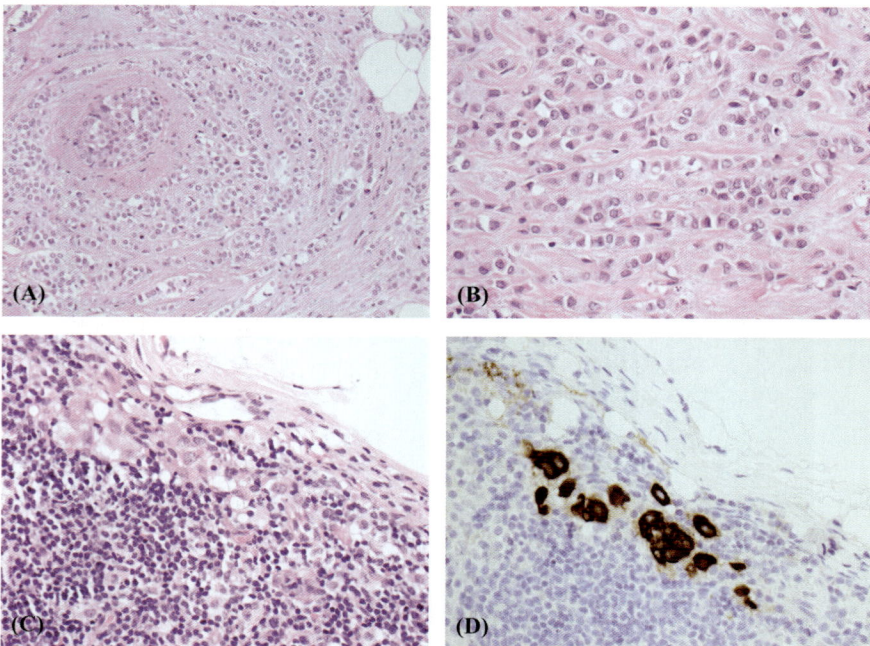

Figure 26

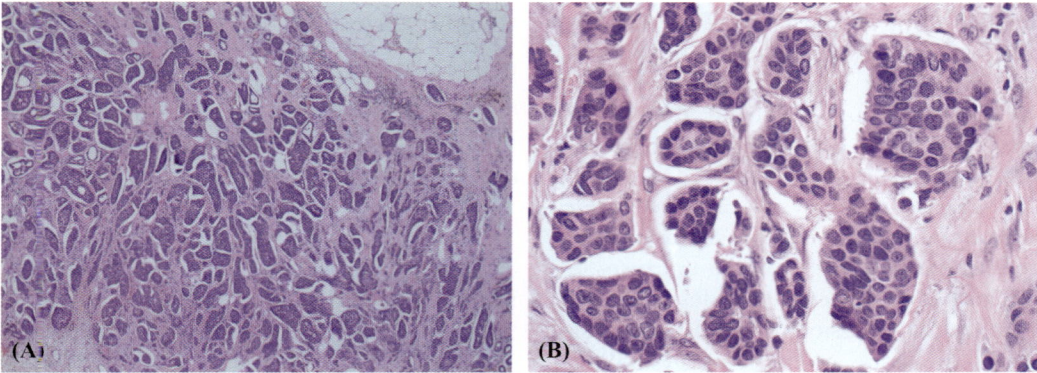

Figure 27

power), B (high power)]. There were several satellite foci and associated DCIS. One of the two sentinel lymph nodes harvested on the right contained a micrometastasis on standard H&E sections (Fig. 26C), which was confirmed on staining with anticytokeratin Cam5.2 antibody (Fig. 26D).

Left: An invasive carcinoma (grade II) of micropapillary subtype with associated high nuclear grade cribriform DCIS (with comedo necrosis) [Fig. 27A (low power), B (high power)]. The aggregate diameter of invasive and noninvasive components was 21 mm, and there was evidence of lymphovascular invasion. None of the four sentinel lymph nodes on the left side contained metastases.

Multidisciplinary Review 3

It was recommended that the patient undergo a completion axillary lymph node dissection on the right side on the basis of a focus of micrometastasis in one out of two sentinel lymph nodes. Radiotherapy to the chest wall was not indicated, and tamoxifen with an early switch (2–3 years) to an aromatase inhibitor was prescribed as adjuvant systemic hormonal therapy NPI (Nottingham Prognostic Index): $(0.2 \times 2.3) + 2 + 2 = 4.46$].

Treatment and Progress

It was explained to the patient that there was a relatively low probability (~15%) of finding further disease in the nonsentinel nodes. Furthermore, at the age of 81 years, any completion axillary dissection was unlikely

to impact on either regional disease control or overall survival. The patient initially accepted the recommendation of the multidisciplinary team and a date for further surgery was arranged. However, upon reflection and discussion between the patient and her family, she decided not to proceed with formal axillary dissection. She was an otherwise fit and active person for her age and did not wish to risk incurring significant morbidity from further surgery.

Discussion

In a seminal study involving more than 20,000 breast cancers, only 3.7% of cases were found to be bilateral, of which one-third were synchronous and two-thirds were metachronous (1). Though the incidence of bilateral synchronous carcinoma is low (1.2%), this case illustrates the benefit of MRI examination, which can detect not only ipsilateral multifocal disease but also clinically occult contralateral breast cancer. The latter occurs in 4% to 8% of patients with a prior carcinoma, and for younger patients, there is a greater chance of clinical manifestation in their remaining lifetime. Moreover, MRI is a more sensitive investigation than mammography in the relatively dense breast tissue of premenopausal women (2). In the case described, MRI detected multifocal disease in both breasts, which was not readily apparent on either mammography or ultrasound examination of the breasts. The threshold for undertaking breast MRI examination should be much lower in younger patients. This elderly patient was potentially faced with bilateral axillary surgery for staging purposes. Within the older age group (≥70 years), the risks of axillary surgery are proportionately greater and the benefits less.

The disease-free survival of some older patients is unlikely to be improved by axillary surgery when there are competing causes of death and life expectancy is less. Similar arguments for omission of axillary staging apply to the issue of completion axillary dissection following a positive sentinel lymph node biopsy. For some patients, the risk-benefit ratio for detection of nonsentinel lymph node–positive cases may not justify any delayed procedure. The chance of non-sentinel lymph node involvement is related to the volume of disease in the sentinel node; when only micrometastatic deposits (>0.2 mm and ≤2 mm) are present in the sentinel node, the risk of nonsentinel node involvement is 15% compared with 25% to 50% for macrometastases (>2 mm) (3). Axillary recurrence remained relatively low (2% at 3 years follow-up) when completion axillary dissection was selectively omitted in a group of more than 200 sentinel node–positive patients who either refused axillary dissection or were considered to be at low risk of relapse (4). The low rates of axillary relapse are unlikely to translate into any meaningful reduction in long-term survival among an older group of patients. The Cambridge Breast Unit has recently elected to omit completion axillary dissection in the following group of patients:

- Micrometastases only in sentinel node
- Age ≥70 years
- Tumor size ≤3 cm
- ER positive
- Grade I or II (consider grade III)

The morbidity from further axillary surgery could be quite significant for this older group of patients. It has been suggested that the lower age limit for this policy be reduced to 60 years (grade I and II, ≤2 cm). However, some of the patients in this group might receive chemotherapy in the event of further nodal involvement.

Related Cases

Bilateral breast cancer—*Case Studies 22, 23, and 32*

Preoperative MRI—*Case Studies 6 and 8*

Completion axillary dissection—*Case Studies 10 and 13*

Learning Points

1. The incidence of bilateral synchronous breast cancers increased in the 1970s, soon after bilateral mammography was introduced for the evaluation of women with primary breast cancer. The incidence of bilateral breast cancers is likely to increase even further in the years ahead, as the use of breast MRI increases.
2. Axillary lymph node dissection decreases the risk of local (axillary) recurrences, but is associated with significantly greater morbidity than sentinel node biopsy alone. Axillary recurrences are of less concern in the elderly because they often have tumors with a better prognosis and also because competing causes of mortality might intervene before regional recurrence becomes a threat.

References

1. Wanebo HJ, Senofsky GM, Fechner RE, et al. Bilateral breast cancer: risk reduction of contralateral biopsy. Ann Surg 1985; 201: 667–677.
2. Warren R. New radiological techniques: digital mammography, MRI scintimammography, PET and some more for "Tomorrow's World". In: Querci della Rovere G, Warren R, Benson JR, eds. Early Breast Cancer. London and New York: Taylor and Francis, 2006: 175–199.
3. Cserni G, Gregori D, Merletti F, et al. Non-sentinel node metastases associated with micrometastatic sentinel nodes in breast cancer: metaanalysis of 25 studies. Br J Surg 2004; 91:1245–1252.
4. Naik AM, Fey J, Gemignani M, et al. The risk of axillary relapse after sentinel lymph node biopsy for breast cancer is comparable with that of axillary lymph node dissection: a follow up study of 4008 procedures. Ann Surg 2004; 240:462–471.

Inflammatory Breast Cancer

CASE STUDY 25

History

A 39-year-old woman presented to the breast clinic having noticed a reddened area over the medial aspect of the right breast for the preceding six weeks. The area was tender to palpation and the patient had been prescribed a course of antibiotics by her general practitioner. However, the erythematous area failed to respond and indeed extended to involve much of the right breast. The patient was not aware of any discrete lump or change in consistency of the right breast. She was otherwise well and reported no weight loss or unusual cough or back pain. There had been no previous breast problems, but there was a strong history of breast cancer in the family; her mother had been recently diagnosed with breast cancer in her 60s and the patient's maternal grandmother died from bone secondaries relating to a primary breast cancer. The patient had 3 children (eldest aged 9 years) and underwent menarche at the age of 10 years. She had used the oral contraceptive pill for a cumulative period of four years prior to her first pregnancy and remained premenopausal.

Clinical Findings

Examination revealed gross swelling of the right breast with extensive erythema, edema, and peau d'orange. No discrete mass lesion was palpable but the consistency of the right breast was much firmer than the left side. There was an ill-defined mass in the right axilla, which clinically may have represented either lymphadenopathy or a mass in the axillary tail of the right breast (E5) (Fig. 1).

Clinical Assessment

The history and findings were highly suggestive of an inflammatory carcinoma of the right breast. The patient was informed of the likely diagnosis and probable management with primary chemotherapy.

Investigations

Mammography

Extensive edema and thickening of the right breast tissue was evident with no focal mass lesion (R5) (Fig. 2A, B).

Breast/Axillary Ultrasound

Sonographic assessment of the right breast corroborated the mammographic findings and showed edema of the tissues with no discernable mass lesion (Fig. 3A). Malignant appearing nodes were seen in the right axilla (U5) (Fig. 3B, C).

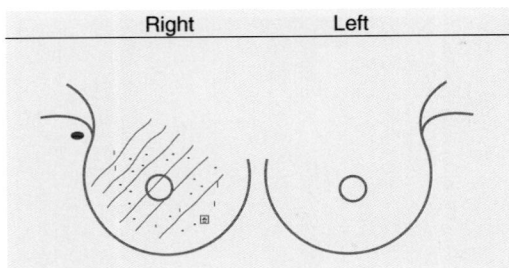

Figure 1

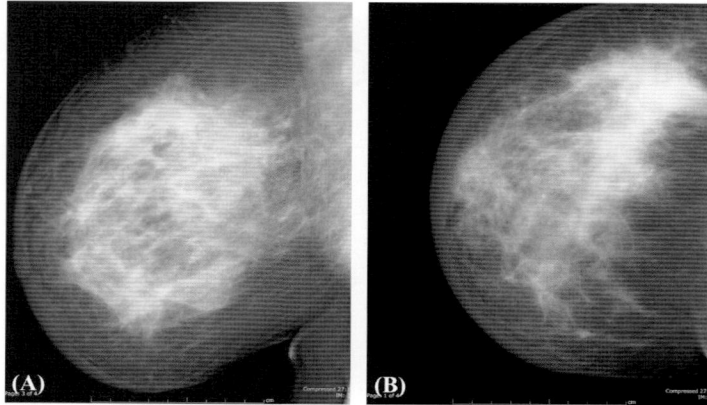

Figure 2

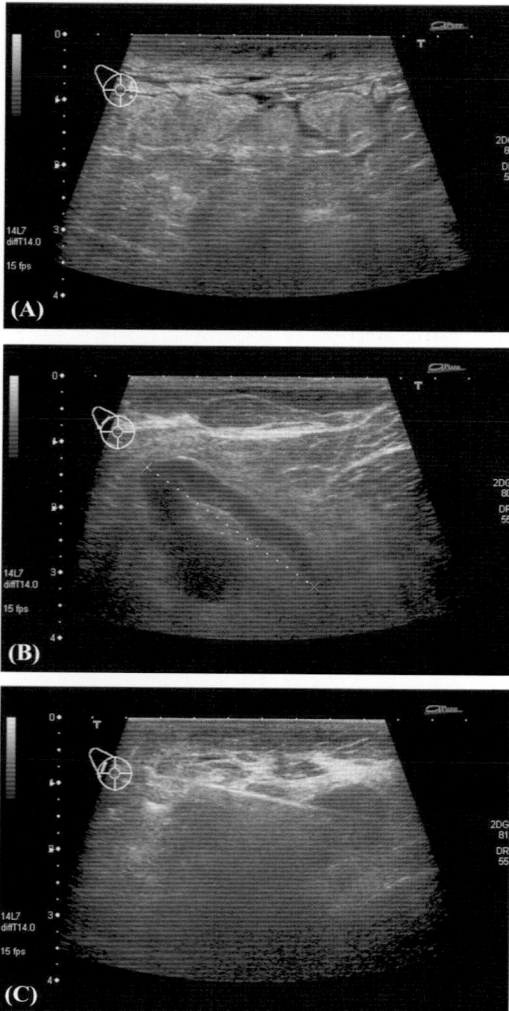

Figure 3

Core Biopsy

Ultrasound-guided core biopsy (16-gauge needle) of the right axillary mass confirmed an invasive carcinoma (grade III, ER negative) [Fig. 4A (low power), B (high power)]. Epithelial elements were more readily visualized on immunohistochemical staining with anticytokeratin antibody (5D3) compared with H&E staining (Fig. 5).

Diagnosis

Inflammatory cancer of the right breast in a premenopausal patient (T4dN1)

Multidisciplinary Review 1

Following multidisciplinary discussion, it was recommended that full staging investigations be carried out, including chest X ray, liver function tests, calcium, CT chest/abdomen/pelvis, and bone scan. In the absence of any evidence of distant metastases, the patient would be offered neoadjuvant chemotherapy followed by a right modified radical mastectomy (without immediate breast reconstruction) and irradiation of the chest wall and supraclavicular fossa. HER2 status was requested as this was not routinely done on core biopsy at time of this patient's diagnosis.

Treatment and Progress

The patient commenced chemotherapy within 10 days of tissue confirmation of a

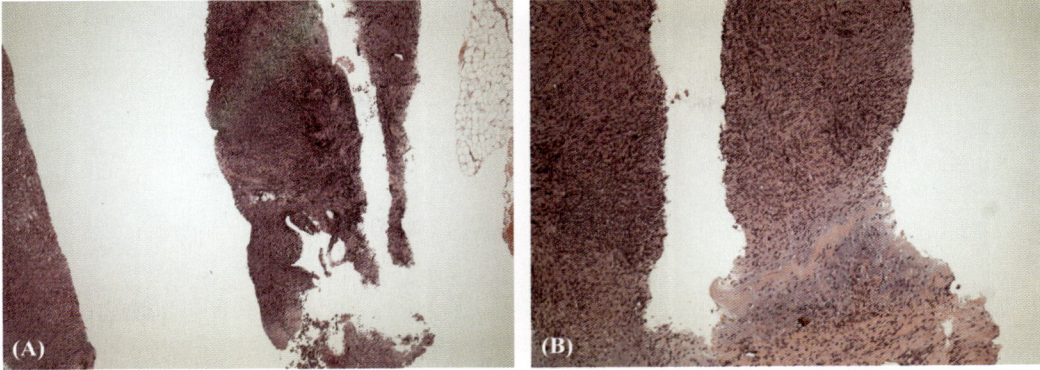

Figure 4

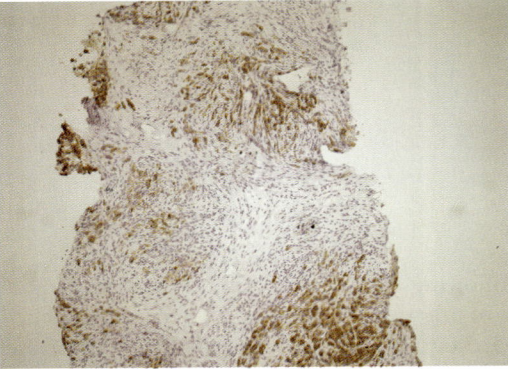

Figure 5

breast cancer diagnosis. She received four cycles of epirubicin/cyclophosphamide followed by four cycles of taxanes (EC/docetaxel—see Appendix III). The patient tolerated treatment well with partial resolution of the inflammatory changes in the right breast and a complete clinical response in respect of the right axillary nodes. Breast imaging with MRI after the eighth cycle of chemotherapy revealed a mass lesion in the upper inner quadrant of the right breast measuring 4.2 cm. Interestingly, this was the first accurate measurement of the dimensions of the right breast cancer—at the time of previous assessment, the margins of the tumor were masked by the inflammatory component.

It was noted at the time of further breast imaging that some inflammatory changes had developed in the contralateral breast, with erythema and peau d'orange (Fig. 6). However, there was no radiological evidence of malignancy in the left breast on MRI (opinion of a second radiologist sought). It was proposed to carry out a skin biopsy of the left breast at the time of definitive surgery of the right breast cancer or alternatively random core biopsies of the left breast (fan-shaped distribution). The patient proceeded to a right modified radical mastectomy six weeks after completion of the final cycle of docetaxel (blood counts satisfactory).

At the time of surgery, there was much edema of the breast and evidence of some skin infiltration by tumor. A wide skin incision was therefore performed together with a level III axillary lymph node dissection (macroscopic evidence of nodal disease in right axilla with at least two frankly malignant nodes).

The patient made an excellent postoperative recovery and arrangements were made for core biopsies of the left breast to be undertaken prior to discharge home.

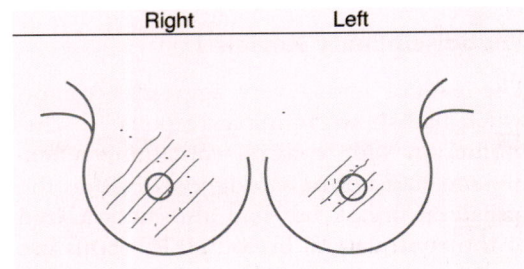

Figure 6

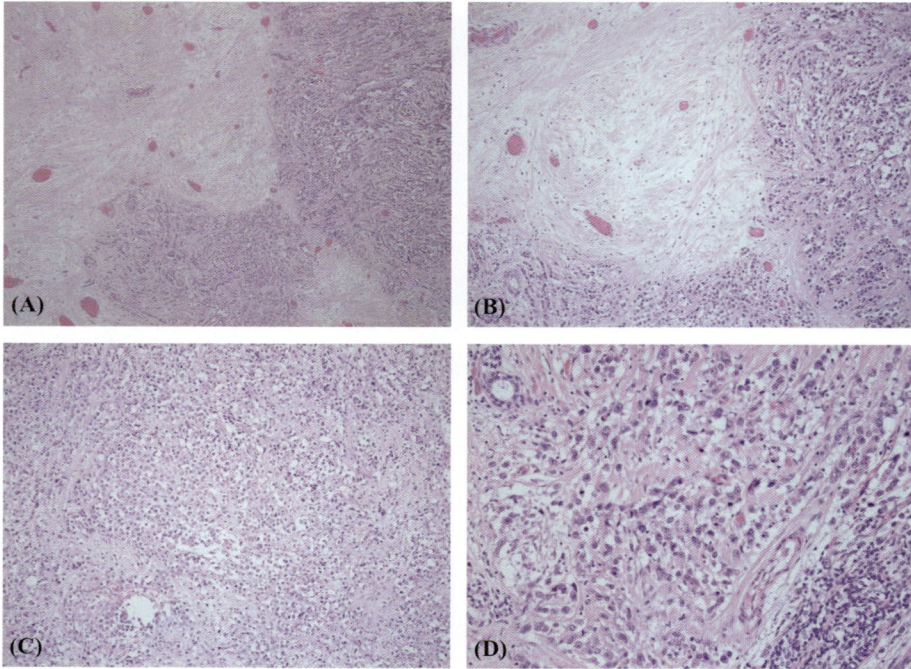

Figure 7

Definitive Histology

This revealed characteristic chemotherapy effects at the site of the tumor [Fig. 7A (magnification 5×), B (magnification 10×)], but extensive viable tumor was evident within the right breast measuring 110 mm in maximum diameter [Fig. 7C (low power), D (high power)]. There was also tumor in random sections taken from other parts of the breast with lymphovascular invasion of dermal lymphatics. Thirteen out of 15 nodes contained metastatic carcinoma with extracapsular extension. All core biopsies taken from the left breast showed invasive carcinoma, which was metastatic from the right breast.

Multidisciplinary Review 1

The patient had a very aggressive tumor, which had shown minimal response to chemotherapy with a taxane-containing schedule and had not only progressed within the ipsilateral breast, but had also metastasized to the contralateral breast. HER2 status was positive and it was recommended the patient be immediately commenced on Herceptin following assessment of left ventricular ejection fraction (LVEF) with a baseline echocardiogram. A repeat ultrasound scan of the liver showed no evidence of metastases. It was anticipated that locoregional control would be a potential problem; in addition to receiving radiotherapy to the right chest wall and supraclavicular fossa, consideration would be given to primary radiotherapy of the left breast (depending on response to Herceptin).

Treatment and Progress

The patient underwent irradiation of the right chest wall and supraclavicular fossa within four weeks of surgery. She developed a right chest wall recurrence shortly after completion of radiotherapy and was commenced on capecitebine (concurrent with three-weekly Herceptin). Further staging CT scan showed no evidence of distant metastases. Almost 12 months following surgery, the patient started a course of taxol combined with the antiangiogenic agent avastin (bevacizumab). This was associated with grade II nausea and vomiting, which settled with ondansetron. The patient otherwise remains generally well in herself and continues to be active and to care for her three young children.

Discussion

Inflammatory carcinoma is one of the most aggressive forms of breast cancer, which historically constitutes about 1% to 5% of all breast cancers and has been associated with a poor prognosis (1,2). It is a form of locally advanced breast cancer, though it remains unclear whether these reflect an advanced breast cancer continuum or represent distinct clinicopathological entities. Inflammatory cancers are usually high-grade lesions with fewer than half staining positive for either ER or PR. Between 30% and 50% overexpress HER2 together with e-cadherin and p53. With single modality therapies, the five-year survival rate for surgery alone was 2% to 10% and not much better for primary radiotherapy (3%) (2). Multimodality therapy with a combination of chemotherapy, radiotherapy, and surgery has significantly improved both local control and disease-free survival (approximately 50% 5-year survival) (3–5). The majority of patients with inflammatory carcinoma are in the younger age group and are managed with a sequence of primary chemotherapy followed by mastectomy (with axillary dissection) and irradiation of the chest wall and supraclavicular fossa. The latter reduces locoregional recurrence by two-thirds. Those patients who are HER2 positive receive Herceptin and most chemotherapy regimens incorporate a taxane. Many surgeons are reluctant to offer immediate breast reconstruction to this group because of the relatively high risk of locoregional relapse. Delayed reconstruction may be considered if patients are alive and disease-free after 18 to 24 months. When there is overt evidence of tumor progression after initial chemotherapy, patients can be treated with radiotherapy prior to surgery.

Complete staging investigations should be carried out prior to initiation of chemotherapy as these patients have a high risk of distant metastases. Moreover, treatment planning for this group of patients must be undertaken in a multidisciplinary setting with surgeon, radiation, and medical oncologist. Patients with a complete clinical response to initial chemotherapy have a disease-free survival rate of almost 50% at 15 years compared with only 9% for those with a partial response (6). Inflammatory breast cancer can be mistaken clinically for a benign inflammatory condition of the breast such as periductal mastitis or a breast abscess. This patient's general practitioner had initially prescribed a course of antibiotics and it was the failure to respond to these that prompted referral to a breast unit. The patient had not noticed any lump or change in consistency of the breast herself, though clinical examination revealed marked erythematous changes with edema, peau d'orange, and a generalized firmness of the breast. Breast imaging likewise failed to show any focal mass lesion, but revealed extensive edema and thickening of the breast tissue. A mass lesion subsequently became evident on MRI after the final cycle of chemotherapy; the inflammatory components of the tumor had precluded assessment of margins at the time of previous breast imaging.

A variety of preoperative chemotherapy schedules have been employed for treatment of inflammatory breast cancer. Most of these incorporate an anthracycline (doxorubicin or epirubicin) with complete and partial response rates averaging 12% and 60%, respectively (7,8). It is better to switch to a taxane than continuing with chemotherapy. If there is no response to an anthracycline-based chemotherapy, then patients should switch to docetaxol (4 cycles). In this particular case, the standard preoperative schedule of EC/docetaxel was used though a related schedule is eight cycles of TAC (docetaxel, adriamycin, and cyclophosphamide). There was only minimal response to chemotherapy and the tumor not only progressed within the ipsilateral breast but had metastasized to the contralateral breast. Further systemic therapy included Herceptin together with capecitebine for chest wall recurrence postmastectomy. The patient subsequently received taxol combined with an antiangiogenic agent. This case illustrates the potential problems with local control for inflammatory cancers when patients have not succumbed from distant disease. Occasionally uncontrolled local disease can lead to "cancer en cuirasse," which can restrict respiratory movements and be very distressing for the patient. The histopathological features of the right breast cancer were typical for an inflammatory carcinoma; high grade, ER negative, and HER2 positive with extensive infiltration of lymphovascular spaces, dermal lymphatics, axillary nodes, and extranodal fatty tissue. In addition, the tumor had metastasized throughout much of the contralateral breast. The presence of dermal lymphatic invasion does not predict response to treatment. Refractory cases of inflammatory breast cancer can be managed with the tyrosine kinase inhibitor, lapatinib, which is a dual inhibitor of both EGFR and HER2, though in reality functions mainly as an inhibitor of HER2 (9).

Related Cases

Inflammatory breast cancer—*Case Study 26*

Taxane-based neoadjuvant chemotherapy—*Case Studies 25–29*

Herceptin—*Case Studies 8, 11, 26, and 27*

Postmastectomy radiotherapy—*Case Studies 2, 3, 26, and 28*

Learning Points

1. Inflammatory breast cancer is the most aggressive manifestation of primary breast cancer. These patients are treated with neoadjuvant (preoperative) chemotherapy, which generally includes anthracyclines and taxanes. This is followed by locoregional treatment (mastectomy and radiotherapy) and then hormonal intervention for those with ER-positive disease.

2. A pathological complete response (pCR) indicates no histological evidence of tumor after neoadjuvant chemotherapy. pCR is a favorable prognostic factor, and these patients have better survival rates.

References

1. Levine PH, Steinhorn SC, Ries LG, Aron JL. Inflammatory breast cancer: the experience of the Surveillance, Epidemiology and End Results (SEER) program. J Natl Cancer Inst 1985; 74:291–297.
2. Jaiyesimi IA, Buzdar AU, Hortobagyi GN, et al. Inflammatory breast cancer: a review. J Clin Oncol 1992; 10:1014–1024.
3. Pisansky TM, Schaid DJ, Loprinzi CL, et al. Inflammatory breast cancer: integration of irradiation, surgery and chemotherapy. Am J Clin Oncol 1992; 15:376–387.
4. Brun B, Otmezquine Y, Feuilhade F, et al. Treatment of inflammatory breast cancer with combination chemotherapy and mastectomy versus breast conservation. Cancer 1988; 61:1096.
5. Fein DA, Mendenhall NP, Marsh RD, et al. Results of multimodality therapy for inflammatory breast cancer: an analysis of clinical and treatment factors affecting outcome. Ann Surg 1994; 60:220–225.
6. Hortobagyi GN, Buzdar AU. Treatment of metastatic breast cancer. In: Singletary SE, Robb GL, eds. Advanced Therapy of Breast Disease. Ontario: BC Decker Inc., 2000:281–289.
7. Rouesse J, Friedman S, Sarrazin D, et al. Primary chemotherapy in the treatment of inflammatory breast cancer: a study of 230 cases from the Institute Gustave-Roussy. J Clin Oncol 1986; 4:1765–1771.
8. Smith IE, Walsh G, Jones A, et al. High complete remission rates with primary neoadjuvant infusional chemotherapy for large early breast cancer. J Clin Oncol 1995; 13:424–429.
9. Gluck S. Management of inflammatory breast cancer. Miami Breast Cancer Conference, Orlando, Florida, 2008, February 20–23.

CASE STUDY 26

History

A 52-year-old woman underwent a routine screening mammogram that showed a carcinoma of the left breast radiologically. On direct inquiry, the patient reported a lump in the left breast, which had been present for a relatively short period of two weeks. She had no previous breast problems and no family history of breast or ovarian cancer. The patient had two children and was aged 26 years at the birth of her first child. She

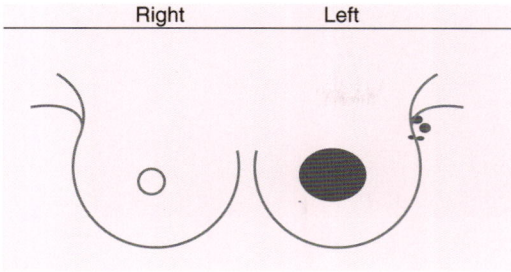

Figure 8

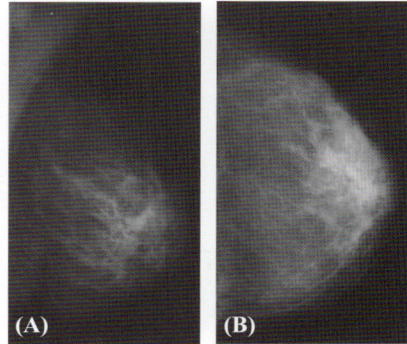

Figure 9

had used the oral contraceptive pill for a brief period of 12 months.

Clinical Findings

On examination there was a firm irregular mass in the upper outer quadrant and retro-areolar regions of the left breast. There was associated peau d'orange but no erythema of the breast and with slight indrawing of the left nipple. There were hard, but mobile nodes in the left axilla (E5) (Fig. 8).

Clinical Assessment

The clinical signs were suggestive of a carcinoma of the left breast with an inflammatory component.

Investigations

Mammography

An asymmetric density was apparent in the upper outer quadrant of the left breast measuring 80 mm in maximum diameter. There were multiple clusters of coarse granular microcalcifications highly suspicious for malignancy (R5) (Fig. 9A, B).

Breast and Axillary Ultrasound

A solid mass lesion was seen on ultrasound examination measuring 60 mm in maximum diameter (Fig. 10A). The echo pattern was hypoechoic with posterior acoustic attenuation. Multiple pathological nodes were visualized in the left axilla, the largest measuring 29 mm in its longitudinal axis. In addition there was radiological evidence of

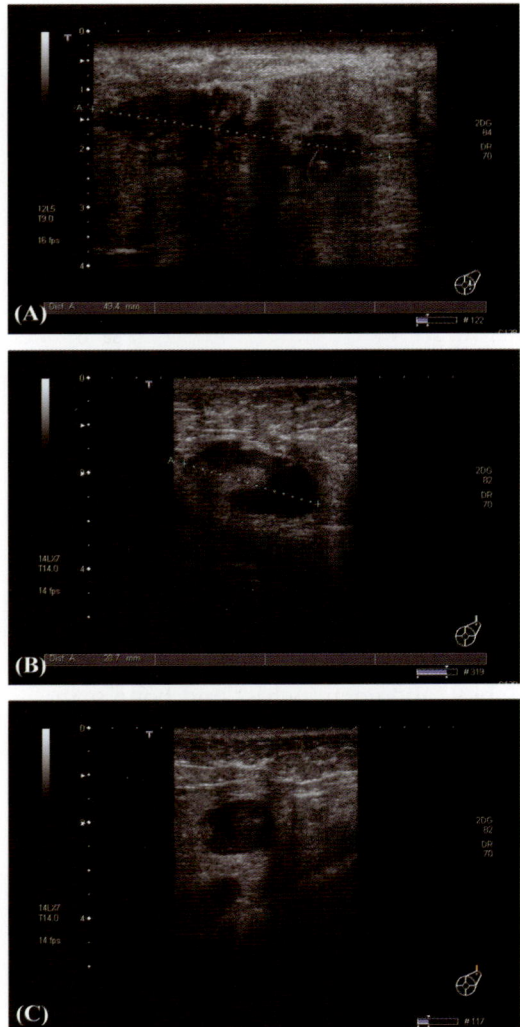

Figure 10

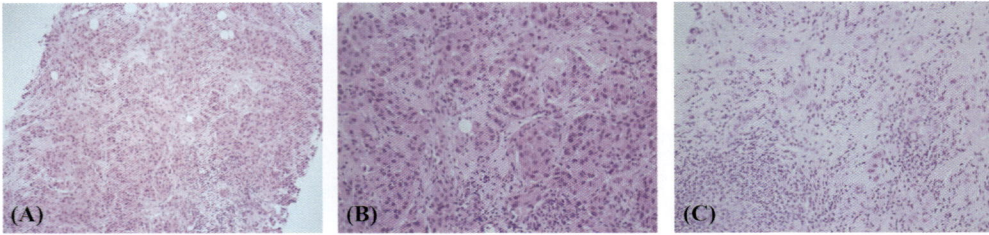

Figure 11

lymphedema with skin thickening (U5) (Fig. 10B, C).

Core Biopsy

Image-guided core biopsy of the breast mass confirmed an invasive carcinoma (grade III, ER negative, HER2 positive) [Fig. 11A (low power), B (high power)]. There was histological evidence of nodal involvement from percutaneous biopsy of the largest axillary node (Fig. 11C).

Diagnosis

Large inflammatory carcinoma of the left breast (T4dN1).

Multidisciplinary Review 1

It was recommended that the patient undergo neoadjuvant chemotherapy followed by a left modified radical mastectomy and radiotherapy to the chest wall and supraclavicular fossa (documented nodal disease prechemotherapy). The presence of an inflammatory component contraindicated immediate breast reconstruction. Staging investigations were requested including CT (chest/abdomen/pelvis) and bone scan.

Treatment and Progress

The patient was very distressed upon being informed of the diagnosis of breast cancer and the need for mastectomy following chemotherapy. She appeared particularly upset at being told that immediate reconstruction would not be offered and enquired about delayed reconstruction. Staging investigations revealed no evidence of distant metastatic disease, though CT imaging showed a questionable sclerotic area in one of the vertebral bodies but a subsequent bone scan was normal.

The patient commenced a course of four cycles of epirubicin/cyclophosphamide (EC) followed by four cycles of taxotere with Herceptin given concurrently (see Appendix III). The patient tolerated chemotherapy well with a partial tumor response. After seven cycles of chemotherapy, the tumor was much softer and measured 3 to 4 cm clinically and 32 mm sonographically. There was no peau d'orange or erythema of the breast and the palpable nodes in the left axilla had reduced in size. The patient was reviewed surgically and operative management discussed further. Despite having been informed at the time of diagnosis that a left modified radical mastectomy would be undertaken without reconstruction, the patient was adamant that she would not contemplate removal of the entire breast without immediate reconstruction. At no time had the patient ever been led to believe that she might be eligible for breast conservation. Inflammatory carcinoma is not an absolute contraindication to immediate breast reconstruction and it was the impression of various health professionals (breast/plastic surgeons, oncologist, breast care nurse) that the psychological benefits of reconstruction for this particular patient outweighed any potential disadvantages in this scenario. The patient was aware that she was at higher than average risk for locoregional recurrence and was prepared to accept this. She was referred to the plastic surgeon for discussion of reconstructive options and received appropriate psychological support from a senior nurse practitioner. It was considered that reconstruction with a latissimus dorsi flap and implant would be most appropriate for this patient based on the following factors:

1. Patient's age
2. Need for postoperative radiotherapy
3. Proposed wide skin excision (inflammatory component)

The patient proceeded to surgery six weeks after completion of the final cycle of chemotherapy. A left modified radical mastectomy was performed with removal of much of the breast skin that had originally shown peau d'orange changes. A correspondingly large island of skin was taken from the donor site on the back. The patient made an uneventful recovery and was discharged home on the seventh postoperative day. She was very pleased with the final cosmetic result (Fig. 12A, B).

Definitive Histology

There was invasive carcinoma (grade III) within the breast extending over an area of 60 mm, though this represented low volume residual disease (Fig. 13A, B). Tumor was clear of all margins and 5 out of 10 nodes contained metastatic carcinoma [Fig. 13C (magnification 5×), D (magnification 10×)].

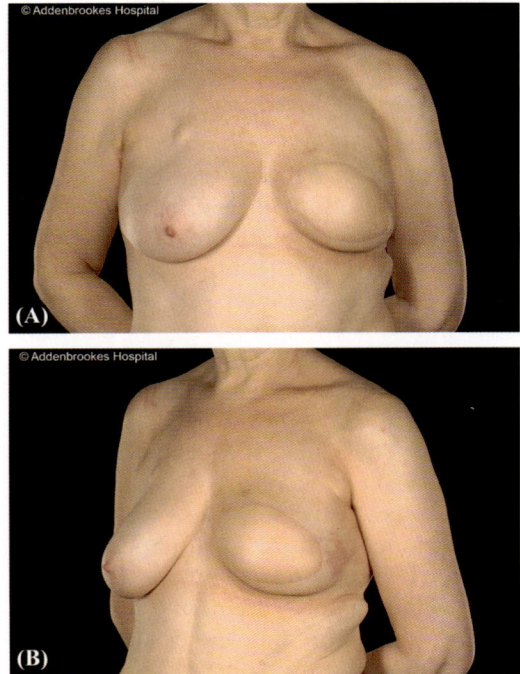

Figure 12

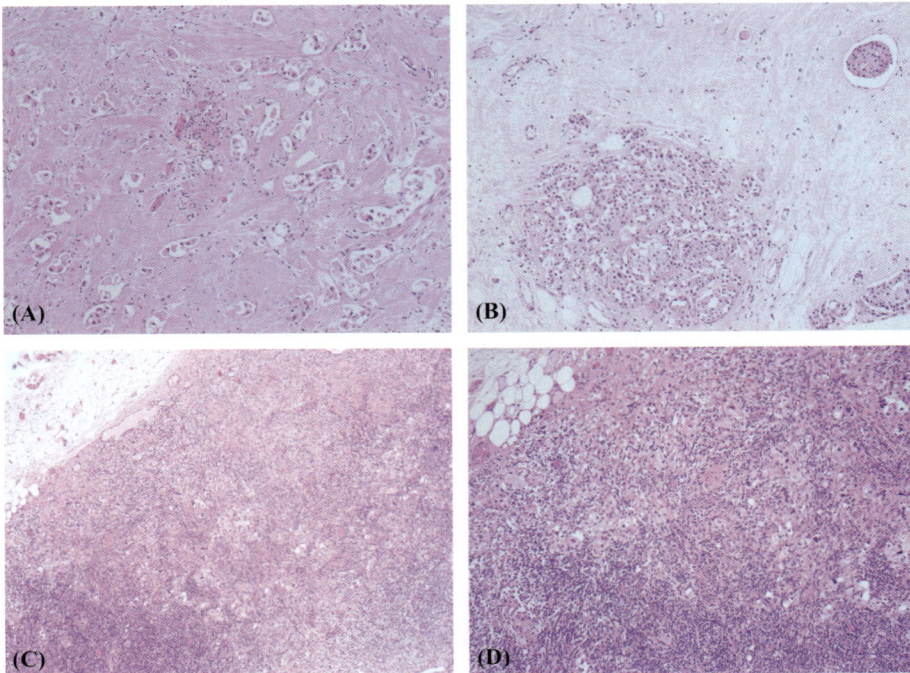

Figure 13

Discussion

This case illustrates how a diagnosis of inflammatory breast cancer may not be straightforward and this can generate dilemmas in the clinical decision making process. Inflammatory carcinoma is a clinical entity and not a histological type. It represents a superficial manifestation of an underlying carcinoma within the breast parenchyma. These cutaneous features are often associated with dilated vascular spaces and invasion of dermal lymphatics by carcinoma cells (tumor emboli). This patient had no signs of erythema at the time of initial clinical presentation. There were signs of peau d'orange but minimal edema of the skin and subcutaneous tissues. However, there was radiological evidence of breast lymphedema with skin thickening; the patient was diagnosed as an inflammatory carcinoma on the basis of the radiological appearances. This would not have presented any practical issues unless the patient had not been insistent on immediate breast reconstruction. Inflammatory carcinoma is a relative contraindication to immediate breast reconstruction and would not have been offered routinely in this particular case. However, the patient was very insistent on reconstruction as an immediate procedure and would not even consider a delayed procedure. It was felt on balance that the psychological benefits of immediate breast reconstruction in this particular case outweighed any disadvantages in terms of increased risk of locoregional relapse. The cancer was not typically inflammatory, though there was a transient episode of erythema of the breast after completion of the final cycle of chemotherapy.

From an oncological point of view, it was mandatory to perform a wide skin excision that incorporated the area of peau d'orange and also that of the transient erythema. The area of skin removed was more than for a conventional (non–skin sparing) mastectomy and this was replaced with a large skin island from the donor site. Therefore performing immediate breast reconstruction with a latissimus dorsi flap (and implant) had facilitated a wide surgical clearance. Final histology of the resected specimen

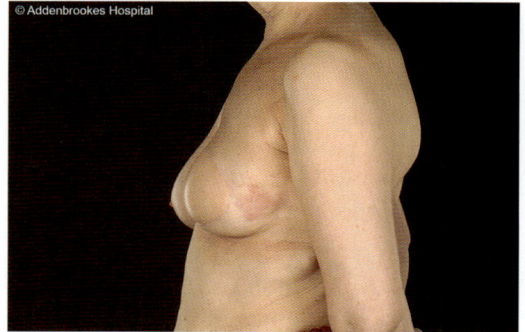

Figure 14

had revealed no evidence of tumor cells within the dermal tissues at the edge of the specimen. Residual tumor, though extending over a large area, appeared to have been excised with satisfactory margins. Though this together with radiotherapy would minimize the chance of local recurrence, the patient was carefully monitored clinically for any signs of locoregional relapse. Unfortunately she developed an area of erythema over the lateral aspect of the reconstructed breast for which a punch biopsy revealed invasive carcinoma. This patch of erythema was initially attributed to post-radiotherapy changes, but its persistence and texture raised an element of clinical suspicion (Fig. 14).

Despite development of local recurrence in the native mastectomy flap, the patient was pleased with the outcome of surgery and did not regret having undergone immediate breast reconstruction. In retrospect, the decision to undertake immediate breast reconstruction appears to have been justified from the patient's perspective. Herceptin had been resumed two weeks postoperatively and the local recurrence was managed initially with further systemic therapy (capecitebine).

Related Cases

Inflammatory breast cancer—*Case Study 25*

Taxane-based neoadjuvant chemotherapy—*Case Studies 22, 25, 27, 28, and 29*

Herceptin—*Case Studies 8 and 11*

Postmastectomy radiotherapy—*Case Studies 2, 3, 22, 25, 27, and 28*

Locally recurrent disease—*Case Study 20*

Learning Points

1. Inflammatory breast cancer is a clinical diagnosis based upon the following features: diffuse erythema, edema involving more than two-thirds of the breast, peau d'orange, tenderness, induration, warmth, enlargement, and diffuseness of the tumor on palpation.

2. About 1% to 6% of all breast cancer patients present with inflammatory breast cancer. In the United States, the incidence of inflammatory breast cancer is higher among African Americans than other ethnic groups.

3. Women with inflammatory breast cancer are at increased risk for locoregional recurrence, so immediate breast reconstruction is discouraged.

Neoadjuvant Chemotherapy

8

Part I: Mastectomy Postchemotherapy

CASE STUDY 27

History

A 25-year-old woman sought a second opinion following initial assessment of a lump in the right breast, which was erroneously diagnosed as a sebaceous cyst. No preliminary investigations such as breast imaging had been undertaken, and the patient was scheduled for excision of the lump under local anesthetic as a day case. At the time of her attendance for surgery it was noted that the breast lesion was clinically more ominous than a simple sebaceous cyst and formal breast assessment was arranged. The lump had been present for approximately two months and had progressively increased in size. There was no fluctuation in size with the menstrual cycle, and no associated nipple discharge. The patient had no previous history of breast problems and no family history of breast or ovarian carcinoma. She was nulliparous and had used the oral contraceptive pill continuously since the age of 18 years. The patient's general health was otherwise good, and she reported no unusual cough, back pain, or weight loss. Interestingly, she had been treated for a Wilm's tumor of the right kidney at the age of four years and received adjuvant treatment with both radiotherapy and chemotherapy. There was no evidence of any disease recurrence at a recent routine follow-up.

Clinical Findings

Examination revealed a large tumor occupying much of the right breast and measuring approximately 5 to 6 cm in maximum diameter. There was a small area of skin involvement in the upper inner quadrant, which presumably corresponded to the area considered to be a "sebaceous cyst" on initial clinical assessment elsewhere. There was no evidence of any inflammatory component, and soft, mobile nodes were palpable in the right axilla. Much of the right breast was firm and hard to palpation (E5). There were soft mobile nodes palpable in the right axilla, which were not suspicious clinically (Fig. 1).

Clinical Assessment

Locally advanced cancer of the right breast in a young woman.

Investigations

Breast and Axillary Ultrasound

Sonographic assessment of the clinical carcinoma was difficult due to the generalized hardness of the tissues. The main tumor mass measured at least 4.8 cm, and several

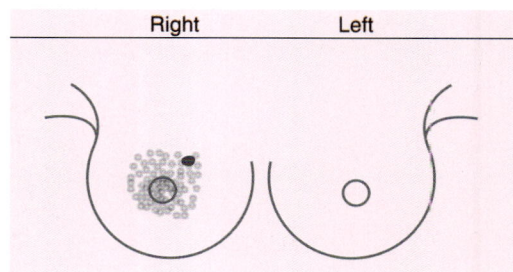

Figure 1

146

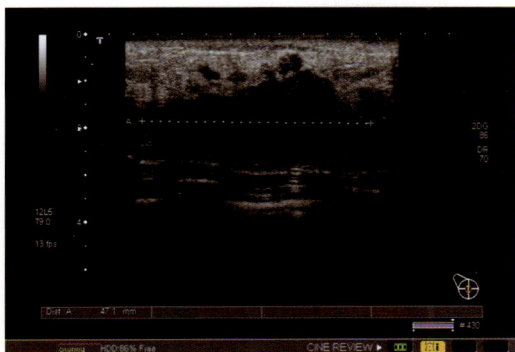

Figure 2

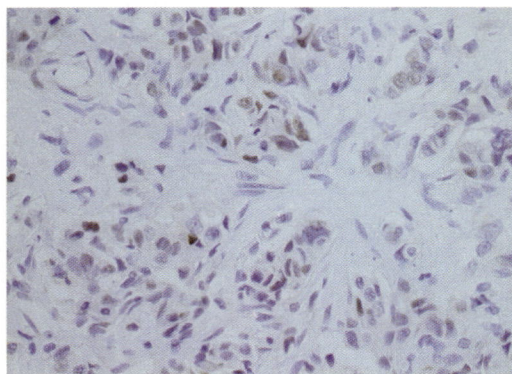

Figure 3

satellite foci were detected each measuring 5 mm (U5) (Fig. 2).

Core Biopsy

Review of pathology from the ultrasound-guided core biopsy (14-gauge needle) of the right breast mass performed originally confirmed an invasive carcinoma (grade III, ER negative).

Multidisciplinary Review 1

Following multidisciplinary review, full staging investigations were undertaken and HER2/neu status was requested. In addition, ER immunohistochemical assay was repeated at the secondary referral center. There were concerns about possible compromised renal function as a consequence of treatment for a previous Wilm's tumor. It was recommended the patient undergo neoadjuvant chemotherapy followed by surgery. The patient was informed that breast conservation surgery would not be feasible whatever the response to primary chemotherapy. However, she would be eligible for immediate breast reconstruction in the absence of any inflammatory component.

Further Investigations

1. CT scan of head/chest/abdomen/pelvis—this showed no evidence of distant metastatic disease in the lungs, liver, or brain (or elsewhere)
2. Routine blood tests—full blood count, urea and electrolytes, liver function tests, and calcium were all within the normal range
3. Repeat ER assay—Allred score of 4/8 (weakly positive) (Fig. 3)
4. HER2/neu assay—positive (Fig. 4).

Diagnosis

Locally advanced but operable right breast cancer (T4N1M0).

Treatment and Progress

The patient commenced a modified regimen of chemotherapy considered to be

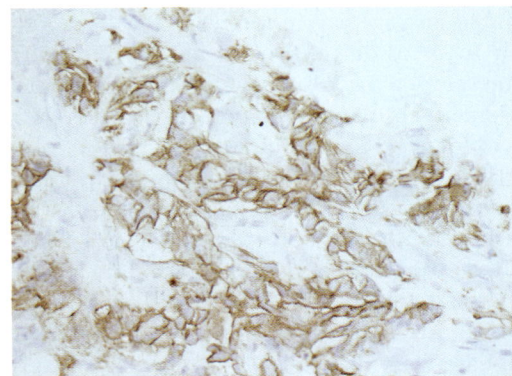

Figure 4

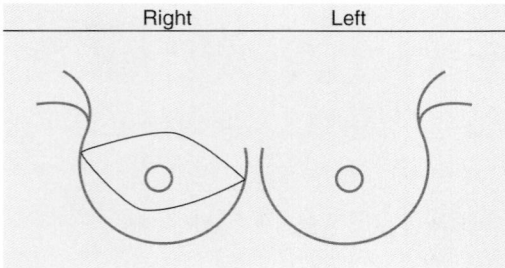

Figure 5

compatible with previous chemotherapy for a Wilm's tumor. This consisted of six cycles of docetaxel and carboplatin combined with Herceptin. She had an excellent clinical response and repeat imaging at three months showed a dramatic response with reduction of tumor size by more than 50%. The patient proceeded to a right modified radical mastectomy with level II axillary lymph node dissection upon completion of chemotherapy (the patient declined immediate breast reconstruction, see discussion below) (Fig. 5). She made an excellent postoperative recovery and Herceptin was continued throughout the perioperative period. Herceptin had been withheld from the final cycle of chemotherapy due to a fall in left ventricular ejection fraction (LVEF) from 52% to 38%. Cardiac function subsequently recovered and Herceptin was recommenced.

Definitive Histology

Extensive sampling of the mastectomy specimen revealed no evidence of any residual viable invasive carcinoma (Fig. 6A). A nodular focus of dense hyaline fibrosis (Fig. 6B) surrounded by tissue containing numerous pigment-containing macrophages (Fig. 6C) and mast cells was identified as the presumed site of pretreatment invasive tumor. Neither in situ carcinoma nor any intravascular tumor was found, and none of the 20 lymph nodes removed contained any metastases but showed fibrosis suggestive of previous nodal involvement and downstaged disease (Fig. 6D and E).

Multidisciplinary Review 2

Despite a complete pathological tumor response, it was recommended the patient undergo irradiation of the right chest wall in view of the initial tumor size at presentation. The patient had elected to undergo a subsequent contralateral prophylactic mastectomy with bilateral breast reconstruction at the same time (i.e., immediate breast reconstruction on the left side and delayed breast reconstruction on the right). Herceptin was continued for a minimum period of 12 months and tamoxifen commenced as adjuvant systemic hormonal therapy. The option of ovarian suppression was discussed (patient of young age, though still nulliparous).

Discussion

Though this 25-year-old patient had no family history of breast cancer, she was inadequately assessed at the time of her initial presentation to a neighboring breast unit. There was failure to appreciate clinically that the patient had an extensive tumor extending throughout much of the right breast. This had directly infiltrated the skin and led to the erroneous diagnosis of a sebaceous cyst (1). No breast imaging had been undertaken, and some might omit any radiological investigation when there is a confident clinical diagnosis of a skin lesion with no intraparenchymal abnormality. This case illustrates the importance of excluding the latter with appropriate imaging. This patient had a history of Wilm's tumor that was treated with chemotherapy (doxorubicin and ifosfamide) and radiotherapy. This potentially compromised both cardiac and renal function (nephrectomy), and a modified neoadjuvant regimen was employed consisting of docetaxel and carboplatin together with Herceptin.

The underlying rationale for neoadjuvant chemotherapy is based on several potential advantages and opportunities. These include improved overall survival, increased chance of breast preservation and assessment of individual tumor sensitivity to particular

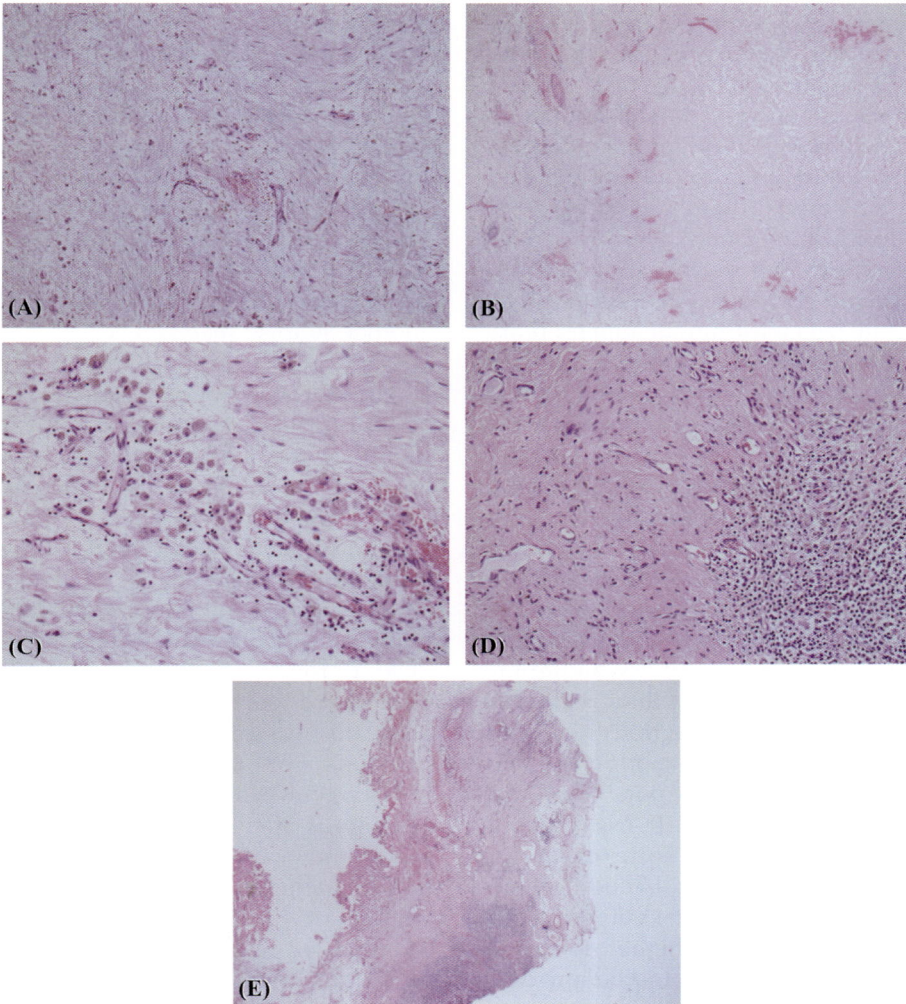

Figure 6

chemotherapeutic agents, and eventual correlation of tumor response to long-term outcome (2,3). Neoadjuvant or primary chemotherapy was originally employed for management of inoperable, locally advanced cancers that could be rendered technically operable (4). Neoadjuvant approaches have increasingly been advocated for operable breast cancers with the expectation of improved outcomes and possible breast conservation (5,6). Though there is evidence of increased overall survival from preoperative chemotherapy in a rat model of breast cancer, this has not translated into any clinical

gains (2). A meta-analysis of neoadjuvant versus adjuvant systemic therapy for early-stage breast cancer reveals that overall and disease-free survival are comparable for the two schedules (7). If the act of surgery itself causes a systemic perturbation that can be offset by induction chemotherapy, this would provide biological underpinning for neoadjuvant therapy. Nonetheless, it is perhaps naïve to assume that a modest shift in the timing of chemotherapy relative to surgery would have any significant clinical impact (2). There is some evidence that patients with a complete pathological response to neoadjuvant chemotherapy have a more favorable longer-term outcome. However, only about 10% of patients achieve such a response and are difficult to identify prospectively (5,8). In an analysis of six retrospective case series of neoadjuvant chemotherapy, a complete pathological response was observed among only 300 out of 2584 patients with invasive ductal carcinoma (9).

For patients with a large unifocal tumor, which is situated away from the nipple-areolar complex, neoadjuvant chemotherapy can downstage the tumor and permit breast conservation (10,11). Clinical trials suggest this may be accomplished in 25% to 50% of cases that would otherwise have required mastectomy. Tumors do not necessarily shrink in a concentric manner in response to chemotherapy. Even if no viable cancer cells remain at the site of the original tumor periphery, this zone may contain unstable epithelium that is prone to malignant change (12). Furthermore, tumor regression is difficult to assess radiologically, and clinicoradiopathological correlation in the neoadjuvant setting is generally poor (even with use of MRI). The NSABP B-18 trial randomized patients between four cycles of doxorubicin and cyclophosphamide chemotherapy given before or after surgery. Rates of local recurrence are higher following breast conservation postchemotherapy compared with primary breast-conserving surgery (15% and 7%, respectively) (13). This particular patient would not have been suitable for breast-conserving surgery whatever the response to chemotherapy. Despite a complete pathological response, the tumor occupied much of the central portion of the breast, and the tissue in this area had to be excised at the time of surgery.

Neoadjuvant chemotherapy allows serial core biopsies to be undertaken, which provide potential information on pathological and molecular predictors of response. Together with imaging parameters, this enables nonresponders to be identified early on and therapy changed accordingly.

This patient opted to undergo a contralateral prophylactic mastectomy as a delayed procedure. Despite absence of any family history of breast cancer, this patient had a significant lifetime risk of developing a further contralateral breast cancer. As younger patients are being treated more successfully for breast cancer, they are living long enough to develop another cancer—whether this be a contralateral breast cancer or a de novo cancer in the ipsilateral breast. The risk of a further malignancy is approximately 1% per year. If a patient is treated at the age of 25 years for a breast cancer and survives for another 30 to 40 years, she will likely develop another breast cancer.

The decision to undergo this contralateral prophylactic procedure influenced the timing of the ipsilateral breast reconstruction. Moreover, the requirement for chest wall radiotherapy (based on initial tumor size) was a factor in the final surgical management plan. The chance of severe capsular contracture following irradiation of an implant (with a latissimus dorsi flap) is up to 20% at four years (14). Women should be warned of this if they are likely to need postmastectomy radiotherapy. Some surgeons now prefer to delay definitive breast reconstruction until approximately 12 months after radiotherapy. Skin-sparing mastectomy can be undertaken with insertion of a temporary tissue expander (subcutaneous or submuscular) that remains for the duration of radiotherapy. Transposition of an autologous flap and insertion of a definitive implant can be carried out as a delayed procedure (15). There is a risk that the quality of the skin flaps may be compromised under these circumstances and an alternative option is to perform immediate breast reconstruction in all patients and perform implant exchange in those cases affected by capsular contracture after radiotherapy. Increasing numbers of women are receiving postmastectomy radiotherapy, and this is often routine after neoadjuvant chemotherapy for a large primary tumor (with or without supraclavicular irradiation) (16).

Trastuzumab or Herceptin is a humanized recombinant monoclonal antibody that targets the HER2/neu receptor (17). This is expressed in normal and malignant breast epithelial cells, but overexpressed in 20% to 30% of all breast cancers (18). In the preclinical studies, overexpression of the

HER2/neu oncogene results in increased rates of proliferation and a more tumorigenic phenotype in vivo with greater metastatic potential. Recent trials have shown that the use of Herceptin for one to two years following standard chemotherapy regimens in HER2-positive patients prolongs disease-free survival and reduces rates of relapse by up to 50% (19,20). The relative magnitude of gains from Herceptin is similar across all subgroups and there is less than a 20% chance that these benefits will be lost with more prolonged follow-up. There is compound cardiotoxicity from combined therapy with Herceptin and taxanes that should be sequenced when baseline LVEF is suboptimal. This patient received concomitant chemotherapy with docetaxel/carboplatin and Herceptin. Measurement of LVEF fell from 52% to 38% during treatment, and Herceptin was withheld temporarily until resumption of satisfactory left ventricular function. Cardiac function is particularly susceptible to the combination of an anthracycline, taxane, and herceptin. Current recommendations are for combination of herceptin with the nonanthracycline component of chemotherapy (usually a taxane).

This patient's repeat ER assay revealed an Allred score of 4/8. She was therefore eligible for hormonal treatment. Options for premenopausal women include both tamoxifen and ovarian suppression. A meta-analysis by the Early Breast Cancer Trialists Collaborative Group confirmed that the proportional benefits from tamoxifen were similar in pre- and postmenopausal women, though the former are susceptible to a supraphysiological surge of estrogens secondary to competitive blockade of the estrogen receptor (21). Tamoxifen is additive to chemotherapy in premenopausal women (22). However, it remains unclear whether ovarian suppression confers any additional benefits over and above the combined effects of chemotherapy and tamoxifen. There is evidence that women under 35 years of age who become amenorrheic after chemotherapy have a better prognosis. Ovarian suppression should probably be recommended after chemotherapy for the majority of higher-risk ER-positive premenopausal women under the age of 40 years. Most of these women will resume ovarian function after chemotherapy, while fewer than 50% of those over this age will do so. The use of LHRH agonists allows preservation of ovarian function and the possibility of subsequent conception (23). However, if the anticipated survival gains from ovarian suppression are modest, it is preferable to use tamoxifen alone in hormone-sensitive women. For those higher-risk women under 35 years of age who do not become amenorrheic (or whose menses resume) after chemotherapy, ovarian suppression is mandatory. Chemotherapy alone is insufficient for this group of patients.

Related Cases

Neoadjuvant chemotherapy—*Case Studies 23, 28, and 29*

Ovarian suppression—*Case Studies 8 and 23*

Contralateral prophylactic mastectomy—*Case Study 39*

Capsular con tracture—*Case Studies 3 and 18*

Herceptin—*Case Studies 8, 11, and 26*

Chest wall radiotherapy—*Case Studies 2, 3, 22, and 26*

Learning Points

1. In patients with locally advanced or inflammatory breast cancers, neoadjuvant chemotherapy reduces tumor burden, thereby facilitating mastectomy. For patients with large tumors, the rate of breast-conserving surgery is increased with neoadjuvant chemotherapy.

2. In theory, neoadjuvant chemotherapy might allow for the in vivo assessment of tumor response, enabling oncologists to tailor chemotherapy to achieve maximum response. Several clinical trials are further evaluating this approach, but there is as yet no evidence that neoadjuvant chemotherapy results in improved survival.

References

1. Argy O, Hughes KS, Roche CA. Managing the patient with a breast mass. In: Jatoi I, ed. Manual of Breast Disease. Wilkins, Williams: Lippincott, 2002, 135–148.
2. Davidson NE, Morrow M. Sometimes a great notion—an assessment of neoadjuvant systemic therapy for breast cancer. J Natl Cancer Inst 2005; 97:159–161.
3. Wolff AC, Davidson NE. Primary systemic therapy in operable breast cancer. J Clin Oncol 2000; 18:1558–1569.
4. Gilles R, Guinebretiere JM, Toussaint C, et al. Locally advanced breast cancer: contrast-enhanced subtraction MR imaging of response to preoperative chemotherapy. Radiology 1994; 191:633–638.
5. Bonadonna G, Valagussa P, Bramnilla C, et al. Primary chemotherapy in operable breast cancer: eight year experience at the Milan Cancer Institute. J Clin Oncol 1998; 16:93–100.
6. Smith IE, Walsh G, Jones A, et al. High complete remission rates with primary neoadjuvant infusional chemotherapy for large early breast cancer. J Clin Oncol 1995; 13:424–429.
7. Mauri D, Pavlidis N, Ioannidis JP. Neoadjuvant versus adjuvant systemic treatment for breast cancer: a meta-analysis. J Natl Cancer Inst 2005; 97: 188–194.
8. Fisher B, Brown A, Mamounas E, et al. Effect of preoperative chemotherapy on locoregional disease in women with operable breast cancer: findings from the National Surgical Adjuvant Breast and Bowel Project. B-18. J Clin Oncol 1997; 15: 2483–2493.
9. Katz A, Saad ED, Porter P, et al. Primary systemic chemotherapy of invasive lobular carcinoma of the breast. Lancet Oncol 1997; 55–62.
10. Bonadonna G, Veronesi U, Brambilla C, et al. Primary chemotherapy to avoid mastectomy in tumours with diameters of three centimeters or more. J Natl Cancer Inst 1990; 82:1539–1545.
11. Makris A, Powles TJ, Ashley SE, et al. A reduction in the requirements for mastectomy in a randomized trial of neoadjuvant chemoendocrine therapy in primary breast cancer. Ann Oncol 1998; 9:1179–1184.
12. Veronesi U, Bonadonna G, Zurrida S, et al. Conservation surgery after primary chemotherapy in large carcinomas of the breast. Ann Surg 1995; 222:612–618.
13. Wolmark N, Wang J, Mamounas E, et al. Preoperative chemotherapy in patients with operable breast cancer: nine-year results from the National Surgical Adjuvant Breast and Bowel Project. B-18. J Natl Cancer Inst Monogr 2001; 30:96–102.
14. Behranwala KA, Dua RS, Ross GM, et al. The influence of radiotherapy on capsule formation and aesthetic outcome after immediate breast reconstruction using biodimensional anatomical expander implants. J Plast Reconstr Aesthet Surg 2006; 59:1043–1051.
15. Kronowitz S. Delayed-immediate reconstruction in patients who might require postmastectomy radiation therapy. Miami Breast Cancer Conference, Orlando, Florida, February 20–23, 2008.
16. Recht A, Edge SB, Solin SJ, et al. Post-mastectomy radiotherapy: clinical practice guidelines of the American Society of Clinical Oncology. J Clin Oncol 2001; 19:1539–1569.
17. Slamon DJ, Clark GM, Wong SG, et al. Human breast cancer: correlation of relapse and survival with amplication of the HER-2/neu oncogene. Science 1987; 235:177–182.
18. Slamon DJ, Leyland-Jones B, Shak S, et al. Use of chemotherapy plus a monoclonal antibody against HER2 for metastatic breast cancer overexpresses HER2. N Engl J Med 2001; 344:783–792.
19. Romond EH, Perez EA, Bryant J, et al. Trastuzumab plus adjuvant chemotherapy for operable HER2 positive breast cancer. N Engl J Med 2005; 353:1659–1684.
20. Piccart-Gebhart MJ, Procter M, Leyland-Jones B, et al. 2 year follow up of trastuzumab after adjuvant chemotherapy in HER2 positive breast cancer. N Engl J Med 2005; 353:1659–1672.
21. Early Breast Cancer Trialists Collaborative Group. Tamoxifen for early breast cancer: an overview of the randomized trials. Lancet 1998; 351:1451–1461.
22. Albain KS, Green SJ, Ravdin PM, et al. for SWOG, ECOG, CALGB, NCCTG and NCIC-CTG. Adjuvant chemohormonal therapy for primary breast cancer should be sequential instead of concurrent: initial results from the Intergroup Trial 0100 (SWOG-8814). Proc Am Soc Clin Oncol 2002; 21 (abstr 143).
23. Recchia F, Sica G, de Filippis S, et al. Ovarian protection with goserilin during chemotherapy for early breast cancer: long term results of a phase II study. Proc Am Soc Clin Oncol 2002; 21 (abstr 62).

CASE STUDY 28

History

A 46-year-old woman of Eastern European extraction was referred to the breast clinic with altered breast contour and dimpling of her right breast. The patient reported a lump in the right breast, which had been present for almost five years. She attributed this to an innate "structural" or anatomical abnormality, but the lump had increased in size during the preceding four weeks. There was no associated nipple discharge, and the patient was otherwise well with no unusual back pain, cough, or weight loss. There was no family history of breast or ovarian cancer, and the patient had two children both of whom were breast-fed. She underwent menarche at the age of 12 years and had used the oral contraceptive pill for a brief period of six months prior to her first pregnancy.

Clinical Findings

There was an ill-defined mass in the lower outer quadrant of the right breast measuring approximately 3 cm. There was dimpling of the overlying skin and retraction of the right nipple. The mass was mobile on the chest wall and two enlarged hard nodes were palpable in the right axilla (E5) (Figs. 7 and 8A–C).

Clinical Assessment

Locally advanced clinical carcinoma of the right breast with nodal involvement.

Investigations

Mammography

An irregular spiculate opacity was seen in the lower outer quadrant of the right breast measuring 30 mm in maximum diameter (R5) (Fig. 9A and B).

Breast Ultrasound

The sonographic correlate of this opacity was a 32-mm heterogeneous solid mass with a hypoechoic pattern (no acoustic enhancement or attenuation) (U5) (Fig. 10). Three

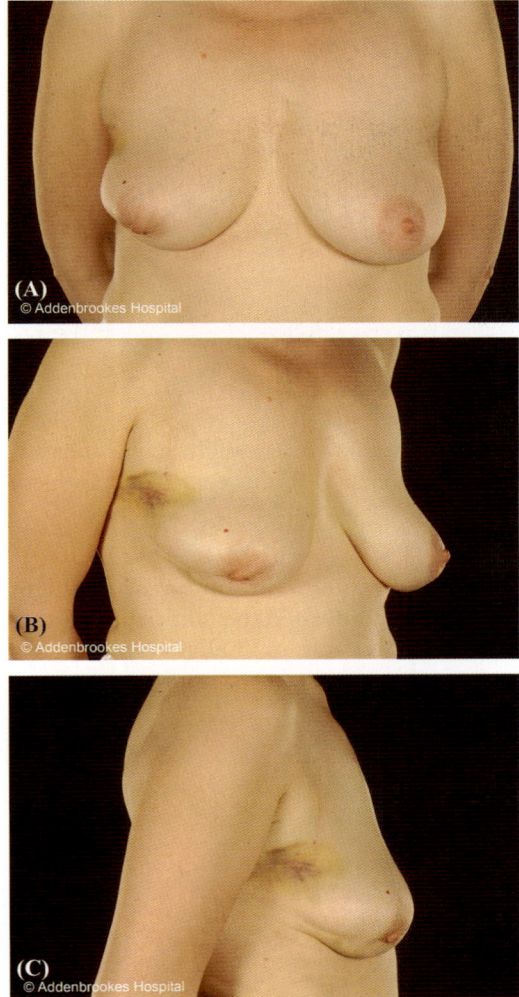

Figure 8

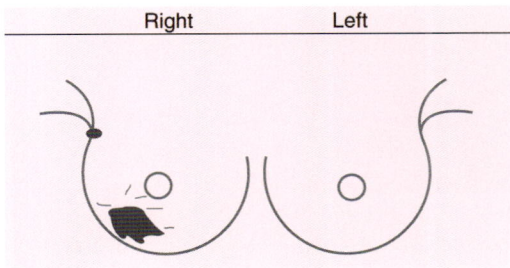

Figure 7

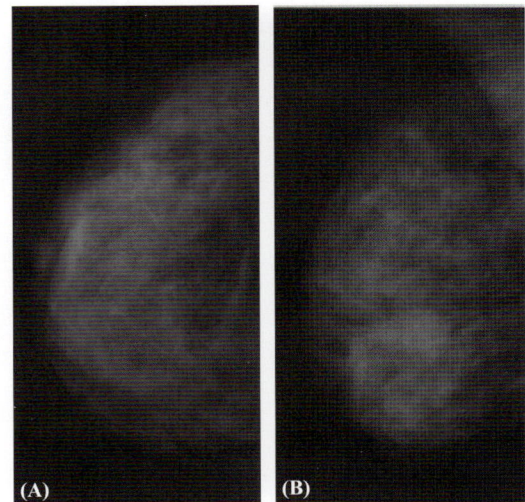

Figure 9

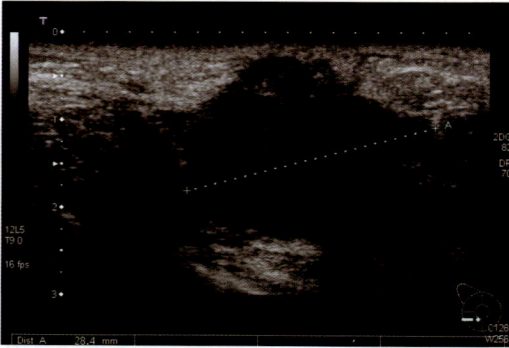

Figure 10

nodes were seen in the right axilla measuring no more than 8 mm each.

Core Biopsy

Ultrasound-guided core biopsy of the right breast mass confirmed the clinical and radiological impression of malignancy with an

invasive carcinoma (grade II, ER positive,[a] HER2 negative) [Fig. 11A (magnification 10×) and B (magnification 20×)]. Core biopsy of a right axillary node showed metastatic carcinoma (Fig. 11C).

Diagnosis

Locally advanced cancer of the right breast (T4bN1).

Multidisciplinary Review 1

Following multidisciplinary review, it was recommended that the patient undergo primary chemotherapy within the NEOTANGO trial. She would require right mastectomy and axillary dissection after completion of chemotherapy together with irradiation of the chest wall and supraclavicular fossa. It was likely the patient would be rendered postmenopausal by chemotherapy (aged 45 years) and be eligible for hormonal

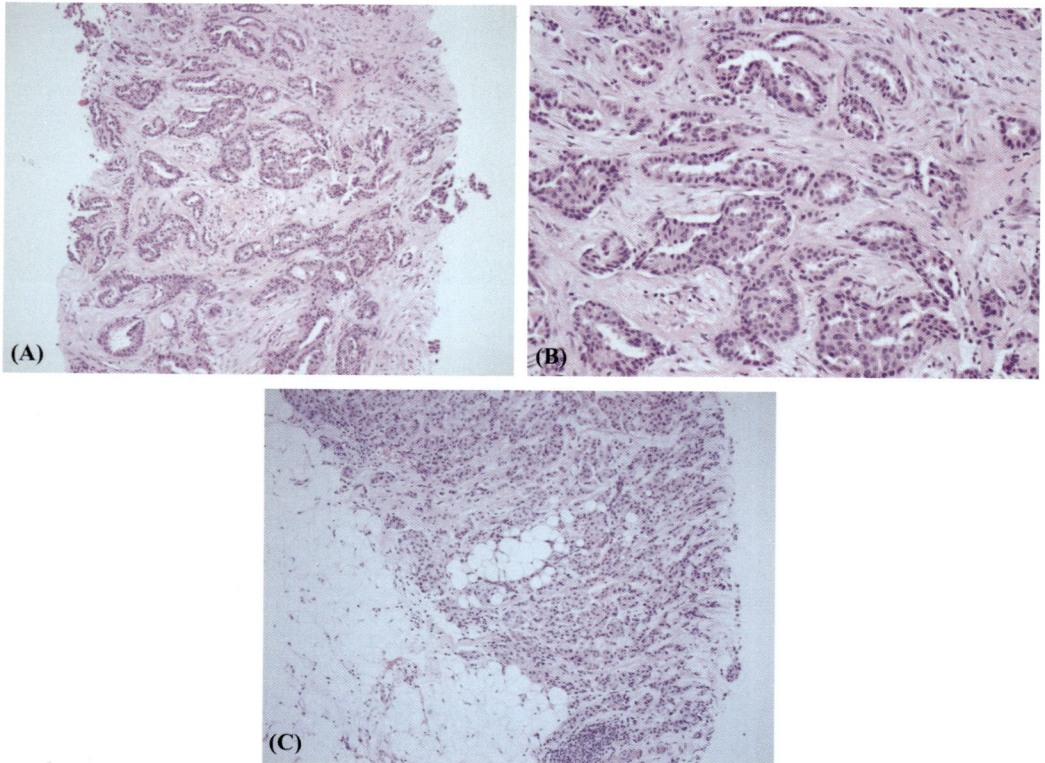

Figure 11

---

[a] Allred score 8/8

therapy with tamoxifen for two to three years followed by an early switch to an aromatase inhibitor.

Further Investigations

Breast MRI

Initial MRI examination revealed the tumor measuring 30 mm in maximum diameter, which corresponded to the mammographic and sonographic estimates.

CT Chest/Abdomen/Pelvis

No evidence of distant metastases.

Treatment and Progress

Chemotherapy was discussed with the patient both within the context of the NEOTANGO trial and standard regimens (see below). The patient was keen to participate in the trial and was provided with relevant information. Chemotherapy was commenced one week later. Following three cycles of Taxol, the tumor in the right breast had become softer but remained approximately 3 cm in size. The patient suffered mild nausea and arthralgia (grade I) as side effects of treatment. A repeat MRI scan confirmed that the tumor had reduced in size to 22 mm and was unifocal. However, simultaneous ultrasound showed a persistent abnormality at the site of the original MRI lesion, suggesting that there had not been concentric shrinkage of the tumor. It was, therefore, reaffirmed that the patient should proceed to a right modified radical mastectomy (with level II axillary lymph node dissection) and would not be suitable for breast-conserving surgery. The patient underwent a skin sparing mastectomy

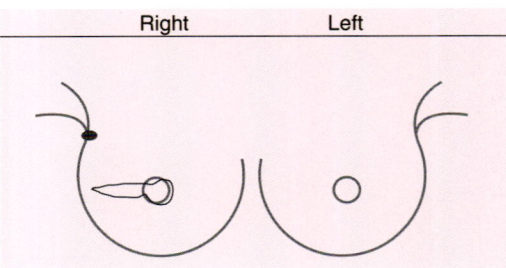

Figure 13

and immediate reconstruction with latissimus dorsi flap and implant after completion of chemotherapy. At the time of operation, a modified periareolar incision was made to encompass the area of skin dimpling just lateral to the nipple (Figs. 12 and 13). The patient made an excellent recovery and was discharged home on the fifth postoperative day.

Definitive Histology

This revealed significant residual invasive ductal carcinoma, measuring at least 50 mm and extending to the deep surface of the nipple. There was a central area of sclerosis consistent with a chemotherapy response (<50%) (Fig. 14A and B). No definite lymphovascular invasion was seen, and focal perineural invasion was present. Four out of 14 lymph nodes contained metastatic carcinoma (Fig. 14C).

Multidisciplinary Review 2

Following further multidisciplinary review, it was recommended the patient be prescribed tamoxifen as adjuvant systemic hormonal therapy and be offered ovarian suppression. She would receive irradiation of the chest wall and supraclavicular fossa as part of the neoadjuvant protocol (≥4 nodes positive).

Treatment and Progress

The patient proceeded to laparoscopic bilateral salpingo-oophorectomy five weeks following mastectomy. There was no evidence of any intra-abdominal nor pelvic malignancy at the time of laparoscopic exploration. A

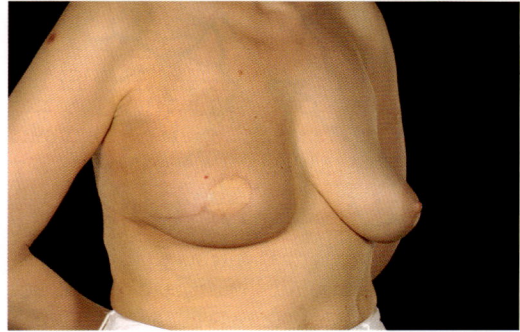

Figure 12

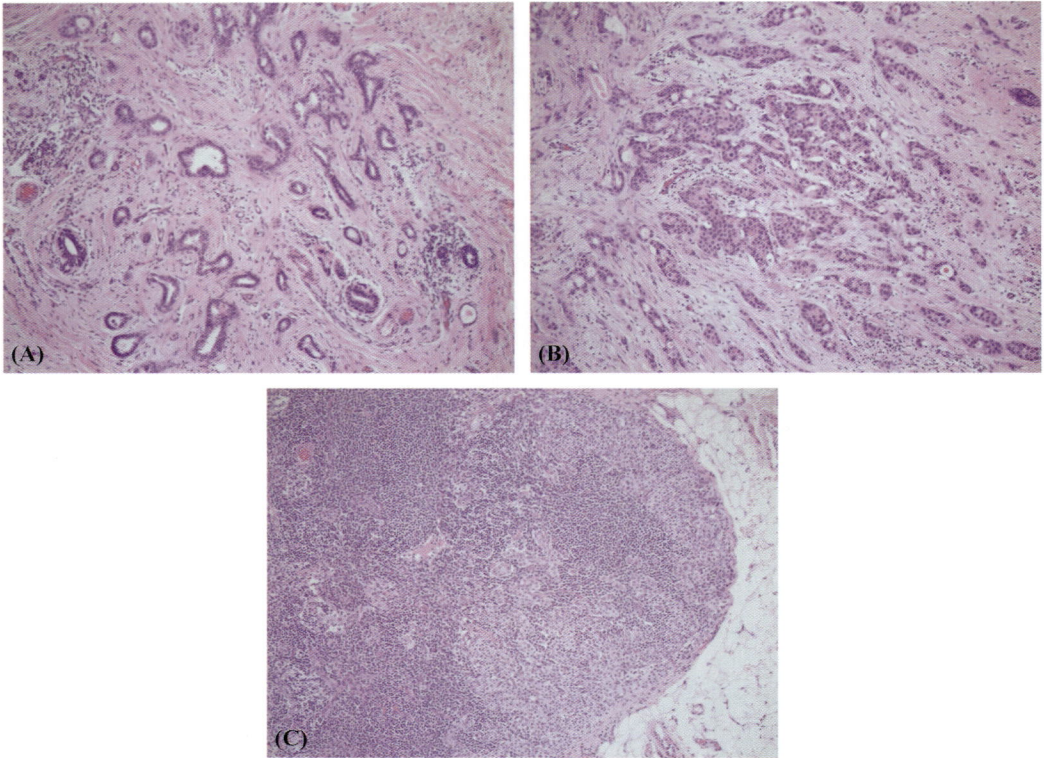

Figure 14

course of radiotherapy to the chest wall and supraclavicular fossa followed shortly thereafter, and hormonal therapy was completed with tamoxifen for five years. The patient had an excellent cosmetic result three months following completion of radiotherapy (Fig. 15A and B).

Discussion

This relatively young patient presented with a locally advanced breast cancer with histo-logically confirmed nodal involvement. Locally advanced tumors encompass those that exceed 5 cm in size or that involve the skin or chest wall (T3 or T4). This classification also includes patients with fixed (N2 or N3) axillary nodes but not supraclavicular nodal disease. Approximately 20% to 30% of all breast cancer patients have locally advanced disease at the time of presentation, though this figure is falling with heightened public awareness and screening programs. Indeed, among women who undergo regular

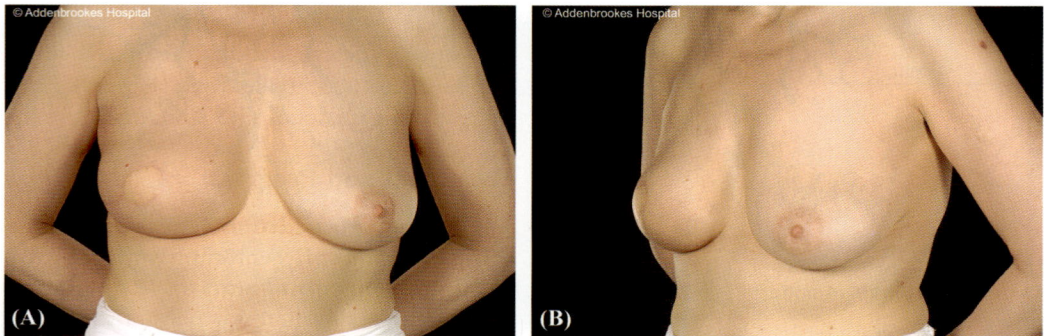

Figure 15

screening, fewer than 5% are diagnosed with locally advanced disease (1). Single modality therapies in the past yielded poor results with five-year survival rates from surgery and radiotherapy alone of 41% and 29%, respectively (2). This group of patients are now managed with a combination of surgery, radiotherapy, and systemic therapy (3). These patients are likely to have disseminated micrometastatic disease at the time of presentation, and primary chemotherapy is a more rationale approach and has improved outcomes significantly. Younger patients (≤50 years) usually have induction chemotherapy irrespective of hormone receptor status. Preoperative chemotherapy reduces tumor volume that can facilitate subsequent surgical excision. In selected cases, breast conservation surgery rather than mastectomy may be feasible (4), but often mastectomy is indicated based on initial tumor size, location, and involvement of skin and/or chest wall musculature. These patients are at greater risk of local recurrence, which is minimized by mastectomy and irradiation of the chest wall. Radiotherapy has been combined with chemotherapy for more than 50 years, and all trials have shown that postmastectomy radiotherapy reduces the proportional risk of local failure by two-thirds to three-quarters (5). Most of this effect is seen in the first five years, and a recent meta-analysis by the EBCTCG confirms that for women with node-positive disease, there is also a mortality gain of 5.4% at 15 years (6). Furthermore, for patients with ≥4 nodes positive, the incidence of supraclavicular failure is sufficiently high to recommend routine irradiation of the supraclavicular fossa in this group. For those with one to three positive nodes, it remains unclear whether supraclavicular irradiation is justified, and this issue is being addressed in the ongoing SUPREMO study (7).

Patients with locally advanced and inflammatory cancers will often be given chest wall and supraclavicular irradiation after mastectomy. However, for less-advanced tumors, the extent of nodal involvement prechemotherapy may be unclear; core biopsy or sentinel lymph node biopsy may confirm that at least one node is positive. This may be insufficient to warrant either chest wall radiotherapy or supraclavicular fossa irradiation in some patients with T1/T2 tumors. Nodal downstaging can occur following neoadjuvant chemotherapy, and sometimes it is possible to discern pathologically those nodes that previously were "positive" but no longer contain viable tumor. This patient was offered primary chemotherapy within the NEOTANGO trial, which is a four-arm randomization to a preoperative schedule of sequential epirubicin, cyclophosphamide, and paclitaxel with or without gemcitabine (Table 1). She was given the option of having a standard neoadjuvant regimen (EC/docetaxel or FEC/docetaxel) but opted for trial entry. Patients who have operable tumors who failed to respond to an anthracycline-based regimen and/or taxanes can undergo immediate mastectomy. For those patients with inoperable tumors who do not respond to induction systemic therapy, primary radiotherapy is an option. It is important that patients are provided with adequate verbal information that can be supplemented with leaflets. Patients should understand why they are being offered primary chemotherapy, particularly when breast conservation surgery is improbable whatever the response to induction chemotherapy.

At the age of 46 years, it is likely that this patient would be rendered postmenopausal by chemotherapy. She would, therefore, be eligible for treatment with an aromatase inhibitor as part of systemic adjuvant hormonal therapy (ER-positive tumor).

Table 1   NEOTANGO Trial Schema

ARM **A1**	4 cycles EC	Followed by 4 cycles Paclitaxel
ARM **A2**	4 cycles Paclitaxel	Followed by 4 cycles EC
ARM **B1**	4 cycles EC	Followed by 4 cycles Paclitaxel + Gemcitabine
ARM **B2**	4 cycles Paclitaxel + Gemcitabine	Followed by 4 cycles EC

Abbreviations: E, epirubicin; C, cyclophosphamide.

Related Cases

Locally advanced tumors—*Case Studies 27, 30, and 31*

Neoadjuvant chemotherapy—*Case Studies 27 and 29*

Aromatase inhibitors—*Case Studies 1, 8, 9, 10, 19, and 22*

Supraclavicular irradiation—*Case Studies 2 and 22*

Learning Points

1. In patients with locally advanced breast cancers, preoperative chemotherapy reduces tumor burden, thereby facilitating mastectomy.
2. Even though locally advanced tumors are often downstaged following preoperative chemotherapy, these patients should still receive postmastectomy radiotherapy to minimize the risk of locoregional recurrence.
3. In some patients with locally advanced breast cancer, preoperative chemotherapy might result in a substantial reduction in tumor burden, making breast-conserving surgery feasible. However, these patients will have a significantly greater risk of local recurrence, when compared to patients who undergo breast-conserving surgery followed by adjuvant chemotherapy.

References

1. Seidman H, Gelbs K, Silverberg E, et al. Survival experience in the Breast Cancer Detection Demonstration Project. CA Cancer J Clin 1987; 37:258–290.
2. Hortobagyi GN. Comprehensive management of locally advanced breast cancer. Cancer 1990; 66:1387–1391.
3. Swain SM, Sorace RA, Bagley CS, et al. Neoadjuvant chemotherapy in the combined modality approach of locally advanced nonmetastatic breast cancer. Cancer Res 1987; 47:3889–3894.
4. Singletary SE, Mcnees MD, Hortobagyi GN. Feasibility of breast conservation surgery after induction chemotherapy for locally advanced breast carcinoma. Cancer 1992; 69:2849–2852.
5. Early Breast Cancer Trialists' Collaborative Group. Effects of radiotherapy and surgery in early breast cancer: an overview of the randomized trials. N Engl J Med 1995; 333:1444–1455.
6. Early Breast Cancer Trialists Collaborative Group. Effects of radiotherapy and of differences in the extent of surgery for early breast cancer on local recurrence and 15 year survival: an overview of the randomized trials. Lancet 2005; 366:2087–2106.
7. SUPREMO breast cancer trial. Selective Use of Postoperative Radiotherapy after Mastectomy. Available at: www.supremo-trial.com. Accessed November 17, 2008.

Part II: Breast Conservation Surgery Postchemotherapy

CASE STUDY 29

History

A 51-year-old woman presented with a two-month history of a lump in the left breast. She noticed this shortly after sustaining mild trauma to the breast after a fall. There was no bruising of the breast at the time, but she became aware of the lump immediately afterward. The lump was nontender and there was no associated nipple discharge.

The patient had no previous breast problems and had not yet undergone a first round screening mammogram in the NHS program. There was neither family history of breast nor ovarian cancer. She had two children (3 pregnancies) both of whom were breast-fed and gave birth to her eldest child at the age of 25 years. The oral contraceptive pill had been used for a cumulative period of 10 years both before and after pregnancy.

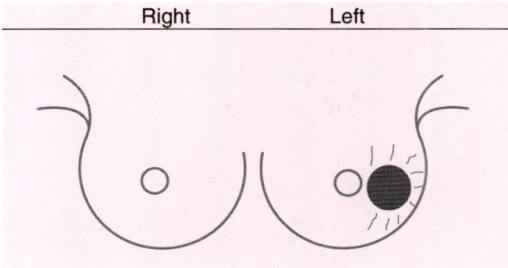

Figure 16

Clinical Findings

There was a large mobile mass in the lower outer quadrant of the left breast, which was firm and quite hard on palpation (E5). It measured at least 5 to 6 cm clinically and was associated with distortion of the outer aspect of the breast, but no erythema or peau d'orange. There was palpable left axillary lymphadenopathy. Some minor bruising was evident overlying the mass (Fig. 16).

Clinical Assessment

Large clinical carcinoma of the left breast.

Investigations

Mammography

Bilateral mammography showed a well-circumscribed 5-cm opacity in the lower outer quadrant of the left breast at the level of the nipple (right side normal) (R4/5) (Fig. 17A and B).

Breast and Axillary Ultrasound

The mammographic opacity corresponded to a heterogeneous mass measuring 52 mm in maximum dimension with areas of enhanced vascularity (Fig. 18A). A 2-cm node was seen in the left axilla with focal cortical thickening. The overall radiological appearances were suspicious for carcinoma (U5) (Fig. 18B).

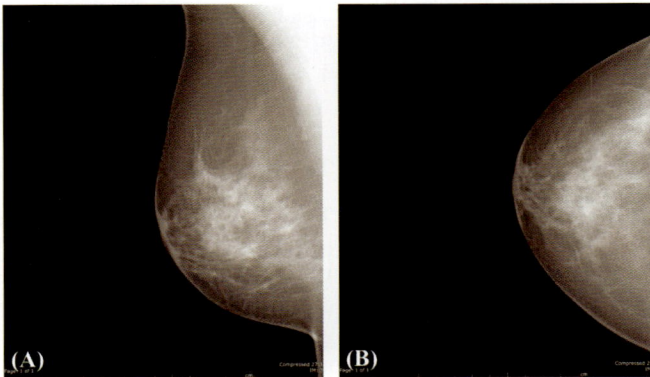

Figure 17

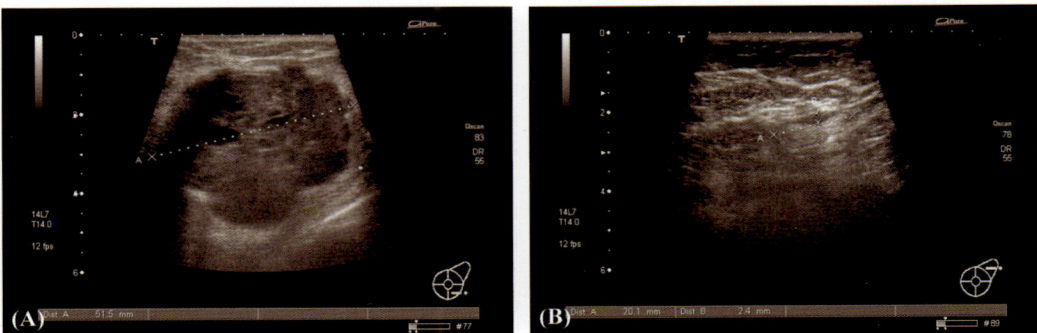

Figure 18

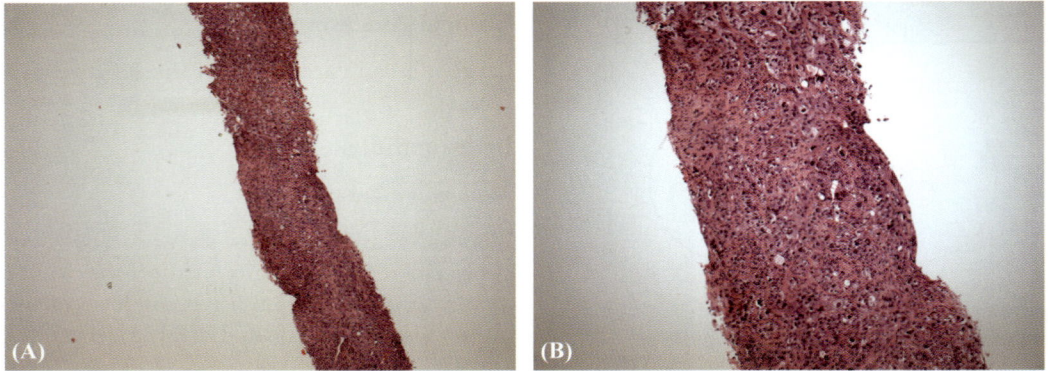

Figure 19

Core Biopsy

Image-guided core biopsy (14-gauge needle) of the breast mass confirmed an invasive carcinoma (grade III, ER/PR negative) [Fig. 19A (low power) and B (high power)]. Biopsy of the left axillary node showed reactive changes only (lymphoid hyperplasia).

Diagnosis

Early-stage left breast cancer (T3N1).

Multidisciplinary Review 1

Following multidisciplinary review, it was recommended that the patient be managed with neoadjuvant chemotherapy that might downstage the tumor permitting breast conservation at a later stage. Though the tumor measured up to 5 cm on imaging, it appeared unifocal and away from the nipple-areolar complex. The patient was very keen to preserve her breast and avoid mastectomy if possible. A final decision on surgical management would be made after assessment of response to chemotherapy. Despite a negative axillary node core biopsy, sentinel lymph node biopsy was not advised prechemotherapy due to primary tumor size (5 cm). The patient would therefore undergo axillary lymph node dissection at the time of definitive surgery irrespective of breast conservation or mastectomy.

Further investigations were requested including an MRI examination of the breasts, liver ultrasound, bone scan, and HER2 status. These were considered appropriate in view of the primary tumor size at presentation (no evidence of nodal involvement).

1. Breast MRI—this confirmed that lesion in the lower outer quadrant of the left breast was unifocal
2. Liver ultrasound—normal
3. Isotope bone scan—normal
4. HER2 status—negative

Treatment and Progress

The patient proceeded with four cycles of epirubicin/cyclophosphamide (EC) followed by four cycles of taxotere, which were well tolerated (see Appendix III). After six cycles of chemotherapy, there had been an excellent clinical response with no obviously palpable tumor in the left breast and no axillary lymphadenopathy. Repeat imaging at this stage with ultrasound confirmed the impression of a dramatic clinical response and showed a residual tumor focus measuring 7 mm. A coil was inserted for future reference to identify the site of the original tumor in the event of breast conservation surgery. At subsequent surgical review, the tumor was now deemed amenable to a guidewire localized wide local excision. The residual tumor (and coil) lay more than 2 cm from the nipple-areolar complex, and there were no areas of skin dimpling or alteration of breast contour.

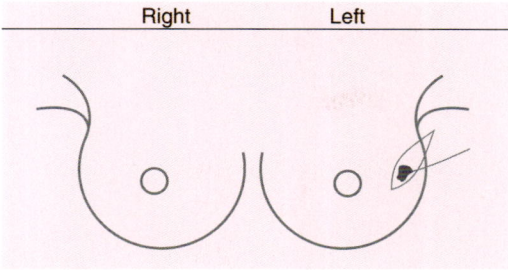

Figure 20

The patient underwent a left quadrantic style resection with removal of the axillary nodes (level II dissection) in continuity with the breast excision (single radial incision). At the time of operation, there was no macroscopic evidence of any tumor, and a wide area of tissue around tip of the wire was excised down to the pectoral serratus anterior fascia (Fig. 20). A specimen radiograph confirmed a satisfactory margin of tissue around the wire tip (about 2 cm) together with the presence of the coil. The patient made an uneventful postoperative recovery and required aspiration of seroma from the left axilla on two occasions.

Definitive Histology

There was no evidence of any residual tumor (invasive or in situ) in the breast excision specimen, and all 16 nodes retrieved were free of metastases. There was evidence of reactive stromal changes and collections of foamy macrophages consistent with tumor response to induction chemotherapy [Fig. 21A–C (magnification 20×)]. This area of tissue did not reach the radial margins of the excised specimen, but was present at the deep margin. Moreover, there was no evidence of any previous metastases within any of the lymph nodes [Fig. 22 (magnification 40×)]. Therefore, a complete pathological response had occurred in a tumor initially measuring in excess of 5 cm.

Treatment and Progress

The patient received radiotherapy to the breast but no further systemic therapy in view of having a "triple negative tumor" (hormone receptor negative and HER2/neu negative). A follow-up mammogram at 12 months revealed no evidence of

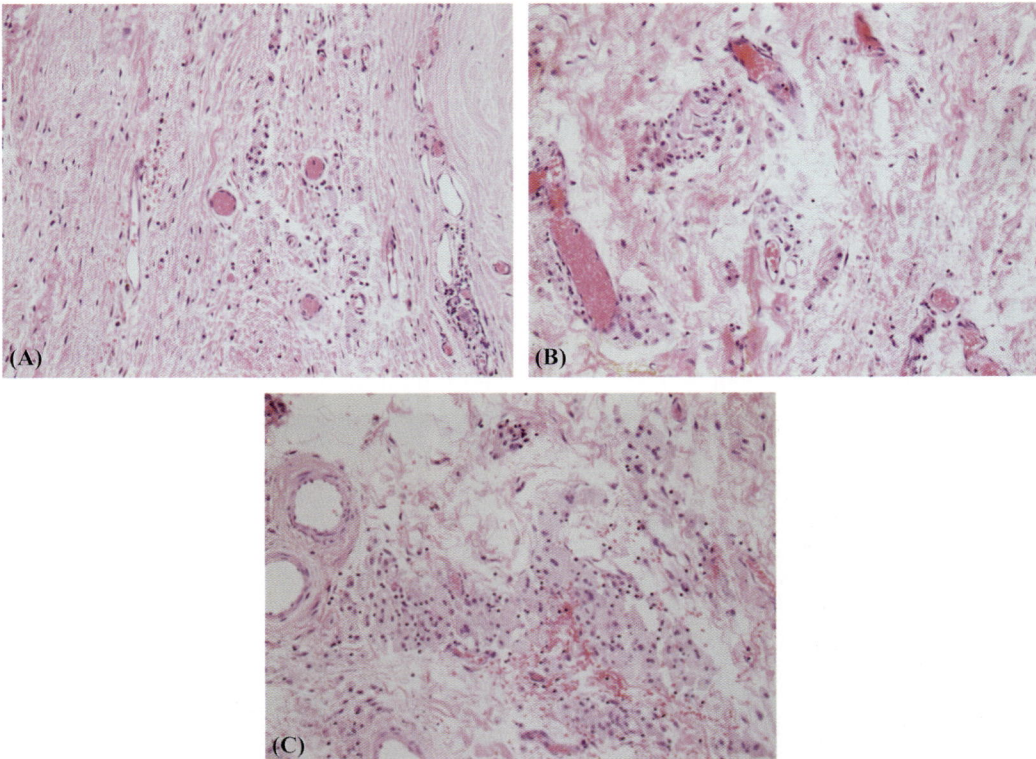

Figure 21

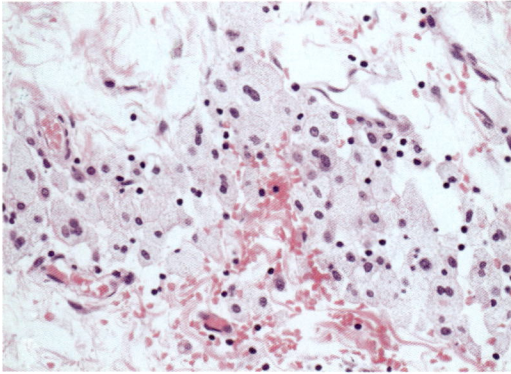

Figure 22

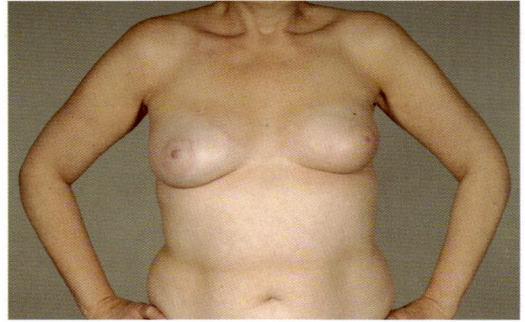

Figure 24

recurrent disease (Fig. 23A and B) and the patient had a very good cosmetic result with an inconspicuous scar in the lateral aspect of the left breast (Fig. 24).

Discussion

A lump that turns out to be a breast cancer may be noticed by a patient following an episode of trauma to the breast. Patients often erroneously conclude that trauma has a causative role in development of the breast cancer; this is not the case and the bruising and discomfort associated with the trauma draw the patient's attention to the lump that has often been present for some time.

This patient had a large T3 cancer located in the lower outer quadrant of the left breast away from the nipple-areolar complex. She was very keen to preserve her breast at the outset, and downstaging with preoperative chemotherapy was the desired objective. The tumor was too large initially for breast-conserving surgery and imaging confirmed the lesion to be unifocal. Neoadjuvant chemo-

therapy increases rates of breast conservation and is the only clear benefit of primary versus adjuvant chemotherapy after almost 25 years of managing patients with upfront systemic treatments. Makris and colleagues reported a decrease in rates of mastectomy from 22% to 11% after neoadjuvant chemotherapy (1). Rates of subsequent mastectomy are generally reduced by 25% to 50% after induction chemotherapy, which is associated with response rates of 80% to 90% (2). This patient had a dramatic clinical response to a standard preoperative regimen (4 cycles of epirubicin and cyclophosphamide followed by 4 cycles of taxotere), with residual tumor measuring less than 1 cm radiologically after six cycles. Despite initial placement of a coil at the site of the tumor and re-excision of positive margins when indicated, rates of local recurrence remain higher when breast-conserving surgery follows rather than precedes chemotherapy (3). Tumor regression may be "honeycombed" rather than concentric with viable tumor cells remaining some distance from the residual tumor (corresponding to the periphery of the original tumor) (4).

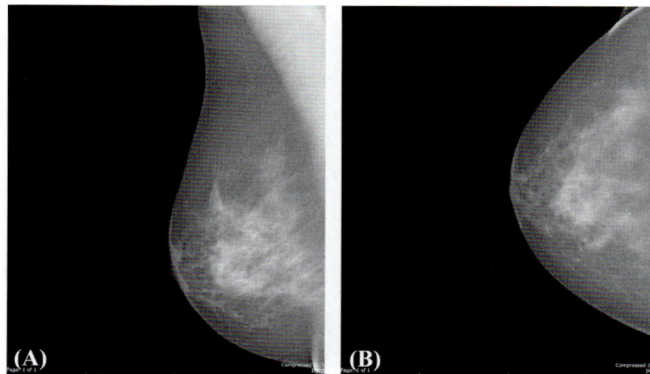

Figure 23

This patient had a complete pathological tumor response with no evidence of any residual invasive or noninvasive disease. Though a complete pathological response appears to be associated with a better clinical outcome, there remain uncertainties about the longer-term prognosis of patients receiving breast conservation surgery after neoadjuvant chemotherapy. Though initial response rates for neoadjuvant chemotherapy exceed 80%, clinical response rates are in general poorly correlated with disease-free and overall survival (5,6). It is now acknowledged that local recurrence can act as a determinant of distant metastases and adversely affect overall survival (7). It is essential that women receive fully informed consent when being offered breast-conserving surgery after a course of primary chemotherapy—particularly if there is a poor response or concerns about the true extent of disease based on ultrasound, CT, or MRI of the breast. When there is residual tumor present, mastectomy must be considered when margins would remain compromised after re-excision or there is multifocal disease in the excision specimen. The optimal regimen for neoadjuvant chemotherapy remains to be determined, but usually contains an anthracycline and a taxane—in this case epirubicin and taxotere. Other schedules include

1. 5-Fluorouracil, epirubicin, cyclophosphamide (FEC) × 4 cycles + weekly paclitaxel × 12
2. Adriamycin and docetaxel (AT) × 4 cycles
3. Adriamycin and cyclophosphamide (AC) × 4 cycles + weekly paclitaxel × 12 cycles

The use of epirubucin rather than doxorubicin is associated with less cardiotoxicity and fewer gastrointestinal symptoms such as nausea and vomiting. This allows for an escalation of dose for epirubicin, which may have advantages in the neoadjuvant setting. Epirubucin is more commonly employed in Europe and the preferred choice of anthracycline. Preoperative EC-taxotere is a popular off-trial neoadjuvant schedule that is similar to the American NSABP B-27 study of preoperative AC-docetaxel (switch of anthracycline only) (6).

New treatment strategies must focus on achieving complete pathological response in a much higher proportion of patients (8). Neoadjuvant schedules incorporating both chemotherapy and Herceptin have shown promising results in respect of complete pathological response rates, which appear higher among ER-negative patients. However, within the large NSABP B-27 study, increased rates of pathological response were not associated with improved overall survival (6). Though identification of this group will allow amended regimens with shorter courses of treatment and perhaps reduced dosages of chemotherapeutic agents, complete pathological response may not be the best way of tailoring treatments. Multivariate models incorporating tumor size, proliferative indices (Ki67), and ER can help predict those patients who will relapse and may benefit from chemotherapy. Moreover, molecular profiling of tumors with assessment of changes in gene expression over a two-week period may identify short-term predictors of longer-term outcomes. There is some evidence that neoadjuvant chemotherapy may cause differential downstaging between sentinel and nonsentinel lymph nodes (9). For this reason, it has been argued that sentinel lymph node biopsy should be undertaken prior to commencing chemotherapy to minimize the risk of a false-negative result (this would occur if the sentinel node responded to chemotherapy but not the nonsentinel nodes). This patient's tumor size precluded sentinel lymph node biopsy (>5 cm), and a formal axillary dissection was carried out at the time of surgery (previous axillary node core biopsy revealed reactive changes only).

When the sentinel lymph node biopsy is positive prior to chemotherapy, there is no quantification of metastatic load in the regional nodes. If these are subsequently downstaged by chemotherapy, it remains unclear whether the patient falls into nodal category 1 to 3 or ≥ 4 nodes. (the latter would receive chest wall radiotherapy after mastectomy and supraclavicular irradiation). Of course, some patients will receive postmastectomy radiotherapy based on primary tumor size, grade, and status of the deep margin. It is customary to consider that the nodal status *at presentation* is relevant to prognosis and decisions on adjuvant radiotherapy. However, when nodes are downstaged by chemotherapy (in 30–40% of cases), then patients may be rendered node negative and could avoid full axillary dissection when sentinel node biopsy is carried out postchemotherapy. Identification rates are between 72% and 100% in these circumstances and the overall false-negative rate using a meta-analysis with a pooled estimate is 12% (10). This figure is similar to conventional sentinel node biopsy (9%). When nodes are positive before neoadjuvant chemotherapy, the false negative rate for sentinel lymph node biopsy after chemotherapy is 25%.

Within the Cambridge Breast Unit, sentinel node biopsy is undertaken prechemotherapy. This provides accurate nodal staging before neoadjuvant chemotherapy and helps decision making for radiotherapy. It is helpful if the result is negative, but negative nodes on completion axillary dissection after neoadjuvant chemotherapy and a prior positive sentinel node biopsy are of uncertain significance. It is unclear whether only the sentinel node was originally involved or further nodes that have subsequently been downstaged. Those in favor of sentinel node biopsy after induction chemotherapy maintain that this will spare axillary dissection in up to 40% of patients because of downstaging (10).

Related Cases

Breast conservation surgery before chemotherapy—*Case Studies 8 and 11*

Neoadjuvant chemotherapy—*Case Studies 23, 27, and 28*

Sentinel node biopsy before neoadjuvant chemotherapy—*Case Studies 27 and 28*

Learning Points

1. Preoperative chemotherapy decreases mastectomy rates. However, breast conservation following preoperative chemotherapy might be associated with a greater risk of local recurrence.
2. A pathological complete response (pCR) following preoperative chemotherapy is associated with improved survival rates. However, this improved survival might possibly be attributed to more favorable tumor biology (among patients who experience pCR) rather than to the preoperative chemotherapy itself.

References

1. Makris A, Powles TJ, Ashley SE, et al. A reduction in the requirements for mastectomy in a randomized trial of neoadjuvant chemoendocrine therapy in primary breast cancer. Ann Oncol 1998; 9:1179–1184.
2. Veronesi U, Bonadonna G, Zurrida S, et al. Conservation surgery after primary chemotherapy in large carcinomas of the breast. Ann Surg 1995; 222:612–618.
3. Wolmark N, Wang J, Mamounas E, et al. Preoperative chemotherapy in patients with operable breast cancer: nine-year results from the National Surgical Adjuvant Breast and Bowel Project. B-18. J Natl Cancer Inst Monogr 2001; 30:96–102.
4. Chafare H, Limongelli S, Purushotham AD. Neoadjuvant chemotherapy in breast cancer. Br J Surg 2005; 92:14–23.
5. Mauri D, Pavlidis N, Ioannidis JP. Neoadjuvant versus adjuvant systemic treatment for breast cancer: a meta-analyis. J Natl Cancer Inst 2005; 97:188–194.
6. Bear HD, Anderson S, Smith RE, et al. A randomized trial comparing preoperative (preop) doxorubicin/cyclophosphamide (AC) to preop AC followed by preop docetaxel (T) and to preop AC followed by postoperative (postop) T in patients with operable carcinomas of the breast: results of the NSABP B-27. Breast Cancer Res Treat 2004; 88(suppl):S16.
7. Early Breast Cancer Trialists Collaborative Group. Effects of radiotherapy and of differences in the extent of surgery for early breast cancer on local recurrence and 15 year survival: an overview of the randomized trials. Lancet 2005; 366:2087–2106.
8. Davidson NE, Morrow M. Sometimes a great notion—an assessment of neoadjuvant systemic therapy for breast cancer. J Natl Cancer Inst 2005; 97:159–161.
9. Mamounas E. Sentinel lymph node biopsy after neoadjuvant systemic therapy. Surg Clin N Am 2003; 83:931–942.
10. Mamounas E. When should sentinel node biopsy be done when giving preoperative chemotherapy? Miami Breast Cancer Conference, Orlando, Florida, February 20–23, 2008.

Part I: Mastectomy After Primary Endocrine Therapy

CASE STUDY 30

History

A 71-year-old woman presented with a two-month history of a lump in the right breast associated with altered breast contour and skin dimpling. There was no nipple discharge and the patient had no previous breast problems. She had undergone a screening mammogram several years earlier that was reported as normal. The patient had no family history of breast or ovarian cancer and had two children (eldest aged 40 years). She had used hormone replacement therapy for a brief period of two months only.

Clinical Findings

Examination revealed an ill-defined mass in the upper outer quadrant of the right breast, associated with alteration in contour of the breast laterally. There was overt skin dimpling but no evidence of infiltration or ulceration of the skin. A firm nonmobile node was palpable in the right axilla (E5) (Fig. 1).

Clinical Assessment

Locally advanced right breast cancer with probable nodal involvement.

Investigations

Mammography

This revealed a spiculated mass lesion in the lower outer quadrant of the right breast measuring 35 mm in maximum diameter with the appearances of a carcinoma (Fig. 2A, B).

Breast Ultrasound

The sonographic correlate of this mammographic abnormality was a 25- mm hypoechoic mass lesion with posterior attenuation (U5)

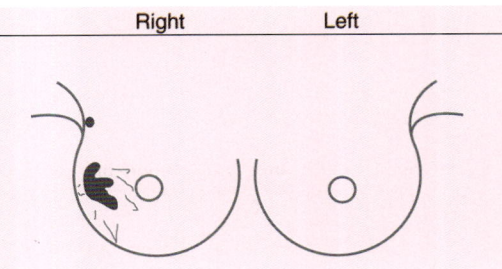

Figure 1

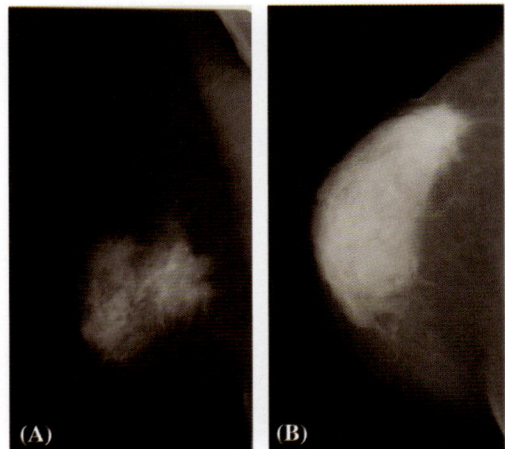

Figure 2

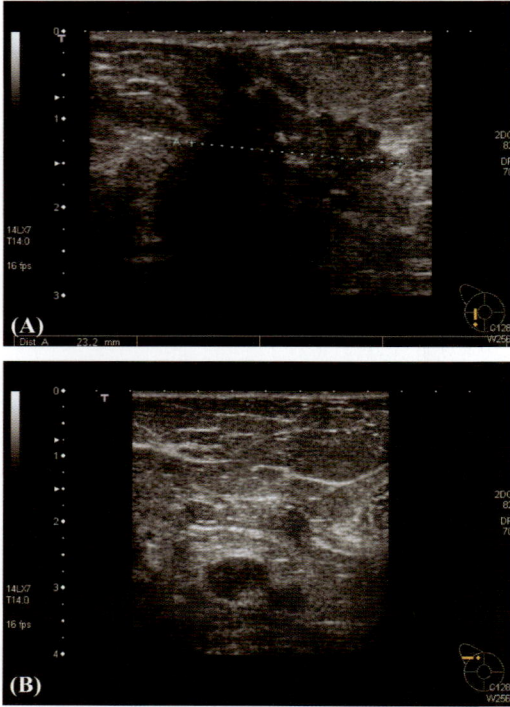

Figure 3

(Fig. 3A). Ultrasound examination of the right axilla confirmed the clinical impression of malignant adenopathy (Fig. 3B).

Core Biopsy

Ultrasound-guided core biopsy (16-gauge needle) of the right breast mass confirmed the clinical and radiological impression of malignancy and showed an invasive ductal carcinoma (grade II, ER positive, HER2 negative) [Fig. 4A (low power), B, C (high power)].

Diagnosis

Locally advanced right breast cancer (T4cN1).

Multidisciplinary Review 1

It was recommended that the patient undergo primary endocrine treatment for a period of four months followed by a right mastectomy and axillary surgery. Ultrasound and possible core biopsy of the right axillary nodes were arranged to determine the pathological node status. In the event of a

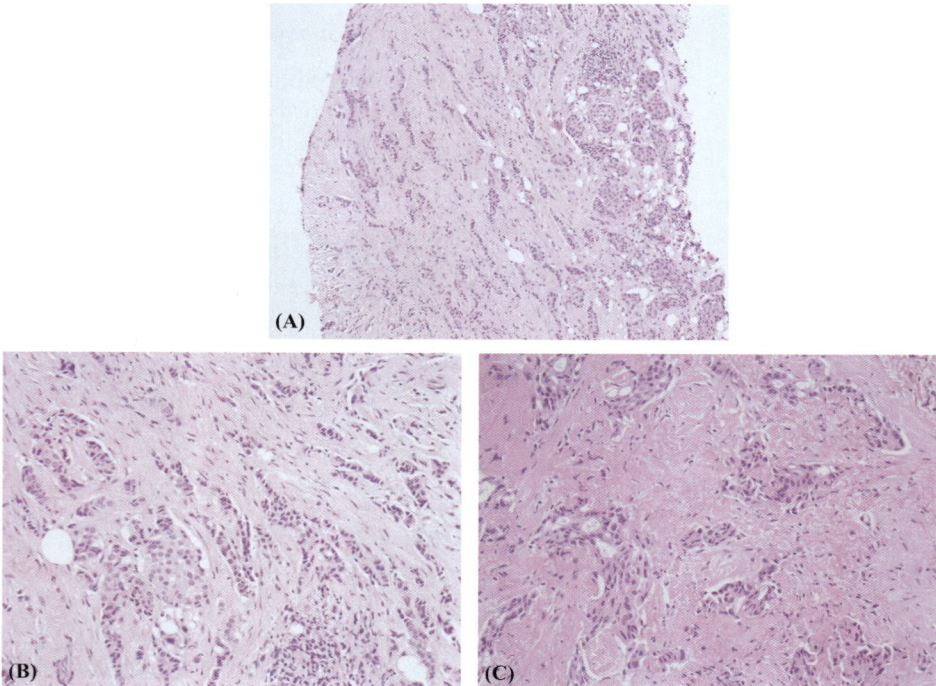

Figure 4

positive axillary node core biopsy, the patient would proceed to a right axillary lymph node dissection (rather than sentinel lymph node biopsy).

Further Investigations

Core Biopsy Right Axillary Node

Metastatic carcinoma was present in a clinically suspicious right axillary node [Fig. 5A (low power), B (high power)].

CT Chest/Abdomen/Pelvis

No evidence of visceral metastases.

Bone Scan

No evidence of bony metastases.

Treatment and Progress

The patient had a strongly ER-positive tumor (8/8) and received primary endocrine

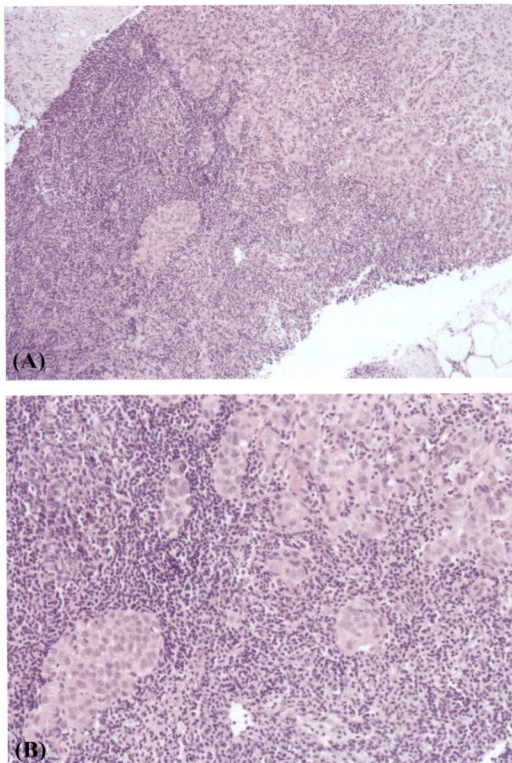

Figure 6

treatment within the context of the MONET study, which randomizes patients to either four months of exemestane or four months of tamoxifen as a preoperative schedule. She subsequently proceeded to a right modified radical mastectomy with a level II axillary lymph node dissection exactly four months after initial presentation. A wide ellipse of skin was removed to incorporate skin overlying the tumor and the area of breast distortion (Fig. 6).

Definitive Histology

This showed a grade III invasive ductal carcinoma measuring 35 mm in maximum diameter with associated DCIS. There was no lymphovascular invasion but perineural invasion was noted (Fig. 7A). Five out of 18 nodes harvested contained metastatic carcinoma and there was evidence of extracapsular spread around one of the nodes [Fig. 7B, C (magnification 5×), D (magnification 10×)].

Discussion

This 74-year-old patient had a locally advanced right breast cancer that was technically operable at presentation. Studies of primary endocrine treatment for locally advanced breast cancers have focused on hormonal manipulation as an alternative to surgery rather than as neoadjuvant therapy. These studies often involved elderly patients who were unfit for surgery, and the aim of treatment was to control the tumor locally without surgical intervention using relatively nontoxic agents. Tamoxifen was initially

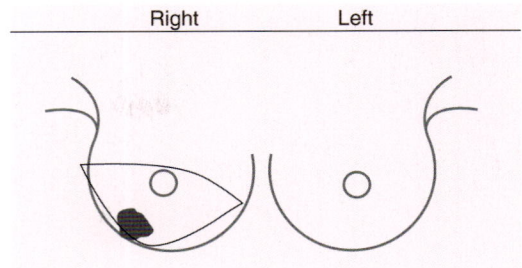

Figure 5

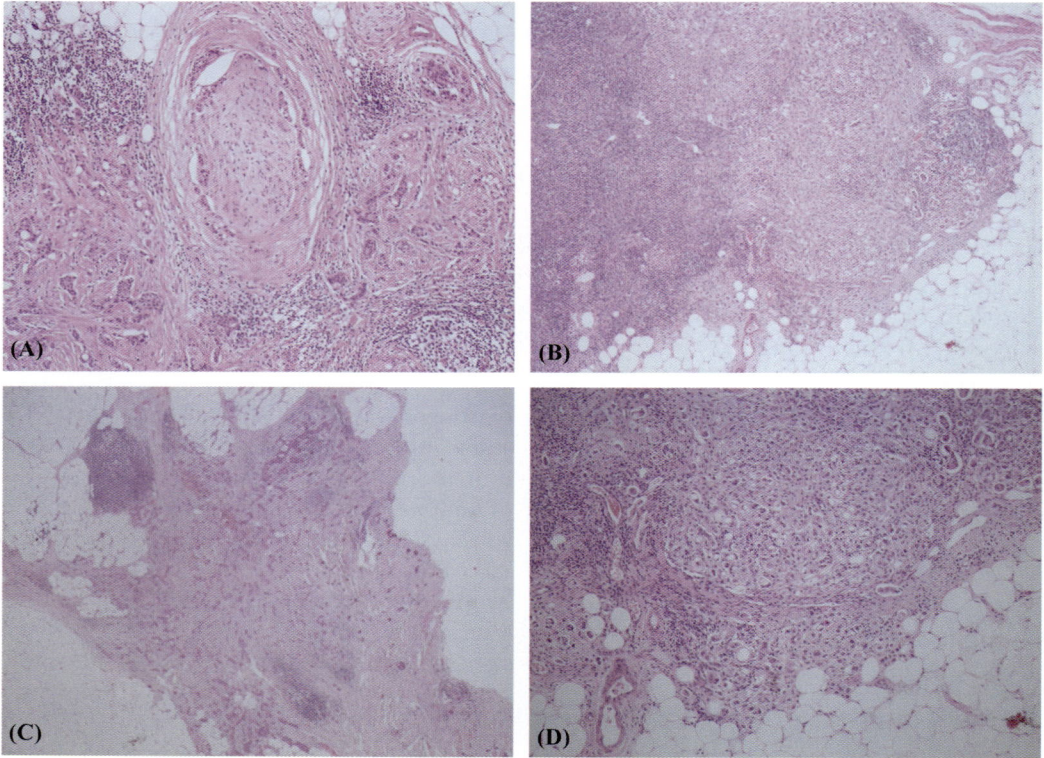

Figure 7

used as primary endocrine therapy for this group of patients with randomization to either tamoxifen alone or surgery (with or without adjuvant tamoxifen) (1,2). A seminal study involving almost 400 patients randomized women over 70 years of age with operable breast cancer to either tamoxifen alone (40 mg) or tamoxifen followed by appropriate surgery (breast conservation or mastectomy). At a median follow-up of 34 months, rates of local failure were higher in the tamoxifen-only group compared with those undergoing subsequent surgery (35% vs. 20.5%) (1). Other studies have also reported higher local relapse rates in the tamoxifen-only group, particularly with longer follow-up (25–80%). However, no differences in overall survival were apparent for primary endocrine treatment versus surgery or combined treatment. The GRETA trial randomized elderly patients with hormone receptor–positive breast cancer to either tamoxifen alone (235 patients) or surgery followed by tamoxifen

(239 patients). The overall response rate was 41.6% (complete clinical response rate 9.2%; partial clinical response rate 32.4%) and median duration of response 19 months. At a median follow-up of 80 months, more than half the patients had died, but there was no difference in overall or breast cancer–survival. Local failure rates were fourfold higher in the tamoxifen-only group (2).

These early studies of tamoxifen as primary endocrine therapy confirmed this to be an acceptable management option in selected patients, especially those considered unfit for surgery. More recent studies have addressed the specific issue of neoadjuvant endocrine therapy in which a preoperative treatment schedule with a hormonal agent forms a component of a planned, multimodality management strategy. Aromatase inhibitors have been compared with tamoxifen in trials of neoadjuvant hormonal therapy and appear superior both in terms of clinical response rates and eligibility for breast conservation surgery (3–5). The MONET study compares tamoxifen with exemestane in a four-month preoperative schedule. Though the possibility of breast-conserving surgery is a potential advantage of neoadjuvant endocrine treatment, some patients will require mastectomy whatever the tumor response. The case described herein was borderline for breast conservation; there was extensive skin tethering with alteration of breast contour. Nonetheless, the initial tumor size was <5 cm and the main tumor mass was not in proximity to the nipple.

It may be feasible to omit surgery in elderly patients who constitute a high anesthetic risk when there has been a good clinical/radiological response to primary endocrine treatment. However, optimal management incorporates surgical excision after a three- to four-month period of hormonal treatment. This strategy will minimize potential problems with local failure in the longer term.

Patients should undergo sonographic assessment of the axilla and any suspicious nodes biopsied. Those patients who are node negative on clinical and ultrasound assessment can proceed to sentinel lymph node biopsy prior to commencement of neoadjuvant endocrine treatment; for those patients who are less fit, a decision can be made on whether to perform a level I or II axillary dissection at the time of surgery based on primary tumor characteristics. It is difficult to justify an additional surgical procedure (and general anesthetic) in this group of older women.

Patients undergoing initial endocrine treatment must be closely monitored and proceed to immediate surgery if there are signs of clinical progression. A second-line hormonal agent can be used if the patient is unfit for surgery. Neoadjuvant endocrine treatment may be an appropriate management option for younger premenopausal women with ER/PR-positive tumors who are either unfit or unwilling to undergo neoadjuvant chemotherapy. An aromatase inhibitor could in theory be combined with an LHRH analogue in this setting to maximize response rates and clinical outcomes.

Related Cases

Primary endocrine treatment—*Case Studies 31, 32, and 33*

Locally advanced breast cancer—*Case Studies 27, 28, 29, and 31*

Learning Points

1. There are several ongoing clinical trials comparing the use of pre- and post-operative endocrine therapy. To date, there is no evidence that preoperative endocrine therapy is associated with a survival advantage.

2. Preoperative endocrine therapy takes longer to achieve an objective response (3–6 months) than preoperative chemotherapy (2–3 months).

3. In patients with ER-positive tumors, preoperative endocrine therapy results in an objective response rate of about 70%, but it generally takes at least three months to achieve a response.

4. Preoperative endocrine therapy has fewer side effects than preoperative chemotherapy. Additionally, the endocrine therapy can be continued during the perioperative period.

References

1. Bates T, Riley DL, Houghton J, et al. Breast cancer in elderly women: a Cancer Research Campaign trial comparing treatment with tamoxifen and optimal surgery with tamoxifen alone. The Elderly Breast Cancer Working Party. Br J Surg 1991; 78:591–594.

2. Mustacchi G, Milani S, Pluchinotta A, et al. Tamoxifen or surgery plus tamoxifen as primary treatment for elderly patients with operable breast cancer: The GRETA Trial. Group for Research on Endocrine Therapy in the Elderly. Anticancer Res 1994; 14:197–200.

3. Eiermann W, Paepke S, Appfelastaedt J, et al. Preoperative treatment of post-menopausal breast cancer with letrozole: a randomized double-blind multicenter study. Ann Oncol 2001; 12:1527–1532.

4. Smith I, Dowsett M, Ebbs SR, et al. Neoadjuvant treatment of post-menopausal breast cancer with anastrozole, tamoxifen or both in combination: the Immediate Preoperative Anastrozole, Tamoxifen or Combined with Tamoxifen (IMPACT) Multi-center Double-Blind Randomized trial. J Clin Oncol 2005; 23:5108–5116.

5. Semiglazov V, Kletzel A, Semiglazov V, et al. Exemestane versus tamoxifen as neoadjuvant endocrine therapy for postmenopausal women with ER positive breast cancer. ASCO Annual Meeting, Orlando, Florida, 2005.

CASE STUDY 31

History

A 57-year-old woman was recalled from routine screening mammography with a large clinical carcinoma of the left breast. The patient suffered from schizophrenia and lived in a nursing home. On direct questioning, the lesion in the left breast had been present for several months and had recently become ulcerated and malodorous. The patient reported no nipple discharge and though she had lost some weight over the preceding few months, there was no history of any unusual cough or back pain. There was no family history of breast cancer and the patient was nulliparous with no prior usage of either the oral contraceptive pill or hormone replacement therapy.

Clinical Findings

There was a large diffuse tumor involving predominantly the lower outer quadrant of the left breast. The tumor measured at least 5 cm clinically and was associated with indrawing of the nipple and general contracture of the breast. A minor degree of ulceration and infection was present close to the nipple. There was no axillary lymphadenopathy and no hepar (E5) (Fig. 8A and B).

Clinical Assessment

Locally advanced left breast cancer presenting through the screening program.

Investigations

Mammography

Mammography was not feasible due to the bulky nature of the tumor and ulceration (patient referred directly from the screening service without mammography being undertaken).

Breast Ultrasound

The size of the tumor precluded accurate sonographic measurement (U5) (Fig. 9).

Core Biopsy

Freehand core biopsy of the large left breast mass confirmed an invasive lobular carcinoma

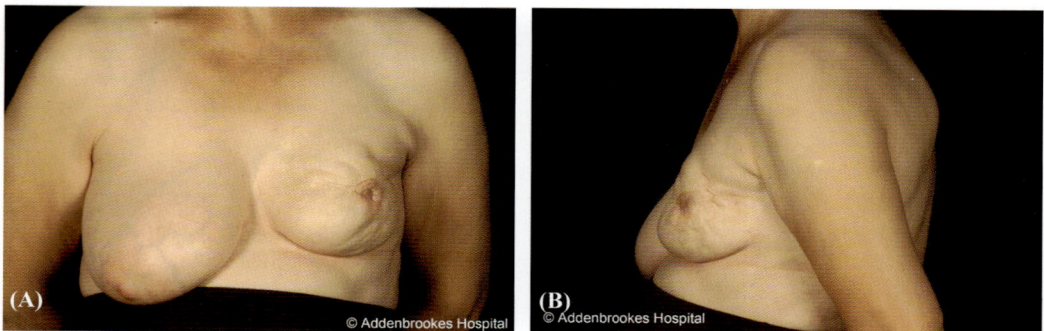

Figure 8

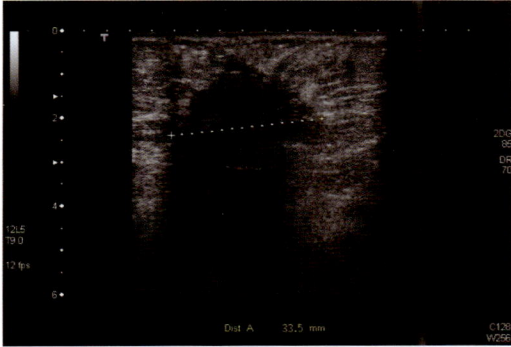

Figure 9

(grade II) [Fig. 10A (magnification 20×)]. This stained positively for ER [Fig. 10B (magnification 20×)].

Diagnosis

Locally advanced left breast cancer (T4cN0).

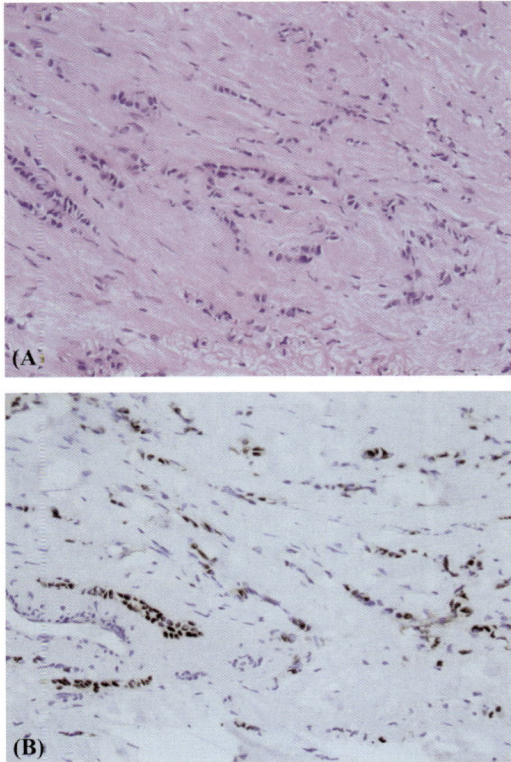

(A)

(B)

Figure 10

Multidisciplinary Review 1

Following multidisciplinary discussion, it was recommended that the patient be commenced on letrozole as primary endocrine treatment. Though technically inoperable at the time of presentation, it was anticipated that the tumor would become amenable to surgery at a future date.

Treatment and Progress

The patient commenced primary endocrine treatment and was monitored three monthly in the breast clinic. It was apparent that the patient was not keen on any form of surgical intervention, whatever the subsequent response of the tumor to endocrine treatment. Upon review after three months, the tumor measured approximately 40 mm in maximum diameter with the impression of a partial response. Letrozole was continued and calcium and vitamin D supplements commenced to prevent bone attrition (bone density scan not undertaken). It is anticipated this patient will undergo mastectomy at an appropriate juncture.

Discussion

In the absence of bony metastases, large locally advanced breast cancers are usually painless and do not interfere with a patient's daily activities. Referral for a medical opinion is often prompted by the offensive odor from secondary infection of an ulcerated, fungating lesion. Occasionally troublesome bleeding from an exophytic tumor causes a patient to seek medical attention.

Breast screening is futile when a patient presents with a clinically advanced lesion. There is now much greater public awareness of breast cancer within the general population, but sometimes there is an element of denial and patients may fear being told a growth is malignant. This patient had a history of mental illness and curiously lived in a nursing home. It is perhaps odd that her carers had not noticed the breast cancer at an earlier stage, which was eventually picked up by radiographers at the time of attendance for routine breast screening.

This patient's tumor was technically inoperable and fixed to the underlying chest wall. It was anticipated that surgical resection would be possible after downstaging with primary endocrine therapy. As the patient was relatively young without evidence of distant metastases, local control of disease was important. It was unlikely that sequential endocrine therapy would adequately control the tumor in the longer term and specific locoregional treatment would be necessary.

By analogy with neoadjuvant chemotherapy, hormonal treatment can be used preoperatively with the intention of downstaging tumors (1–3). This may render inoperable tumors operable and permit breast conservation in patients who might otherwise require mastectomy (4,5). Hormonal therapies are less toxic and potential side effects of chemotherapy can be avoided in elderly patients and those with a poor performance status. This particular patient was relatively young and physically fit, but her schizophrenia was considered a relative contraindication to chemotherapy. Interestingly, patients with hormone receptor–positive disease are less likely to achieve a complete pathological response from the preoperative chemotherapy schedule (6). The aromatase inhibitors have consistently outperformed tamoxifen in the neoadjuvant setting, when endpoints include not only response rates but also breast conservation rates.

In a study of patients with hormonally responsive locally advanced and inoperable breast cancer, letrozole (2.5 mg/day) administered as a preoperative schedule for four months yielded significantly better response rates compared with tamoxifen (20 mg/day) given over a similar period (55% vs. 36%, $p < 0.001$) (7). A significantly higher proportion in the letrozole group was suitable for breast conservation after induction hormonal treatment (45% vs. 35%, $p < 0.022$). The IMPACT study (Immediate Preoperative Arimidex, Tamoxifen or Combined with Tamoxifen) randomized patients to a three-month preoperative schedule of anastrozole, tamoxifen, or a combination of the two. There was no statistically significant difference in response rates (37.2%, 36.1%, and 39.4%,), though anastrozole was more effective at downstaging tumors to permit breast-conserving surgery according to surgeon assessment (8). Therefore, letrozole is associated with higher response rates in the neoadjuvant setting (55% vs. 37.2%), and in vitro studies suggest that letrozole is more than 10-fold potent than anastrozole at inhibiting aromatization. Moreover, letrozole induces a more profound decrease in whole body aromatization and levels of plasma estrogen in postmenopausal breast cancer patients than anastrozole (9). For patients with locally advanced tumors, which demonstrate relatively rapid clinical progression or are bleeding, radiotherapy may help with local control until hormonal therapies have taken effect (2–3 months).

Related Cases

Primary endocrine treatment—*Case Studies 30, 32, and 33*

Locally advanced breast cancer—*Case Studies 27, 28, 29, and 30*

Learning Points

1. Preoperative endocrine therapy may downstage breast cancer, either making inoperable tumors operable or reducing large operable tumors to a size at which breast-conserving surgery rather than mastectomy can be performed.
2. Patients with ER-positive tumors are less likely to achieve a complete pathological response from preoperative chemotherapy than those with ER-negative tumors. Only patients with ER-positive tumors are suitable candidates for preoperative endocrine therapy.
3. In the preoperative setting, better response is generally achieved with the aromatase inhibitors than tamoxifen.

References

1. Veronesi U, Frustaci S, Tirelli U, et al. Tamoxifen therapy in post-menopausal advanced breast

cancer: efficacy at the primary tumour site in 46 evaluable patients. Tumori 1981; 67:235–238.

2. Gazet JC, Ford HT, Coombes RC, et al. Randomised trial of chemotherapy versus endocrine therapy in patients presenting with locally advanced breast cancer (a pilot study). Br J Cancer 1991; 63:279–282.

3. Ellis MJ, Coop A, Singh B, et al. Letrozole is more effective neoadjuvant endocrine therapy than tamoxifen for ErbB-1 and/or ErbB-2 positive estrogen receptor positive primary breast cancer: evidence from a phase III randomized trial. J Clin Oncol 2001; 19:3808–3816.

4. Fisher B, Bryant J, Wolmark N, et al. Effect of preoperative chemotherapy on the outcome of women with operable breast cancer. J Clin Oncol 1998; 16:2672–2685.

5. Wolmark N, Wang J, Mamounas E, et al. Preoperative chemotherapy in patients with operable breast cancer: nine year results from National Surgical Adjuvant Breast and Bowel Project. B-18. J Natl Cancer Inst Monogr 2001; 30:96–102.

6. Buzdar A, Valero V, Theriault RL, et al. Pathological complete response to chemotherapy is related to hormone receptor status. Breast Cancer Res Treat 2003; 82:(abstr 302).

7. Eiermann W, Paepke S, Appfelastaedt J, et al. Preoperative treatment of post-menopausal breast cancer with letrozole: a randomized double-blind multicenter study. Ann Oncol 2001; 12:1527–1532.

8. Smith I, Dowsett M, Ebbs SR, et al. Neoadjuvant treatment of post-menopausal breast cancer with anastrozole, tamoxifen or both in combination: the Immediate Preoperative Anastrozole, Tamoxifen or Combined with Tamoxifen (IMPACT) Multicenter Double-Blind Randomized trial. J Clin Oncol 2005; 23:5108–5116.

9. Geisler J, Haynes B, Anker G, et al. Influence of letrozole and anastrozole on total body aromatization and plasma estrogen levels in postmenopausal breast cancer patients evaluated in a randomized, cross-over study. J Clin Oncol 2002; 20:751–757.

Part II: Breast-Conservation Surgery After Primary Endocrine Therapy

CASE STUDY 32

History

A 56-year-old woman presented with a two-week history of a lump in the right breast. There was no associated nipple discharge and the lump was nontender. Curiously, the patient had undergone a routine screening mammogram two weeks earlier and was awaiting results of this. She had never been recalled from any screening mammograms and had no previous breast problems. The patient had a maternal aunt with postmenopausal breast cancer and was currently taking hormone replacement therapy (total duration of usage 20 years). She had briefly used the oral contraceptive pill for a period not exceeding 12 months in her youth.

Clinical Findings

An ill-defined but firm mass was palpable in the upper outer quadrant of the right breast measuring 3 cm in maximum diameter. There was dimpling of the overlying skin but no nipple abnormalities. A clinically suspicious node was palpable in the right axilla (E5) (Fig. 11).

Clinical Assessment

The clinical impression was highly suggestive of a right breast cancer with an involved axillary lymph node (despite a recent screening mammogram).

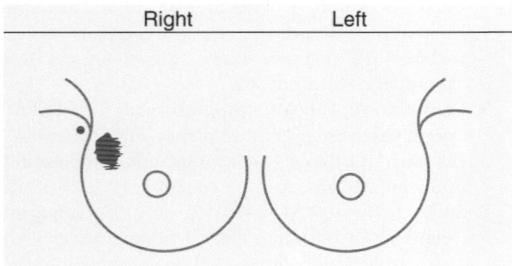

Figure 11

Investigations

Mammography (Right)

A spiculate opacity was seen in the upper outer quadrant of the right breast measuring 28 mm in maximum diameter (R5) (Fig. 12A and B). Previous screening mammograms were requested for review and a left-sided mammogram was not repeated.

Breast Ultrasound

The sonographic correlate of this opacity was a slightly smaller hypoechoic lesion with a maximum diameter of 23 mm. The lesion was heterogeneous with posterior acoustic enhancement and had the radiological features of a carcinoma (U5) (Fig. 13A). The palpable right axillary node was sonographically suspicious (Fig. 13B).

Core Biopsy

Ultrasound-guided core biopsy of the right breast mass confirmed a carcinoma. The

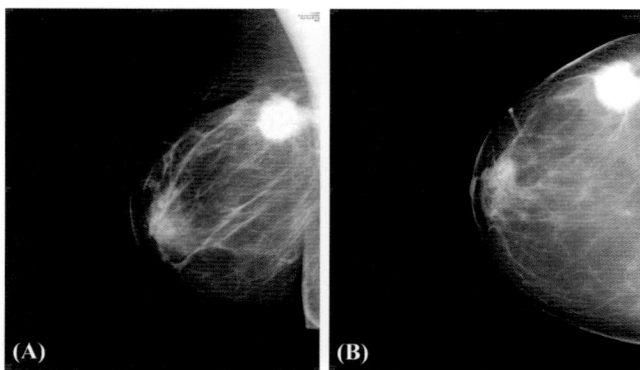

Figure 12

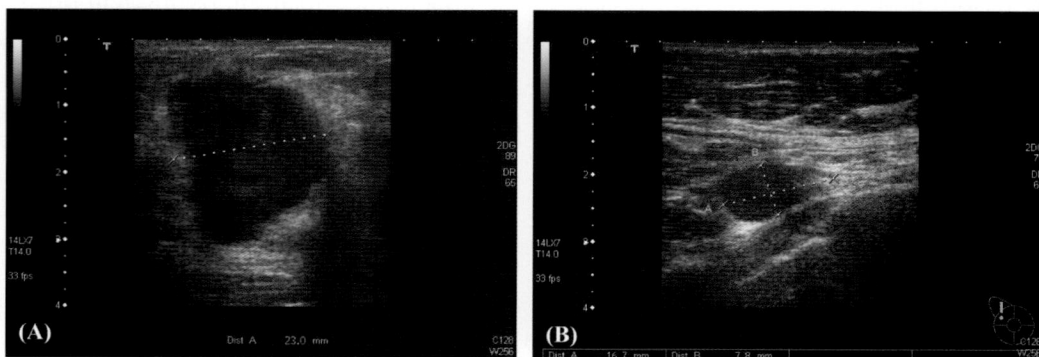

Figure 13

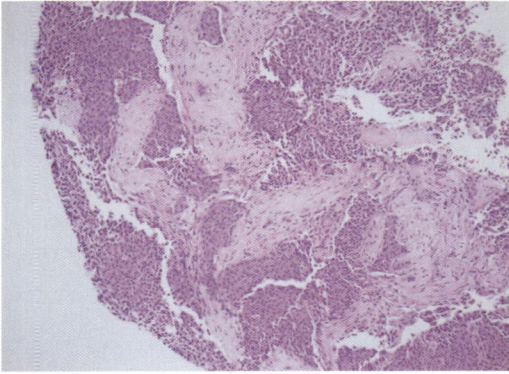

Figure 14

appearances were of a solid papillary lesion with probable areas of focal invasion (ER positive, HER2 negative) (Fig. 14).

Diagnosis

Probable early-stage invasive right breast cancer with nodal involvement (T2N1)

Multidisciplinary Review 1

Recent screening mammograms (performed elsewhere) were reviewed together with results of the right breast core biopsy. Though the core biopsies had not shown unequivocal evidence of invasion, there was palpable right axillary lymphadenopathy. Core biopsy of the right axillary node (with ultrasound guidance) was therefore recommended to confirm invasive carcinoma. In addition to a right-sided breast cancer, the recent screening films revealed a localized area of suspicious microcalcification in the left breast, which required further evaluation and probable biopsy (Fig. 15A–D).

Further Investigations

Arrangements were made for the patient to attend for further investigations as follows:

1. Core biopsy right axillary lymph node—ultrasound-guided core biopsy of the right axillary node revealed extensive

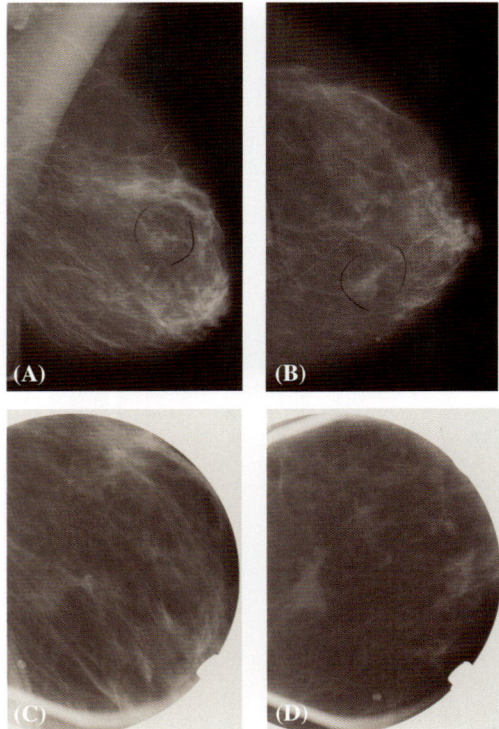

Figure 15

replacement with metastatic carcinoma [Figs. 16A (magnification 10×), B (magnification 20×)].

2. Left breast ultrasound—the area of microcalcification in the left breast was associated with a 4 mm mass lesion (U5) (Fig. 17).

3. Core biopsy left breast—ultrasound-guided core biopsy of the mass/area of calcification showed an invasive carcinoma (grade I, ER positive) [Figs. 18A (magnification 10×), B (magnification 20×)]. There was a single fleck of calcium on specimen radiology (Fig. 19).

Multidisciplinary Review 2

The patient had a histologically documented node-positive breast cancer on the right side and a small 4-mm grade I clinically node-negative cancer of the left breast. After thorough multidisciplinary discussion, it was

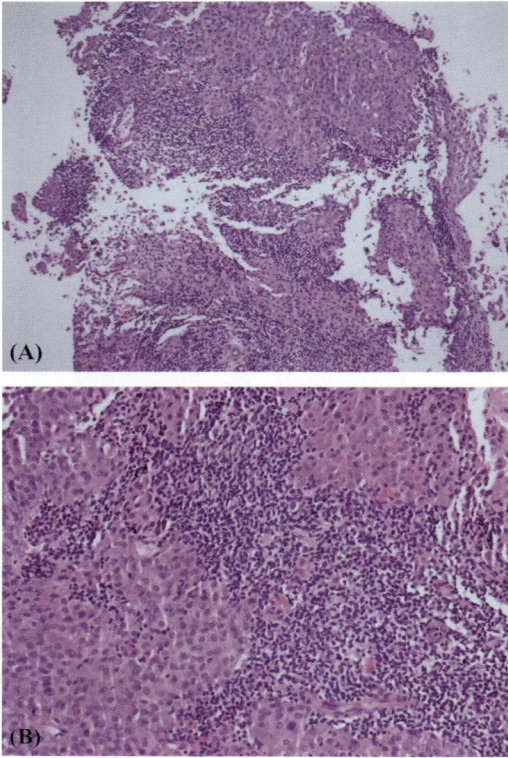

Figure 16

recommended the patient be treated with primary endocrine therapy in the event of HER2 negativity (subsequently confirmed from core biopsy results). The alternative management option was neoadjuvant chemotherapy, but the estimated absolute benefits from chemotherapy were less than 2%, which were insufficient to justify this treatment option. Following induction endocrine treatment, the patient would undergo surgery as follows (*i*) a right wide local excision and axillary dissection and (*ii*) a left guidewire-localized wide local excision. A left sentinel lymph node biopsy would be carried out shortly after commencement of endocrine treatment to stage the left axilla early on.

Treatment and Progress

Bilateral breast coils were inserted to aid subsequent identification of the tumors at the time of surgical excision. A left sentinel

node biopsy was carried out three weeks after commencement of primary endocrine treatment and revealed no evidence of nodal metastases. The patient received primary endocrine treatment within the MONET study, which randomizes older patients with hormone sensitive locally advanced tumors to either exemestane or tamoxifen for a period of four months prior to definitive surgery.

Discussion

This patient with bilateral breast cancers was faced with complex management options, which included primary surgery, primary chemotherapy, or primary endocrine treatment. It is perhaps unusual for a single patient to be potentially suitable for initial treatment with these three modalities. This patient had a moderate sized, node positive, right-sided breast cancer and a small node negative left-sided lesion (both ER positive). Primary surgery would be the conventional management with a right wide local excision and axillary dissection together with a left-sided wire-localized wide local excision and sentinel lymph node biopsy. Though this patient had node-positive disease, her postmenopausal status, tumor size, and negative HER2 status conferred an absolute benefit from chemotherapy of less than 2%. It is inappropriate to give neoadjuvant chemotherapy when a patient is unlikely to derive significant benefit based on known tumor parameters and nodal status.

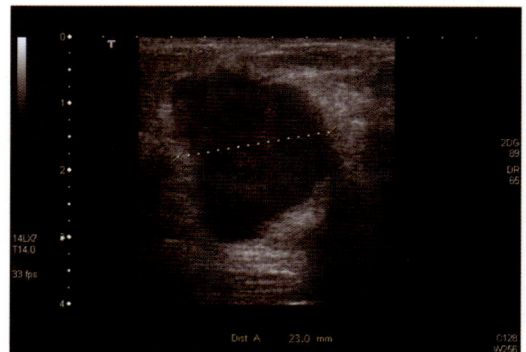

Figure 17

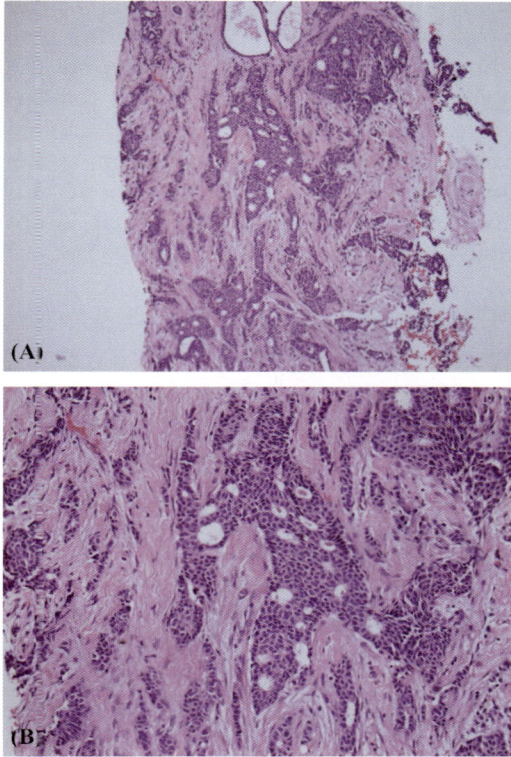

Figure 18

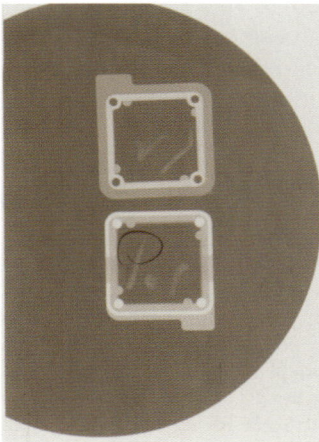

Figure 19

Neoadjuvant endocrine treatment offers several advantages for older, postmenopausal women with hormone receptor–positive breast cancer (1). Like neoadjuvant chemotherapy, primary endocrine treatment permits translational studies on predictive and prognostic markers—the primary tumor remains in situ and is accessible for serial core biopsies. The proliferation marker Ki67 can be measured immunohistochemically and shows a dramatic response to neoadjuvant endocrine treatment (2). Moreover, clinical response can be assessed during induction therapy, which is an indication of the efficacy of a hormonal agent at a biological level, though generally correlates poorly with clinical outcomes. Effective agents in the neoadjuvant setting could be assessed with surrogate predictors of clinical outcome (e.g., Ki67) and incorporated sooner into standard treatment protocols (3). Though this patient had relatively small tumors, larger more locally advanced tumors that invade the skin or chest wall and have extensive nodal involvement can present technical challenges at operation. A period of treatment with primary endocrine therapy can downstage tumors and permit surgical resection. In a recent study involving almost 100 women with T4 tumors, more than 90% became resectable after three to six months of tamoxifen (1).

Primary endocrine treatment with tamoxifen has been used as the exclusive treatment for elderly unfit patients with breast cancer (4,5). Though longer-term local control rates are poorer when surgery does not follow induction endocrine treatment, early response rates are high in ER-positive patients (30–40%) (6). Moreover, disease progression within three to six months is uncommon and neoadjuvant endocrine therapy does not compromise overall survival. Neoadjuvant endocrine therapy can be employed in fit older patients with the aim of improving rates of breast conservation as well as operability (7). Several trials have now confirmed the superiority of aromatase inhibitors in this context, which consistently outperform tamoxifen when endpoints include not only response rates but also breast conservation rates.

These highly favorable response rates for letrozole in the neoadjuvant setting have been exceeded by exemestane in a trial comparing this steroidal aromatase inhibitor with tamoxifen (8). The overall clinical response rates to three months of neoadjuvant exemestane (25 mg daily) or tamoxifen were 76.3% and 40% ($p < 0.05$). MONET is an ongoing study that randomizes postmenopausal women with hormone receptor–positive locally advanced breast cancer (>2 cm ultrasound size) to either four months of exemestane or tamoxifen as a preoperative schedule. This patient had bilateral breast cancers, which were already potentially conservable and could have been managed with bilateral wide local excision. It is possible that a survival advantage might ensue from neoadjuvant endocrine treatment. The act of surgery is associated with a systemic perturbation, which involves the release of various growth factors (vascular endothelial growth factor, epidermal growth factor, insulin-like growth factor) and loss of tumor suppressor factors (angiostatin). Preoperative systemic therapy could theoretically offset any tumor-promoting effects of surgical excision (namely on distant micrometastases) (9).

Therefore primary hormonal therapies in older postmenopausal women with hormone-responsive disease can avoid the potential toxicities of chemotherapy, while achieving good response rates, which in turn translate into improved rates of operability and breast conservation. Tumors are usually more than 3 cm in size, but smaller tumors can be managed with neoadjuvant endocrine treatment, as with the case reported herein. The optimal duration of primary endocrine treatment is unknown, but maximum tumor responses are seen after 12 to 15 months of treatment. In about 20% of cases, maximal responses are seen at 12 months and there is an argument for more prolonged therapy to increase the chance of breast-conserving surgery. Complete pathological responses are uncommon and neoadjuvant endocrine treatment should ideally be incorporated into a preoperative schedule rather than single modality treatment, which might involve sequential endocrine therapies but ultimately poor rates of local control in the longer term. Though rates of tumor regression may be slower with neoadjuvant endocrine treatment compared with chemotherapy, overall response rates appear similar for this group

of ER-positive women. Sentinel lymph node biopsy has been investigated following neoadjuvant endocrine treatment (10), but the optimal timing of this procedure remains unclear; within the MONET study, sentinel lymph node biopsy is undertaken at the beginning of endocrine treatment and involves a separate operation that is not always appropriate in older patients.

Related Cases

Bilateral breast cancer—*Case Studies 22, 23, and 24*

Primary endocrine treatment—*Case Studies 30, 31, and 33*

Learning Points

1. Prior to preoperative systemic therapy, metal clips are often inserted within the tumor (at time of core biopsy). After preoperative systemic therapy, these clips enable the radiologist to visualize the site of the original tumor mammographically, thereby facilitating placement of a wire to aid in wide local excision.
2. Longer follow-up of clinical trials is needed to determine if there are any differences in local recurrence or survival rates between patients receiving pre- and postoperative endocrine therapy.

References

1. Beresford MJ, Ravichandran D, Makris A. Neoadjuvant endocrine therapy in breast cancer. Cancer Treat Rev 2007; 33:48–57.
2. Ellis MJ, Coop A, Singh B, et al. Letrozole inhibits tumour proliferation more effectively than tamoxifen independent of HER1/2 expression status. Cancer Res 2003; 63:6523–6531.
3. Dowsett M, Smith IE, Ebbs SR, et al. Short-term changes in Ki-67 during neoadjuvant treatment for primary breast cancer with anastrozole or tamoxifen alone or combined correlate with recurrence-free survival. Clin Cancer Res 2005; 11:951s–958s.
4. Allan SG, Rodger A, Smyth JF, et al. Tamoxifen as primary treatment of breast cancer in elderly or frail patients: a practical management. Br Med J 1985; 290:358.
5. Akhtar SS, Allan SG, Rodger A, et al. A 10 year experience of tamoxifen as primary treatment of breast cancer in 100 elderly and frail patients. Eur J Surg Oncol 1991; 17:30–35.

6 Bates T, Riley DL, Houghton J, et al. Breast cancer in elderly women: a Cancer Research Campaign trial comparing treatment with tamoxifen and optimal surgery with tamoxifen alone. The Elderly Breast Cancer Working Party. Br J Surg 1991; 78:591–594.

7. Gazet JC, Ford HT, Coombes RC, et al. Prospective randomized trial of tamoxifen versus surgery in elderly patients with breast cancer. Eur J Surg Oncol 1994; 20:207–214.

8. Semiglazov V, Kletzel A, Semiglazov V, et al. Exemestane versus tamoxifen as neoadjuvant endocrine therapy for postmenopausal women with ER positive breast cancer. ASCO Annual Meeting, Orlando, Florida, 2005.

9. Baum M, Benson JR. Current and future roles of adjuvant endocrine therapy in management of early carcinoma of the breast. In: Senn H-J, Goldhirsch RD, Gelber RD, et al., eds. Recent Results in Cancer Research 140—Adjuvant Therapy of Breast Cancer. Hiedelberg: Springer–Verlag, 1996:215–226 (ISBN 3-540 58454-4).

10. Aihara T, Munakata S, Morino H, et al. Feasibility of sentinel node biopsy for breast cancer after neoadjuvant endocrine therapy: a pilot study. J Surg Oncol 2004; 85:77–81.

Part I: Primary Endocrine Therapy

CASE STUDY 33

History

A 92-year-old woman presented with a four-week history of a lump in the left breast. There was no associated nipple discharge and the patient had no previous breast problems being otherwise fit and active for her age. She had a very weak family history of breast cancer with a paternal cousin having the disease in her 40s. The patient was nulliparous and had never used hormone replacement therapy.

Clinical Findings

Examination revealed a firm, ill-defined mass in the upper outer quadrant of the left breast measuring approximately 2 cm (Figs. 1 and 2A). The mass was mobile on the chest wall with subtle evidence of skin tethering in the vicinity of the lump, which was more evident with the arms elevated (Fig. 2B). No axillary lymph nodes were palpable (E4).

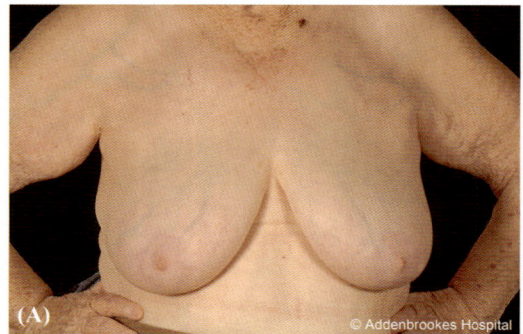

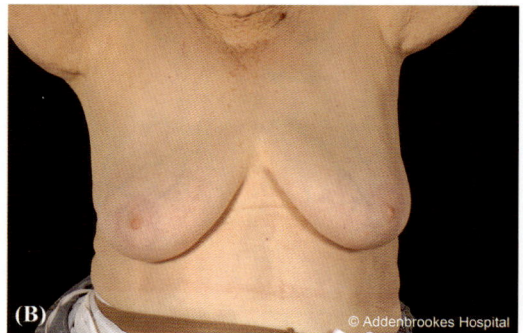

Figure 2

Clinical Assessment

Clinical carcinoma of the left breast without involved axillary lymph nodes.

Investigations

Mammography

A spiculate opacity measuring 20 mm in maximum diameter was seen in the upper

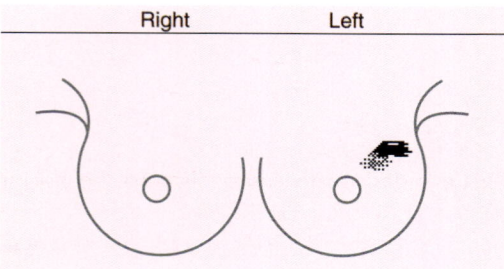

Figure 1

outer quadrant of the left breast corresponding to the palpable lump (Fig. 3).

Breast Ultrasound

The sonographic correlate of this mass was a 20-mm hypoechoic lesion with the radiological features of a carcinoma (U5) (Fig. 4).

Core Biopsy

Ultrasound-guided core biopsy of the breast mass confirmed an invasive carcinoma (grade II) that was strongly ER positive (Fig. 5A (magnification 10×), B (magnification 20×)][a]

Diagnosis

Early-stage left breast cancer (T1N0).

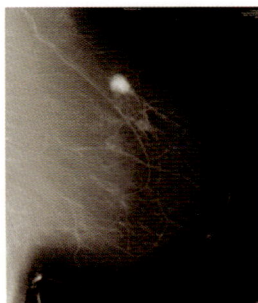

Figure 3

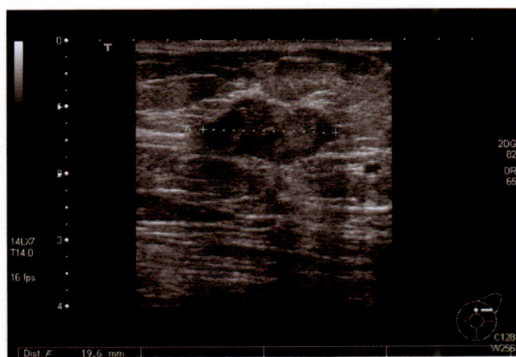

Figure 4

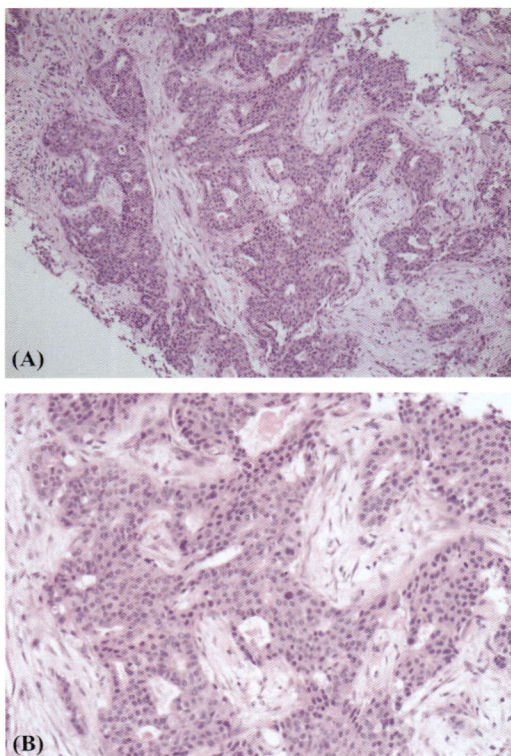

Figure 5

Multidisciplinary Review 1

It was recommended that the patient be managed with primary endocrine treatment. Though the patient was very fit for her age with no significant comorbidities, she was reluctant to embark upon any surgery, and this was considered inappropriate in a nonagenerian.

Treatment and Progress

The patient was initially reviewed four monthly within the breast unit, but subsequently discharged back to the care of her general practitioner for clinical monitoring. This avoided unnecessary visits to the hospital and both the district nurse and general practitioner were able to undertake domiciliary visits.

---

[a] Allred score = 8/8

Discussion

See discussion for Case Study 30.

Related Cases

Breast cancer in the elderly—*Case Studies 24, 34, and 43*

Primary endocrine treatment—*Case Studies 30, 31, and 32*

Learning Points

1. Elderly women with ER-positive breast cancer are sometimes offered endocrine therapy alone (without surgery). This is referred to as primary endocrine therapy.
2. Primary endocrine therapy for ER-positive breast cancers is generally offered to elderly women who are unfit for or refuse surgery.
3. In elderly women with breast cancer, surgery achieves better local control of the tumor than does primary endocrine therapy, but it does not seem to extend survival.

Part II: Primary Radiotherapy

CASE STUDY 34

History

An 87-year-old woman presented with a six-month history of a lump in the left breast. The lump had progressively increased in size and recently had become ulcerated and started bleeding when touched. The patient lived alone and friends had prompted her to seek medical attention due to the malodorous nature of the lesion. There was no associated nipple discharge and no previous breast problems or family history of breast cancer. The patient had not experienced any recent weight loss, unusual back pain, or cough.

Clinical Findings

On examination there was a florid exophytic lesion in the inferior aspect of the left breast, which was ulcerated and infected. The lesion measured at least 5 cm in maximum dimension and was partially fixed to the chest wall. The surface of the lesion was very friable and readily bled. No enlarged nodes were palpable in the left axilla (E5) (Figs. 6 and 7).

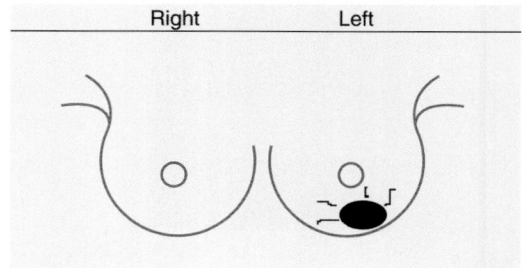

Figure 6

Clinical Assessment

Large fungating cancer of the left breast with ulceration and secondary infection.

Investigations

Mammography

Mammography was precluded by the size and ulceration of the lesion.

Breast Ultrasound

A solid mass was seen in the lower outer quadrant of the left breast, which was ill

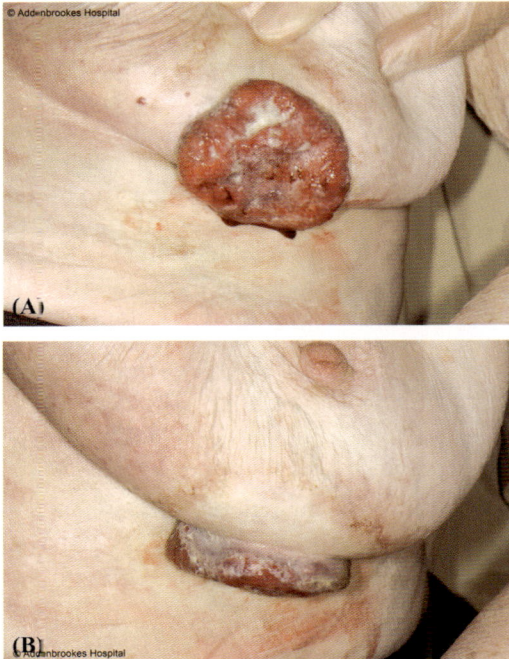

Figure 7

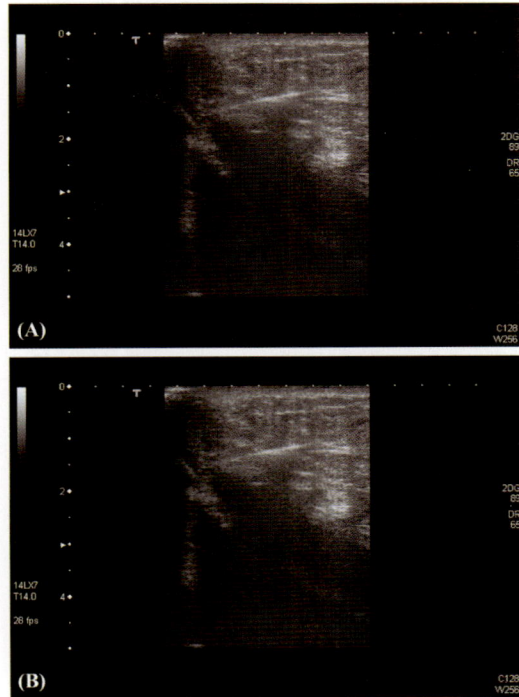

Figure 8

defined and homogeneous. The echo pattern was hypoechoic and the appearances were of a large fungating tumor (U5) (Fig. 8A, B).

Core Biopsy

Freehand core biopsy of the left breast mass confirmed an invasive carcinoma (grade III) that was ER negative (Fig. 9A (low power), B (high power)). The Allred score was 0/8 and this was repeated to reaffirm hormone insensitivity. Interestingly, there was a suggestion histologically that this might be a squamous lesion and this would be consistent with the gross morphology.

Diagnosis

Locally advanced fungating left breast cancer (T4N0).

Multidisciplinary Review 1

Following multidisciplinary discussion, it was felt appropriate to embark on primary radiotherapy. The patient was elderly and unfit for surgery and the tumor was ER negative.

Radiotherapy would help reduce the degree of ulceration and "dry up" the lesion. Arrangements were made for the patient to be seen in the radiotherapy clinic later on that day and for treatment to commence as soon as possible. It was noted that the patient had been admitted as an inpatient since her original attendance in the breast clinic one week earlier. This was attributable to the patient's psychological rather than physical condition and routine blood tests including full blood count, urea and electrolytes, liver function tests, and calcium were within the normal range.

Treatment and Progress

The patient received a single fraction of radiotherapy using a direct field of 260 kV to a dose of 8 Gy. She tolerated this well and clinical review after 14 days showed a marked improvement in the tumor with attainment of hemostasis.

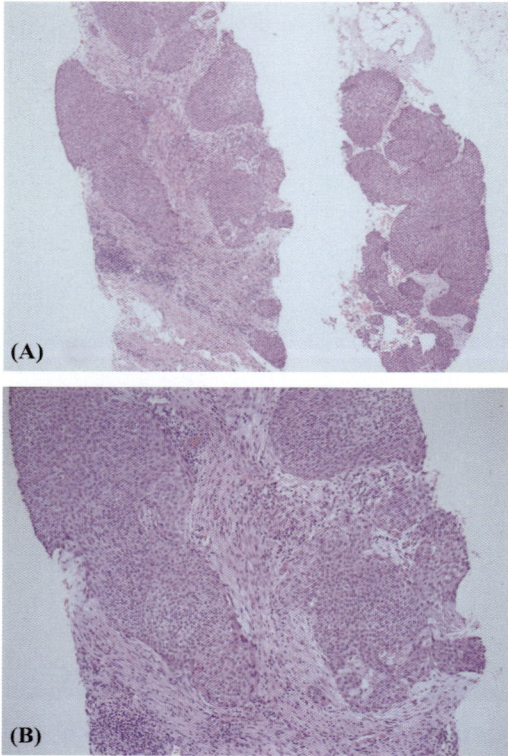

(A)

(B)

Figure 9

Discussion

This elderly patient had a locally advanced carcinoma that had become ulcerated with troublesome bleeding. She was otherwise well with no evidence of any distant metastatic disease and had previously lived alone and independently. She was unfit for any primary surgical intervention and the tumor was hormone receptor negative. She tolerated a short course of radiotherapy to the breast and there was evidence of a marked clinical improvement within two weeks.

Primary radiotherapy for locally advanced tumors is usually a salvage option and employed in lieu of surgery or endocrine treatment for elderly and/or unfit patients (1,2). Studies have shown that relatively high doses of radiation must be used to achieve optimal control (up to 60 Gy) (1) and this can be associated with significant side effects such as skin ulceration and rib necrosis (3).

This patient had a relatively small dose of 8 Gy as a single fraction with the aim of drying up the tumor and preventing further bleeding. More definitive local control is only possible with either much higher doses of radiotherapy or a combination of radiotherapy and surgery, which can result in local control rates of more than 70% to 80% (4). However, combined treatments do not lead to improvements in overall survival compared with either modality alone (5).

Related Cases

Locally advanced breast cancer—*Case Studies 28, 30, and 31*

Breast cancer in the elderly—*Case Studies 24, 33, and 43*

Learning Points

1. Elderly patients with locally advanced ER-negative breast cancers might be offered radiotherapy alone. This is referred to as primary radiotherapy. Elderly women who undergo primary radiotherapy have generally refused or are unfit for surgery.
2. Primary radiotherapy may achieve local control of a locally advanced breast cancer and thereby result in an improved quality of life.

References

1. Harris JR, Sawicka J, Gelman R, et al. Management of locally advanced carcinoma of the breast by primary radiation therapy. Int J Radiat Oncol Biol Phys 1983; 9:345–349.
2. Sheldon T, Hayes DF, Cady B, et al. Primary radiation therapy for locally advanced breast cancer. Cancer 1987; 60:1219–1225.
3. Spanos WJ Jr., Montague ED, Fletcher GH. Late complications of radiation only for advanced breast cancer. Int J Radiat Oncol Biol Phys 1980; 6:1473–1476.
4. Sorace RA, Lippman M. Locally advanced breast cancer. In: Lippman M, Lichter A, Danforth D, eds. Diagnosis and Management of Breast Cancer. Philadelphia: WB Saunders, 1988.
5. Hortobagyi G, Buzdar AU. Locally advanced breast cancer: a review including the MD Anderson experience. In: Ragaz J, Ariel I, eds. High Risk Breast Cancer. Berlin: Springer-Verlag, 1991.

Part I: First Trimester Pregnancy

CASE STUDY 35

History

A 34-year-old woman who was nine-weeks pregnant presented with a lump in the superior aspect of the right breast that had been present for approximately two years. The lump had been previously investigated elsewhere and fine needle aspiration cytology performed—the latter was classified as "C1." The patient felt that the lump had recently increased in size and therefore sought a second opinion. There was no family history of breast or ovarian cancer and this was the patient's first pregnancy. She had used the oral contraceptive pill for a cumulative period of more than 10 years.

Clinical Findings

Examination revealed a rather ill-defined mass in the upper outer quadrant of the right breast measuring 3 cm in maximum diameter. There was an adjacent nodule estimated at no more than 1 cm in size and no skin tethering or axillary lymphadenopathy (E3) (Fig. 1).

Clinical Assessment

Clinically suspicious, though likely benign lump in first trimester of pregnancy.

Investigations

Breast Ultrasound

This showed a dumbbell solid mass in the upper outer quadrant of the right breast measuring 37 mm in maximum diameter. The mass was ill-defined, though homogeneous with a hypoechoic pattern and posterior acoustic enhancement. The appearances were indeterminate and could not distinguish between a possible fibroadenoma or a carcinoma (U3).

Core Biopsy

Ultrasound-guided core biopsy (14-gauge needle) of the right breast mass confirmed an invasive carcinoma (grade II, ER positive) (Fig. 2).

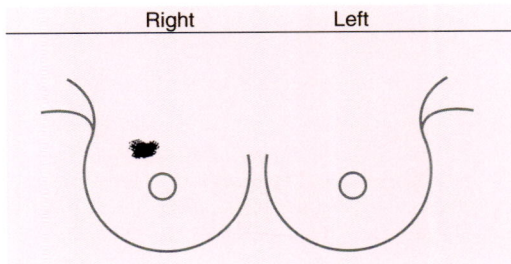

Figure 1

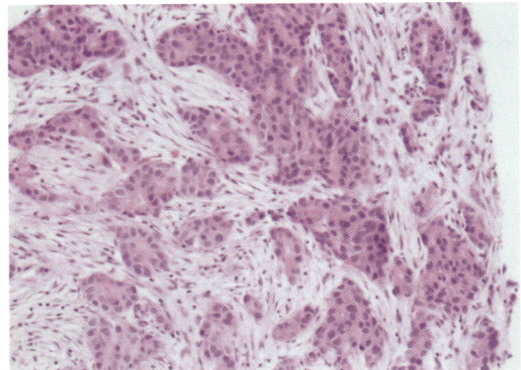

Figure 2

Diagnosis

Early-stage right-sided breast cancer in the first trimester of pregnancy (T2N0).

Multidisciplinary Review 1

The patient was adamant from the outset that she wished to continue with the pregnancy; this was a "cherished" pregnancy in a 34-year-old woman with no existing children. Two potential treatment pathways were outlined and carefully discussed with the patient:

1. Neoadjuvant chemotherapy (commencing at 12 weeks) followed by surgery and a possible course of taxanes postdelivery. It was likely that surgery would involve a right modified radical mastectomy and immediate breast reconstruction could be offered in the postpartum period.
2. Proceed with mastectomy within three- to four-weeks time and prescribe chemotherapy as adjuvant treatment. The patient could subsequently undergo delayed breast reconstruction at a later date.

Treatment and Progress

The patient expressed some reluctance about receiving chemotherapy during pregnancy, but was reassured that there was no evidence for any detrimental effects on the fetus when chemotherapy is given during the second or third trimester (when organogenesis is complete). The patient enquired about the possibility of undergoing primary surgery and delaying chemotherapy until after the birth of her child. It was pointed out that any significant delay in commencing chemotherapy might impact on overall survival. It was suggested that adjuvant chemotherapy, should this be required, could be given in the third trimester. This could be followed by early induction and safe delivery of the baby and completion of chemotherapy thereafter.

After much detailed discussion, including the possibility of breast-conserving surgery after any downstaging by neoadjuvant chemotherapy, the patient opted for primary surgery with a modified radical mastectomy and level II axillary lymph node dissection (level III axillary dissection if evidence of extensive nodal disease at the time of surgery). Surgery was planned for the beginning of the second trimester and a dating scan was carried out at 12 weeks. There were no fetal complications and the patient made an uneventful recovery from surgery. She had a normal full term delivery at 39 weeks.

Definitive Histology

This revealed a grade II invasive ductal carcinoma measuring 15 mm in maximum diameter (Fig. 3A). There was associated DCIS but this did not extend beyond the

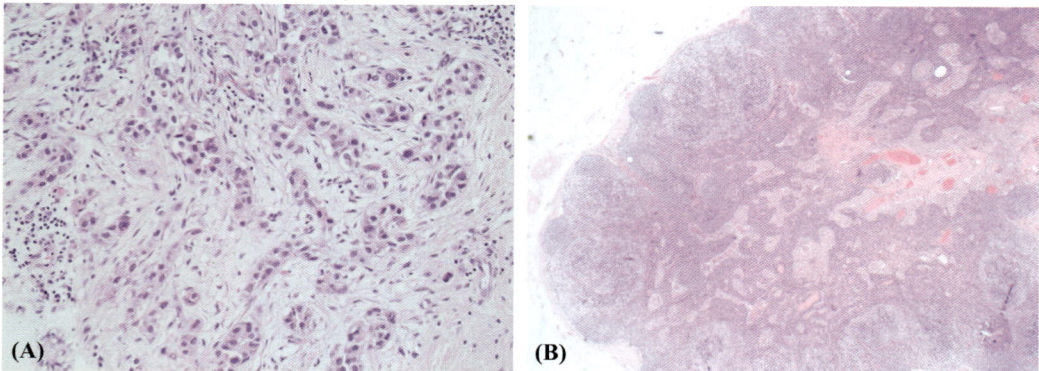

(A)   (B)

Figure 3

invasive component. Lymphovascular invasion was not present and none of the 28 nodes contained metastatic tumor (Fig. 3B).

Multidisciplinary Review 2

The final pathological tumor size was much less than the clinical and sonographic estimate. The calculated NPI was $[0.2 \times 1.5] + 2 + 1 = 3.30$ and the patient would receive an absolute benefit from chemotherapy of <3%. It was therefore recommended that she receive tamoxifen as adjuvant systemic hormonal therapy and ovarian suppression should be discussed (ER-positive tumor).

Treatment and Progress

The patient declined tamoxifen and did not want any form of ovarian suppression. She subsequently become pregnant for a second time and has recently given birth to a second healthy child almost three years after her initial cancer diagnosis. She remains well and will undergo biennial mammography of the contralateral breast until the age of 50 years when she will enter the NHS Breast Screening Programme.

Discussion

It is estimated that pregnancy-associated breast cancer has an incidence of approximately 3% and about 3 out of every 10,000 pregnant women are diagnosed with breast cancer (1). Increasing numbers of women are pursuing careers and deferring childbirth until the fourth or even fifth decade. Not only is this a likely contributory factor to the inexorable rise in incidence of breast cancer, but women will bear children at an age when breast cancer is much more common (2).

This 34-year-old professional woman was diagnosed with breast cancer during the first trimester of her pregnancy. This set of circumstances therefore intensified the emotional impact of a breast cancer diagnosis. Moreover, the lump had been present for almost two years and was previously investigated with an inadequate (C1) cytology specimen, which should have been repeated—or

a core biopsy undertaken. It is possible the patient was falsely reassured by these earlier investigations and did not seek further medical opinion despite persistence of the lump. It was the recent increase in size of the lump that had prompted a second opinion. Perhaps ironically, physiological changes in the breast during pregnancy can obscure a breast mass and cause significant delays (6–12 months) in diagnosis. This applies to both clinical assessment and mammography where the increased breast density and water content reduce the innate sensitivity. The patient was below the age threshold for symptomatic mammography (35 years) but pregnancy itself is not a contraindication to this mode of imaging provided that appropriate abdominal shielding is employed (3). However, many breast units rely exclusively on breast ultrasound examination that can be used to guide percutaneous tissue biopsy (4).

Management options for the pregnant patient with breast cancer can be complex (5); there are potentially two lives at risk with competing priorities for treatment programs. On the one hand the mother's breast cancer must be optimally managed to maximize survival outcome. On the other, the health and viability of the fetus must be preserved and not compromised by cancer treatments (6).

Therapeutic abortion should be considered during the first trimester. This patient presented at nine weeks with a "cherished" pregnancy and adamantly refused to contemplate termination. The options of primary chemotherapy versus primary surgery were discussed and it was explained that there was no evidence for any overall survival difference in the absence of a complete pathological response to induction chemotherapy. The patient was particularly averse to receiving chemotherapy during pregnancy (7,8) and opted for primary surgery with a modified radical mastectomy. No complications were reported among a group of 24 patients treated mainly during the second and third trimesters of pregnancy with 5-fluorouracil, cyclophosphamide, and doxorubicin (4 cycles) (7). If chemotherapy must be given during the first trimester, it is preferable to consider termination. Sentinel lymph node biopsy was not undertaken to avoid the possibility of a delayed axillary dissection. However, there are no documented adverse side effects from injections of radiocolloid or blue dye. The tumor size and grade justified the decision to undertake axillary dissection (>50% chance of nodal involvement with a 37 mm grade III invasive ductal carcinoma in a patient under 40 years of age). Interestingly, the final histology was somewhat discordant with the preoperative assessment; not only was the tumor size less than half the sonographic estimate, but the tumor was downgraded from III to II. The patient had a favorable prognostic index (NPI 3.30) and any benefits from chemotherapy would have been minimal (<3%). Therefore any discussions of possible delayed adjuvant chemotherapy became irrelevant. Despite having a hormonally sensitive tumor, the patient declined both tamoxifen and ovarian suppression and had a further successful pregnancy. In view of this patient's relatively young age and hormone-sensitive tumor, a two-year course of an luteinising hormone releasing hormone (LHRH) agonist immediately following the birth of her first child would have been a reasonable treatment option and may have permitted a subsequent pregnancy (9). Had the patient been at higher risk of relapse, she may have accepted this endocrine option.

When a first trimester pregnancy continues to term, there are potential concerns about the effect of the hormonal milieu of pregnancy (oestrogen friendly) on dormant breast cancer cells, which may persist after surgery. Studies have not revealed any statistically significant differences in 5- and 10-year survival figures for pregnant women compared with stage-matched nonpregnant counterparts. Furthermore, pregnancy subsequent to breast cancer treatment does not have any deleterious impact on recurrence and survival (10,11).

Related Cases

Pregnancy and breast cancer—*Case Studies 36 and 37*

Modified radical mastectomy—*Case Studies 1, 2, and 36*

Adjuvant hormonal therapy—*Case Studies 1, 4, 9, 10, 15, and 19*

Learning Points

1. Although surgery is generally safe during pregnancy, the anesthesia may pose a small risk to the fetus. Therefore, the surgeon, obstetrician, and anesthesiologist should work together to ensure a safe outcome.

2. Radiotherapy is contraindicated during pregnancy, so some surgeons maintain that breast-conserving surgery (which requires radiotherapy) should be avoided during early pregnancy. For women diagnosed with breast cancer late in pregnancy, breast-conserving surgery might be feasible because radiotherapy can be delayed until after delivery of the baby.

3. Most of the internal organs of the fetus develop during the first trimester of pregnancy, so chemotherapy should not be administered during this period.

4. The effects of hormone therapy in pregnant women are largely unknown, but there have been reports linking tamoxifen usage with birth defects.

References

1. Fiorica JV. Special problems. Breast cancer and pregnancy. Obstet Gynecol Clin North Am 1994; 21:721–732.
2. Osteen RT. Unusual presentations of breast cancer. In: Jatoi I, ed. Manual of Breast Diseases. PhiladelphiaLippincott, Wilkins & Williams: 2002:353–364.
3. Liberman L, Geiss C, Dershaw D, et al. Imaging of pregnancy-associated breast cancer. Radiology 1994; 191:245–248.
4. Gupta R, McHutchinson A, Dowle C, et al. Fine-needle aspiration cytodiagnosis of breast masses in pregnant and lactating women and its impact on management. Diagn Cytopathol 1993; 9:156–159.
5. Clark RM, Chua T. Breast cancer and pregnancy: the ultimate challenge. Clin Oncol 1989; 1:11.
6. Theriault RL. Breast cancer during pregnancy. In: Singletary SE, Robb GL, eds. Advanced Therapy of Breast Disease. Ontario: BC Decker Inc., 2000: 167–173.
7. Berry DL, Theriault RL, Holmes FA, et al. Management of breast cancer during pregnancy using a standardized protocol. J Clin Oncol 1999; 17: 855–861.
8. Doll DC, Ringenberg QS, Yarbro JW. Antineoplastic agents and pregnancy. Semin Oncol 1989; 16:337–346.

9. Jakesz R, Hausmaninger H, Samonigg E, et al. Comparison of adjuvant therapy with tamoxifen and goserelin versus CMF in premenopausal stage I and II hormone responsive breast cancer patients: 4 year results of Austrian Breast Cancer Study Group (ABCSG) Trial 5. Proc Am Soc Clin Oncol 1999; 18:67a(abstr 250).

10. Danforth DN. How subsequent pregnancy affects outcome in women with a prior breast cancer. Oncology 1991; 5:23–30.
11. Petrek JA, Dukoff R, Rogatko A. Prognosis of pregnancy-associated breast cancer. Cancer 1991; 67:869–872.

Part II: Third Trimester Pregnancy

CASE STUDY 36

History

A 33-year-old woman presented with a two-week history of a lump in the left breast. She was 36-weeks pregnant with her first child and had noticed a distinctive difference in the consistency of her left breast but no episodes of redness or unusual nipple discharge. There were no previous breast problems and no family history of breast or ovarian cancer.

Clinical Findings

A firm and irregular, though ill-defined mass was palpable in the central zone of the left breast. This measured approximately 4 cm in diameter and was not associated with skin tethering, erythema, or peau d'orange. There was no axillary lymphadenopathy (E4) (Fig. 4).

Clinical Assessment

Clinically suspicious lump in a pregnant patient with no evidence of any inflammatory features.

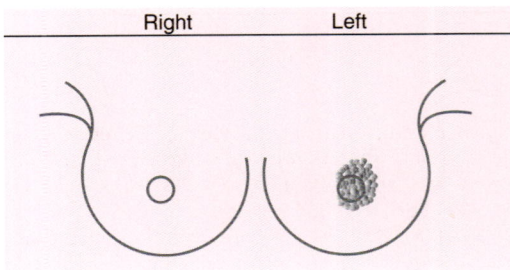

Figure 4

Investigations

Breast Ultrasound

This showed the normal physiological changes of pregnancy with prominent duct dilatation. An echo-poor lesion measuring 2 cm was apparent in the centre of the left breast lying close to the chest wall. This was suspicious for carcinoma (U4). Ultrasound measurement may have underestimated the true size of the tumor that seemed at least twice this size on clinical examination (Fig. 5A, B).

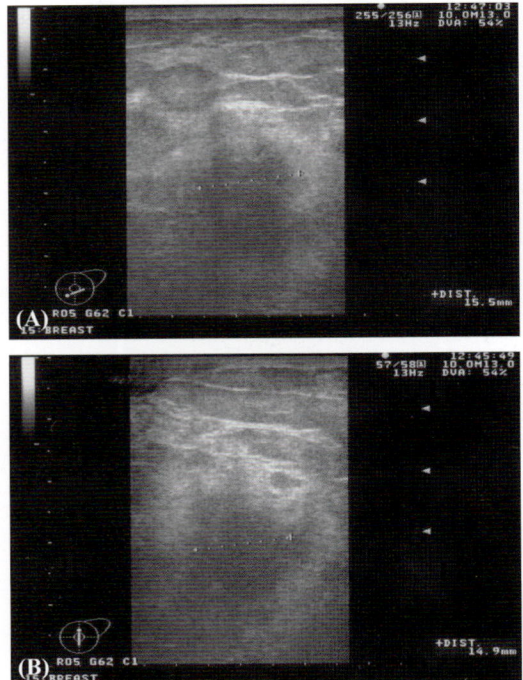

Figure 5

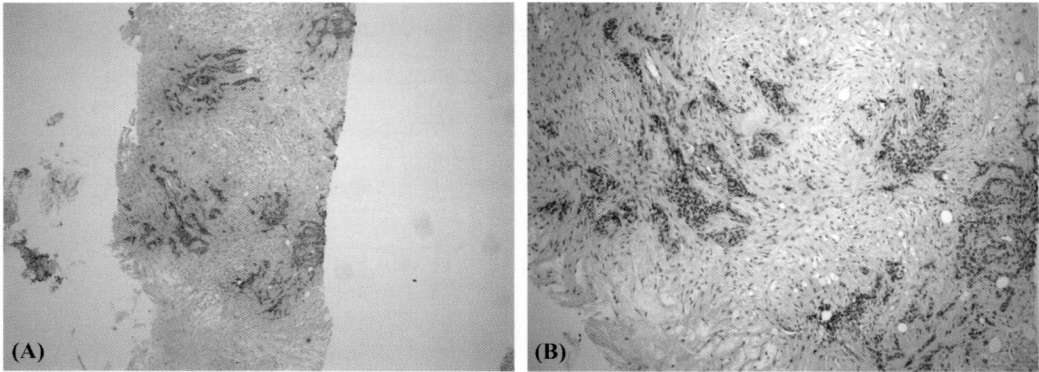

Figure 6

Core Biopsy

Ultrasound-guided core biopsy (14-gauge needle) of the central breast mass confirmed an invasive carcinoma (grade II) with no in situ component [Fig. 6A (low power) and B (high power)]. Immunohistochemical staining for both estrogen receptor (ER) and progesterone receptor (PR) was negative.

Diagnosis

Early-stage noninflammatory left-sided breast cancer in the third trimester of pregnancy (T1/T2N0).

Multidisciplinary Review 1

Following multidisciplinary discussion, it was recommended that the patient be induced at 38 weeks and primary surgery be performed shortly thereafter. The central location of the tumor mandated mastectomy and the patient expressed interest in immediate breast reconstruction. The patient would receive adjuvant chemotherapy on the basis of primary tumor characteristics (2 cm size, hormone receptor negative) and patient's age irrespective of final nodal status. It was considered unlikely that chest wall radiotherapy would be required and this was communicated to the plastic surgeons. The patient's gravida status prevented use of MRI to clarify the extent of the tumor in the left breast (discordance between clinical and sonographic measurements).

Treatment and Progress

The patient was referred to the plastic surgeons for further discussion of reconstructive options and the relevant midwife was contacted and informed of the diagnosis and management plan. The patient expressed some concerns over the longevity of breast implants and preferred a totally autologous reconstruction with a possible free TRAM flap. The plastic surgeons were reluctant to undertake the latter procedure so soon after delivery and considered a delayed reconstruction to be more appropriate if this type was the preferred option.

The patient decided against immediate breast reconstruction and underwent a left modified radical mastectomy two weeks after giving birth to a healthy baby son (Fig. 7). The patient made an excellent recovery with no complications and was discharged home on the fourth postoperative day following removal of both drains.

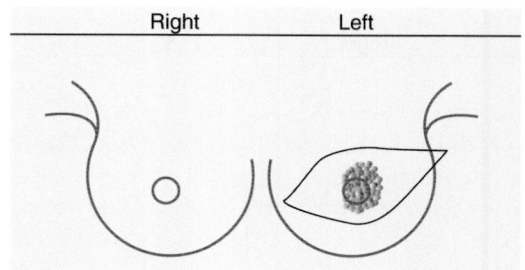

Figure 7

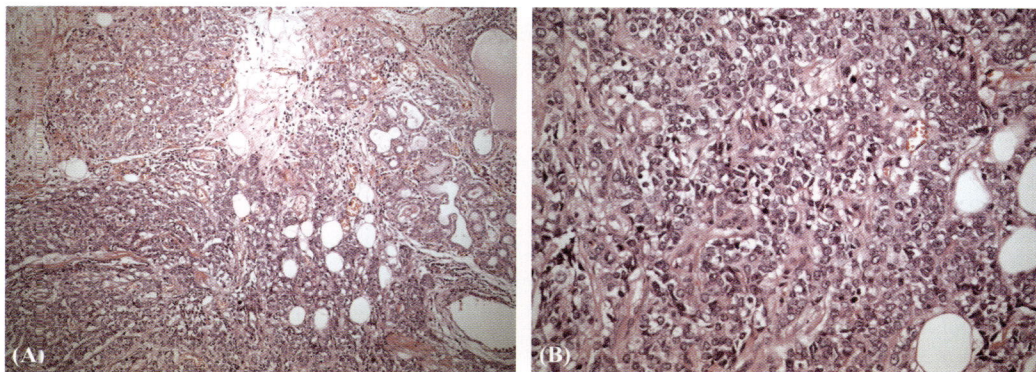

Figure 8

Definitive Histology

This revealed a grade III invasive ductal carcinoma measuring 35 mm in maximum diameter with no in situ component or lymphovascular invasion [Fig. 8A (magnification 10×) and B (magnification 20×)]. The lesion extended to within 1.7 mm of the deep margin, but was otherwise clear of all radial margins by more than 20 mm. None of the 10 lymph nodes retrieved contained metastatic carcinoma.

Multidisciplinary Review 1

Adjuvant chemotherapy was recommended and the patient was eligible for entry into the TANGO trial. This is a randomized phase III trial to determine whether sequential epirubicin (E) and cyclophosphamide (C) (4 cycles) followed by paclitaxel (T) and gemcitabine improves disease-free survival compared with EC-T alone. Women are eligible for entry into the trial who have early-stage breast cancer, but are at higher risk of relapse. She would otherwise receive standard chemotherapy with eight cycles of E-CMF (4 cycles of epirubicin followed by four cycles of cyclophosphamide, methotrexate, and 5-fluorouracil) (see Appendix III). There was no indication for either tamoxifen or ovarian suppression in view of the lack of hormonal receptor expression (<10% of cells stained). Though the tumor was grade III, it was below the size threshold for chest wall radiotherapy in the absence of lymphovascular invasion, involvement of the deep margin or regional nodal involvement.

Treatment and Progress

The patient agreed to enter the TANGO trial and received four cycles of epirubicin/cyclophosphamide followed by four cycles of paclitaxel plus gemcitabine. She experienced some side effects including nausea and vomiting (worse with gemcitabine), neurosensory symptoms (grade I), fatigue, myalgia, and arthalgia. Though the latter were temporary and resolved spontaneously, the patient required a course of a nonsteroidal anti-inflammatory agent for symptom control.

The patient subsequently underwent a delayed reconstruction with a free TRAM flap and was delighted with the final results of reconstructive surgery (Fig. 9).

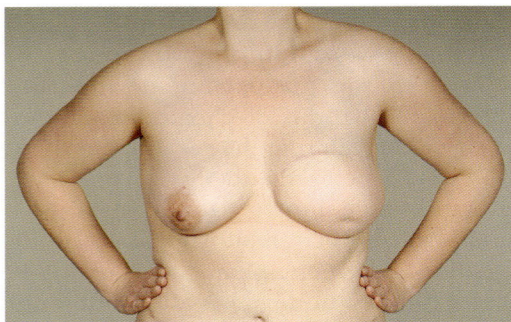

Figure 9

Discussion

This 33-year-old woman was diagnosed with a large tumor in the third trimester of her first pregnancy. The physiological changes within the breast associated with pregnancy may have obscured the mass and delayed initial presentation (1,2). Most breast cancers have been present for several years prior to clinical detection and this patient most likely had a subclinical breast cancer for much of the duration of her pregnancy. Neither clinical examination (E4) or sonographic assessment were diagnostic of breast cancer. Ultrasound can be useful in differentiating discrete solid from cystic lesions and in particular for diagnosing breast cancer against the physiologically altered parenchyma of pregnancy (3). Moreover, ultrasound can provide a confident diagnosis of mastitis when small fluid collections and dilated ducts are present. Nonetheless, a biopsy is required to definitively exclude or confirm an inflammatory cancer (4). Furthermore, the tumor margins were poorly defined on imaging with lack of concordance between the ultrasound measurement and the pathological tumor size.

Definitive treatment of third trimester breast cancers is usually deferred until after induction at, or around, 38 weeks. This removes many of the restrictions on treatment that may apply to women who are concurrently pregnant. Radiotherapy is absolutely contraindicated and cannot be administered during any stage of pregnancy due to fetal radiation exposure (5). Though the effects of radiation on the fetus are greatest during the first trimester, these persist throughout the second and third trimesters when there are risks of sterility/malignancy and radiotherapy must be delayed to the postpartum period (6). Though most forms of chemotherapy can be given safely during the second and third trimesters when organogenesis and limb formation is complete, there remains a small risk of fetal malformation (1.5%) together with spontaneous abortion. It is preferable to undertake all treatments after delivery of the baby if possible, but this may impact on overall survival of the mother. Delays of adjuvant chemotherapy for more than three months from the time of diagnosis have been reported to decrease eight-year relapse-free survival from 77% to 44% (7). For second trimester breast cancers, there would be significant delays in active treatments if the latter were deferred until postdelivery. Both surgery as well as chemotherapy can be safely undertaken after 12 weeks and the longer-term survival of the mother should not be compromised unnecessarily.

The patient had a centrally located tumor measuring 4 cm clinically that precluded breast conservation. Moreover, mastectomy would still be necessary in the event of a response to neoadjuvant chemotherapy. Primary surgical treatment with modified radical mastectomy was considered the most appropriate management option; a level II axillary lymph node dissection was undertaken on the basis of primary tumor size (rather than to avoid any delayed axillary lymph node dissection). There was some discordance between the clinical and sonographic estimates of tumor size and it was not possible to undertake MRI examination to further evaluate tumor dimensions. There are concerns that sentinel lymph node biopsy may be less accurate for tumors exceeding 3 cm in size (8) and trials are ongoing to assess the value of sentinel lymph node biopsy for tumors between 3 and 5 cm in size (9).

Though the patient was keen to undergo immediate breast reconstruction, she preferred to have a free TRAM flap and avoid any implant. The plastic surgeons thought it inappropriate to undertake such a major procedure so soon after delivery. A delayed reconstruction was therefore planned and the patient underwent a conventional mastectomy with an oblique scar on the chest wall. This would remain a nonirradiated field, thus favouring elevation of tissues from the chest wall and subsequent reconstruction. Interestingly, it has been reported that a delayed postpartum TRAM can safely be performed with maintenance of abdominal wall integrity that can withstand the strain of any future pregnancy (10).

The patient was very pleased with the final results of delayed reconstruction (Fig. 9).

Related Cases

Pregnancy and breast cancer—*Case Studies 35 and 37*

Adjuvant chemotherapy—*Case Studies 3, 6, 8, 11, and 37*

Breast reconstruction—*Case Studies 3, 4, 16, 17, and 18*

Learning Points

1. During pregnancy, hormone changes cause the breast to enlarge and become more glandular and tender. These changes may make it difficult to detect a malignant breast lump on clinical examination.

2. Several studies have now shown that certain chemotherapeutic agents can be safely administered during the second and third trimesters of pregnancy (with no increased risk of stillbirths or birth defects). However, the long-term effects of these drugs on the fetus is not known so, if possible, chemotherapy should be administered after delivery.

3. Chemotherapy lowers blood counts and should not be administered within three to four weeks before delivery. Chemotherapy administered during this period may cause bleeding or increase the risk of infection during the perinatal period.

References

1. Anderson BO, Petrek JA, Byrd D, et al. Pregnancy influences breast cancer's stage at diagnosis in women 30 years of age and younger. Ann Surg Oncol 1996; 3:204–211.
2. Noyes RD, Spanos WJ, Montague ED. Breast cancer in women aged 30 and under. Cancer 1982; 49:1302–1307.
3. Frazier TG, Murphy JT, Furlong A. The selected use of ultrasound to improve diagnostic accuracy in carcinoma of the breast. J Surg Oncol 1985; 29:231–232.
4. Hayes R, Mitchell M, Nunnerley HB. Acute inflammation of the breast: the role of breast ultrasound in diagnosis and management. Clin Radiol 1991; 44:253–256.
5. The Steering Committee on Clinical Practice Guidelines for the care and Treatment of Breast Cancer. Breast radiotherapy after breast conserving surgery. CMAJ1998; 158:S35–S42.
6. Brent RL. The effects of embryonic and fetal exposure to X-ray, microwaves and ultrasound. Clin Obstet 1983; 26:484–510.
7. Brufman G, Sulkes A, Biran S. Adjuvant chemotherapy with and without radiotherapy in stage II breast cancer. Biomed Pharmacother 1988; 42:351–355.
8. Benson JR, Querci della Rovere G. Management of the axilla in women with breast cancer. Lancet Oncol 2007; 8:331–348.
9. Gill PG. Sentinel lymph node biopsy versus axillary clearance in operable breast cancer. The RACS SNAC trial, a Multicenter randomized trial of the Royal Australian College of Surgeons (RACS) Section of Breast Surgery, in collaboration with the National Health and Medical Research Council Clinical Trials Center. Ann Surg Oncol 2004; 11:216S–221S.
10. Parodi PC, Osti M, Longhi P, et al. Pregnancy and TRAM flap breast reconstruction after mastectomy: a case report. Scand J Plast Reconstr Surg Hand Surg 2001; 35:211–215.

CASE STUDY 37

History

A 43-year-old woman presented in the 35th week of pregnancy with a four-month history of a lump in the right breast. The lump was nontender with no associated nipple discharge. There was a weak family history of breast cancer with a maternal and paternal aunt having postmenopausal breast cancer. The patient had five other children aged between 18 months and 18 years and was 25 years of age at the time of birth of her first child. She had used the oral contraceptive

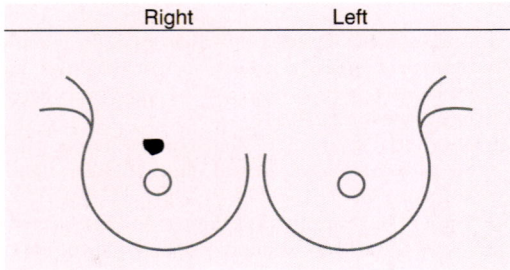

Figure 10

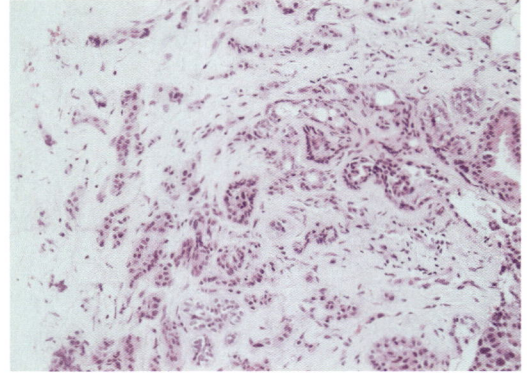

Figure 11

pill for a cumulative period of five years in the past.

Clinical Findings

Examination revealed a smooth mobile lump in the upper outer quadrant of the right breast that had a slightly irregular surface. There was no skin tethering or axillary lymphadenopathy (E3) (Fig. 10).

Clinical Assessment

A clinically indeterminate lump in a pregnant patient.

Investigations

Breast Ultrasound

This showed a cyst in the upper outer quadrant of the right breast measuring 35 mm in maximum diameter. The cyst was aspirated to dryness (non-bloodstained fluid), but a residual lump remained. This appeared sonographically to be a focus of dense breast tissue, but core biopsy was performed as a precaution.

The patient was informed that the findings were consistent with benign disease. She was to return in one week's time for results of core biopsy and arrangements were made for a mammogram to be done postdelivery.

Core Biopsy

Ultrasound-guided core biopsy (14-gauge needle) of the right breast mass confirmed an invasive carcinoma (grade I, ER positive[a], HER2 negative) with no in situ component (Fig. 11).

Diagnosis

Early-stage right-sided breast cancer presenting in the third trimester of pregnancy (T2N0).

Multidisciplinary Review 1

Following histological diagnosis of a right breast cancer, it was recommended that the baby be delivered within the next two weeks and the patient thereafter undergo surgery. Further radiological investigations were requested postdelivery to clarify the extent of disease in the breast and exclude multifocality.

1. Mammography—This revealed moderately dense breast tissue with no focal breast lesion.
2. Breast MRI—This showed the right breast tumor to be more extensive than the original estimate from ultrasound examination alone. The main index lesion in the upper outer quadrant

---

[a] Allred score 7/8.

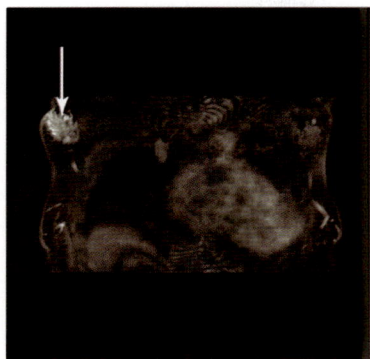

Figure 12

measured 25 mm with several satellite foci yielding an aggregate diameter of 37 mm. In addition, a further enhancing lesion measuring 8 mm in diameter was seen in the retroareolar region. Figure 12 is a coronal MRI section showing a tumour in the upper outer quadrant of the right breast (cardiac artefact is apparent in this relatively early MRI image).

The multifocal nature of the breast cancer mandated mastectomy, but the patient would be eligible for sentinel lymph node biopsy.

Treatment and Progress

The patient was induced at 37 weeks and delivered a healthy child. She had expressed an interest in immediate breast reconstruction on being informed that mastectomy was necessary. Various reconstructive options were discussed with the plastic surgeons and the patient elected to undergo reconstruction with a subpectoral implant only.

She underwent sentinel lymph node biopsy in advance of definitive surgery shortly after giving birth. She was advised to discontinue breastfeeding after sentinel node biopsy, but in the interim period could continue. It was not considered appropriate to be breastfeeding at the time of mastectomy and immediate breast reconstruction.

Sentinel lymph node biopsy was undertaken three weeks postdelivery and showed metastatic involvement in one out of four sentinel nodes [macrometastases (4 mm)] [Fig. 13A (low power) and B (high power)]. The patient proceeded to a right mastectomy with axillary lymph node dissection and immediate breast reconstruction two weeks later. She made an uneventful postoperative recovery.

Definitive Histology

This revealed a grade II invasive ductal carcinoma measuring 42 mm in maximum diameter. There was associated DCIS extending beyond the invasive component yielding a total size of 54 mm [Fig. 14A (magnification 20×) and B (magnification 40×)]. None of the 10 lymph nodes retrieved from completion axillary lymph node dissection contained metastatic carcinoma giving an overall nodal status of 1 out of 14 nodes (1 out of 4 sentinel lymph nodes positive).

Multidisciplinary Review 2

Following multidisciplinary discussion it was recommended that the patient proceed with adjuvant chemotherapy (standard regimen

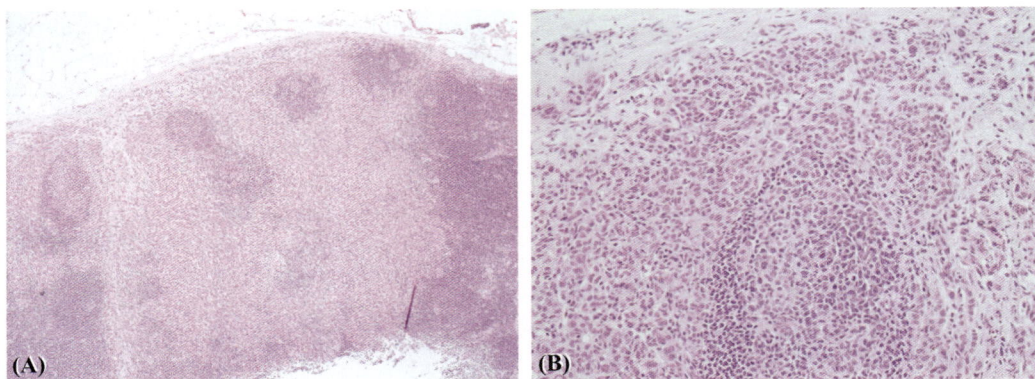

(A)

(B)

Figure 13

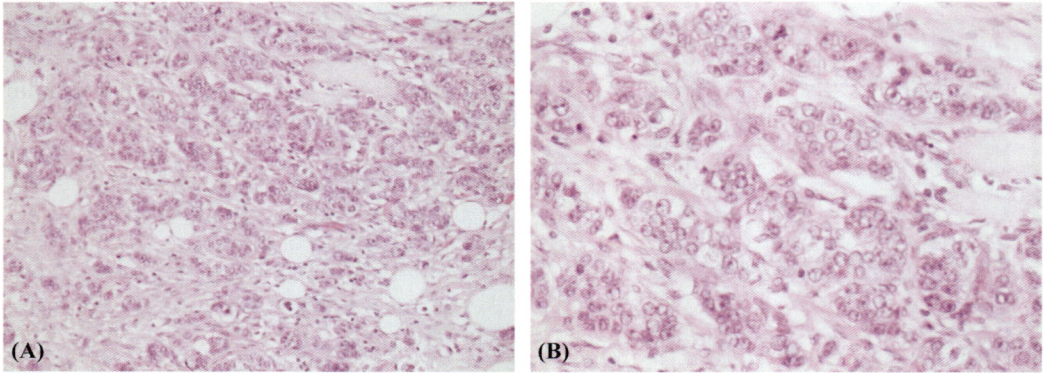

(A)

(B)

Figure 14

of E-CMF—see Appendix III) and thereafter receive radiotherapy to the right chest wall. On completion of chemotherapy, hormonal manipulation would be undertaken in accordance with menopausal status. In view of the patient's age (>40 years), it was likely that she would be rendered postmenopausal by chemotherapy and formal ovarian suppression would be inappropriate. In the event that menses persisted, resumed, or luteinising hormone/follicle stimulating hormone levels remained in the premenopausal range, ovarian ablation could be achieved either surgically by laparoscopic oophorectomy or chemically with an LHRH analogue (for 2–3 years). Irrespective of ovarian suppression, the patient would receive tamoxifen for five years as adjuvant systemic hormonal therapy. Emerging trial data suggest an overall survival benefit in node-positive patients for sequential hormonal therapy with tamoxifen (5 years) followed by the aromatase inhibitor letrozole (2.5 years). The patient's estimated 10-year disease-free survival without additional treatment was 64% and improved to 81% with systemic therapies (chemotherapy/hormonal therapy) (www.adjuvantonline.com).

The patient would receive radiotherapy to the chest wall upon completion of chemotherapy. She had one positive node only and therefore did not qualify for supraclavicular irradiation. Moreover, the patient was HER2 negative and therefore not eligible for Herceptin.

Treatment and Progress

The patient proceeded to chemotherapy with four cycles of epirubicin followed by four cycles of cyclophosphamide, methotrexate, and 5-fluorouracil (E-CMF). Initiation of chemotherapy was delayed by two weeks at the request of the plastic surgeons due to poor wound healing (minor infection). The patient developed profound neutropenia after the second cycle of chemotherapy (neutrophil count 0.8) and required granulocyte colony stimulating factor (GCSF) support. This indicated an extreme sensitivity to epirubicin and the dose for the third cycle of chemotherapy was reduced to 85%. Interestingly, the patient had a family history of neutropenia, but there was no evidence for any primary hereditary hematological abnormality. The neutropenia persisted and the chemotherapy schedule was changed from E-CMF to FEC (5 cycles of the latter).

The patient received a standard schedule of radiotherapy to the chest wall after completion of chemotherapy (commenced approximately 8 months after definitive surgery). This consisted of a total dose of 40 Gy delivered in 15 fractions over a three-week period.

The patient remained premenopausal and underwent laparoscopic oophorectomy 10 months after mastectomy and immediate breast reconstruction; shortly prior to this she had become amenorrheic while taking tamoxifen.

Discussion

This patient's breast cancer might easily have been missed on "triple assessment." She reported having a right breast lump for a period of four months and it remains unclear whether this was considered to be innocent by the patient herself. There was no suggestion that the lump had changed in size over this time period. The palpable mass in the right breast corresponded to a cyst measuring 35 mm; the residual mass post-aspiration was probably not palpable at presentation. Core biopsy was undertaken "as a precaution" and the area of biopsy was considered most likely to represent benign breast tissue. This biopsy yielded invasive carcinoma and a subsequent MRI examination revealed multifocality with an aggregate diameter of 37 mm. The patient therefore required a mastectomy and desired immediate breast reconstruction. Therapy commenced three weeks after delivery, which was induced at 37 weeks. Though sentinel lymph node biopsy was not contraindicated, a formal axillary lymph node dissection at the outset would have been reasonable based on the aggregate tumor size in the context of multifocality. The rationale for undertaking sentinel lymph node biopsy in advance of definitive mastectomy and reconstruction is to avoid a delayed axillary clearance after reconstructive surgery. This can be technically challenging when a latissimus dorsi flap has been used (not an issue in this case). This patient had a positive sentinel lymph node biopsy and proceeded to completion axillary lymph node dissection at the time of mastectomy and immediate breast reconstruction.

A potential disadvantage of immediate breast reconstruction is delay in commencing chemotherapy. Minor infection in the presence of an implant can lead to implant failure (and explantation) when the immune system is suppressed by chemotherapy. The standard adjuvant chemotherapy regimen for patients at average risk of relapse within the Cambridge Breast Unit and several other units within the United Kingdom is E-CMF. The rationale for using this regimen is based on results of two trials designed to specifically address the efficacy of epirubicin as adjuvant treatment for early-stage breast cancer (1). Epirubicin is a more popular anthracycline in Europe and a meta-analysis comparing epirubicin with doxorubicin in the metastatic setting showed the former to be equally efficacious but associated with fewer side effects. The National Epirubicin Adjuvant Trial (NEAT) compared four cycles of epirubicin followed by four cycles of CMF with six cycles of CMF alone. By contrast, the related Scottish Cancer Therapy Network Trial (BR9601) had a slightly amended regimen and compared the same with eight cycles of CMF alone every three weeks. The two trials combined involved more than 2000 patients and at a median follow up of 48 months, relapse free, and overall survival rates were significantly improved in the E-CMF than CMF alone groups. The calculated five-year relapse-free survival rates were 76% versus 69% ($p <$ 0.001) and overall survival rates 82% versus 75%, respectively. The hazard rates for relapse and death from any cause favored epirubicin schedules. This study is the most strongly positive among the few individual trials demonstrating an advantage for anthracycline-based chemotherapy. Moreover, it is anticipated that this schedule will not only prove more effective than dose dense 5-fluorouracil, epirubicin, and cyclophosphamide (FEC) but also be safer in the longer term. It is current policy to offer higher-risk (HER2 positive, $\geq$4 nodes positive) patients FEC-docetaxol as adjuvant chemotherapy (2).

Despite having six children already, this patient enquired about the possibility of a further pregnancy. She initially opted for ovarian suppression with the LHRH analogue with Zoladex for two years, which is potentially reversible. However, upon completion of Zoladex, the patient would be almost 47 years of age (and still remain on tamoxifen). It was considered highly unlikely that she would successfully conceive after completion of chemohormonal therapies. It should be noted that there is no clear evidence that any further pregnancy would increase the risk of breast cancer relapse and adversely influence long-term outcome (3).

This patient was node positive and therefore eligible for extended adjuvant hormonal therapy. Though more than three-quarters of recurrences occur within the first five years, late events do occur and patients remain at chronic risk of relapse. Dormant cancer stem cells can be "kick started" many years after primary treatment of breast cancer. The MA-17 trial randomized 5187 patients who were disease-free upon completion of five-years standard tamoxifen therapy to either letrozole (2.5 mg/day) or placebo for a further five years. All patients had started letrozole within three months of stopping tamoxifen. An interim analysis was carried out at a median follow up of 30 months when the number of events had exceeded a predetermined figure. These initial results showed a significant improvement in disease-free survival for those patients receiving extended adjuvant therapy with letrozole (HR 0.58; 95% CI, 0.45–0.75; $p = 0.0004$). In addition to a reduction in risk of recurrence by 42%, there was also a statistically significant decrease in distant metastases and an increase in overall survival in the node positive group (HR 0.61; $p = 0.04$). An updated analysis of this trial established letrozole as the first aromatase inhibitor to improve outcome after completion of five-years tamoxifen therapy (4). Indeed, the treatment effect was so strong that the trial was unblinded and letrozole was licensed for use as extended adjuvant endocrine therapy. An analysis of this trial post-unblinding revealed a significant improvement in several endpoints for women who switched to letrozole compared with continuation of placebo (5). These included (*i*) disease-free survival (HR 0.31; $p < 0.001$) (*ii*) distant disease-free survival (HR 0.28; $p < 0.002$) and (*iii*) overall survival (HR 0.53; $p < 0.05$). There was also a further reduction in contralateral breast cancer (HR 0.23; $p < 0.012$). Thus extended adjuvant endocrine treatment with letrozole can improve outcomes even when commenced

after a period without adjuvant hormonal therapy. However, this post-unblinding analysis was not based on randomized data and clearly the two arms were not balanced for patient and tumor characteristics. Those patients who were switched from placebo to letrozole were more likely to be younger patients with more aggressive node positive tumors and treated with prior chemotherapy. Thus the group who switched to letrozole from placebo had a greater risk of relapse and a worse prognosis, which has been cited as justification for the decision to unblind. Breast cancer patients remain at chronic risk of relapse, and reintroduction of endocrine therapy at any point along the pathway will improve outcomes. Dormant cancer cells can be activated or "kick started" many years after primary treatment of breast cancer. Examination of hazard rates for recurrence within the extended adjuvant endocrine setting of the MA-17 trial implies that there is a residual risk of recurrence in patients completing five years of tamoxifen. The hazard ratio for recurrence (letrozole:placebo) shows a trend to decrease over time and there is greater benefit from letrozole with more prolonged therapy (6).

Related Cases

Pregnancy and breast cancer—*Case Studies 35 and 36*

Ovarian suppression—*Case Studies 8, 23, and 27*

Fertility issues—*Case Study 23*

Postmastectomy radiotherapy after breast reconstruction—*Case Studies 3 and 18*

Adjuvant chemotherapy—*Case Studies 2, 3, 6, 8, 11, and 36*

Adjuvant hormonal therapy—*Case Studies 1, 4, 9, 10, 15, and 19*

Learning Points

1. Most chemotherapeutic and endocrine therapy agents can enter breast milk and be passed on to the newborn infant. Therefore, if a woman is receiving

chemotherapy or endocrine therapy, she should not breast-feed her baby.

2. During the first seven to nine years following breast cancer diagnosis, women with ER-negative tumors are at greater risk for relapse than those with ER-positive tumors. Thereafter, the risk of relapse is greater for patients with ER-positive tumors. Thus, extended endocrine therapy should be considered for women with node-positive ER-positive tumors as these women are at increased risk for relapse many years after initial breast cancer diagnosis.

References

1. Poole CJ, Earl HM, Dunn JA, et al. For the NEAT and SCTBG Investigators. NEAT (National Epirubicin Adjuvant Trial) and SCTBG BR9601 (Scottish Cancer Trials Breast Group) phase III adjuvant breast trials show significant relapse-free and overall survival advantage for sequential E-CMF. Proc Am Soc Clin Oncol 2003; 22:(abstr 13).

2. Dang CT, Moynahan ME, Dickler MN, et al. Phase II study of dose-dense (DD) 5-fluorouracil, epirubicin and cyclophosphamide followed by alternating weekly paclitaxel (P) and docetaxel (D) in high risk node positive breast cancer: feasibility and efficacy. Proc Am Soc Clin Oncol 2003; 22:(abstr 46).

3. Von Schoultz E, et al. Influence of prior and subsequent pregnancy on breast cancer prognosis. J Clin Oncol 1995; 13:430–434.

4. Goss PE, Ingle JN, Martino S, et al. Randomised trial of letrozole in postmenopausal women after five years of tamoxifen therapy for early stage breast cancer. N Engl J Med 2003; 349:1793–1802.

5. Goss PE, Ingle JN, Palmer MJ, et al. Updated analysis of NCIC CTG MA.17 (letrozole vs placebo to letrozole vs placebo) post unblinding. Breast Cancer Res Treat 2005; 94:S10(abstr 16).

6. Ingle JN, Goss PE, Tu D, et al. Analysis of duration of letrozole extended adjuvant therapy as measured by hazard ratios of disease recurrence over time for patients on NCIC CTG MA.17. Breast Cancer Res Treat 2005; 94:S11(abstr 17).

Prophylactic Mastectomy 12

Part I: Bilateral Prophylactic Mastectomy

History

A 31-year-old woman was referred by the Clinical Genetics Department for discussion of bilateral prophylactic mastectomy. The patient's mother and maternal grandmother both developed breast cancer at 33 and 39 years of age, respectively, and the patient herself was increasingly conscious that she was approaching this age. In addition, to these two relatives, the patient's family history included two maternal great aunts with postmenopausal disease and a maternal grandfather with prostate cancer. Though familial cancer history was incompletely documented, the patients estimated lifetime risk for development of breast cancer was 80% to 85%. There was a high probability of either BRCA-1 or BRCA-2 mutation carriage and genetic testing of the patient's mother and sister was pending at the time of referral. In particular, the patient understood that in the absence of any gene mutation, her risk of developing breast cancer was comparable to an age-matched population. She was keen to pursue prophylactic surgery without information from formal genetic testing (though both the patient and her sister were subsequently confirmed to carry a BRCA-2 gene mutation). This was a carefully considered decision by the patient who had a very balanced and informed point of view. She was a single parent and rather preoccupied with the risk of developing breast cancer and the possible impact on her child. The patient wished to minimize her risk and was provided with quantitative information on risk reduction from prophylactic surgery.

The patient was otherwise fit and healthy; she had undergone excision of a fibroadenoma from the left breast a few years ago. She had one daughter aged four years who was breast-fed and used the oral contraceptive pill for a cumulative period of five years.

Clinical Findings

Examination revealed no discrete or dominant lumps in either breast and no areas of focal nodularity. There was no axillary lymphadenopathy.

Investigations

1. Breast ultrasound—imaging of the breasts with ultrasound was normal (patient too young for mammography) (U1).
2. MRI breasts—normal.
3. Genetic testing—BRCA-2 carrier.

Treatment and Progress

The patient proceeded to bilateral prophylactic surgery almost 12 months after her initial consultation in the breast clinic. By this time, she had received confirmation of BRCA mutation carriage and this strengthened her conviction and provided objective evidence for risk reduction from prophylactic surgery. The patient had discussed reconstructive options with the plastic surgeons and was not keen on autologous tissue transfer. She had smallish-sized breasts and was suitable for an implant-only based technique. Skin-sparing mastectomy was performed without nipple preservation and bilateral subpectoral tissue expanders were inserted at the time of mastectomy. The central defect resulting from excision of the nipple-areolar complex was closed with a transverse incision rather than a purse-string suture (no skin island imported from an autologous tissue flap). The patient made an excellent postoperative recovery and the implants were gradually expanded over the course of the next four to six weeks via a subcutaneous port.

The patient was reviewed in the clinic two weeks following discharge and was relieved to be informed that histological examination of the resected breast tissue had revealed no evidence of hyperplasia, atypia, or malignancy.

Discussion

This patient had both a strong family history of breast cancer and a confirmed mutation in a known breast cancer susceptibility gene (BRCA-2). Though many individuals may possess a relative with breast cancer, only a minority of cases (5–10%) have an autosomally dominant pattern of inheritance consistent with vertical transmission of a high-risk genetic predisposition from one generation to another. The level of genetic risk and probability of carriage of a mutation in a recognized gene is determined by an individual's family cancer history. Contemporary methods of clinical risk assessment involve accurate ascertainment of information relating to the following points:

1. Number of first- and second-degree relatives with cancer—though the history should focus on breast/ovarian cancer, details of other familial malignancies should be sought to identify possible "cancer syndromes." Furthermore, information should be collated from both maternal and paternal relatives. Breast cancer can be inherited through the paternal lineage and cases may be confined to this side of the family.

2. The age at diagnosis (not death) of each affected relative—early-onset breast cancer is arbitrarily defined as development of disease among relatives under the age of 40 years. This patient's mother and maternal grandmother were diagnosed with breast cancer at 33 and 39 years, respectively. It was partly for this reason that the patient wished to pursue a specific interventional procedure around the age of 31 years.

3. Bilateral breast cancer—an inherited genetic predisposition affects all somatic cells and within this setting bilaterality is much more likely to occur than among sporadic cases.

The normal lifetime risk for breast cancer is approximately 10% (1 in 10 women affected). A method termed linkage analysis was previously used to calculate lifetime risk for development of breast cancer based on information from family cancer history (as above). For some individuals the estimated lifetime risk was of the order 80% to 90%, i.e. they were almost certain to suffer the disease assuming they lived for a reasonable period of time and did not succumb from any competing cause of death. This hereditary predisposition is conferred by cancer susceptibility genes, which conform to Knudson's model or "two-hit hypothesis" (1,2). Thus, mutations in both alleles of a gene pair are a prerequisite for cancer development. Individuals with an inherited predisposition already possessed a mutation in one allele (present in all cells) and thus required only one further somatic mutation for tumor formation. Sporadic forms of the cancer were dependent on two somatic mutations, the chances of which were correspondingly smaller for any equivalent mutation rate. Knudson's hypothesis is especially applicable to those tumors arising from loss of function in tumor suppressor genes; usually inactivation of both alleles is essential before levels of the gene product fall sufficiently to induce malignant change. The breast cancer susceptibility genes BRCA-1 and BRCA-2 are tumor suppressor genes located on chromosomes 17q21 and 13q12, respectively and display an autosomal dominant pattern of inheritance with variable penetrance (3,4). Mutations within these two genes account for approximately three-quarters of hereditary breast cancer cases and confer a lifetime risk of 80% to 85% by age 70 years (i.e., a 10-fold increase). At the cellular level, the effects of BRCA-1 and BRCA-2 are recessive and both copies of an allele must be lost or mutated for cancer progression. Individuals with a germline mutation in these genes have a dominantly inherited susceptibility and the second "hit" occurs in the somatic copy. Tumors from genetically predisposed patients show loss of heterozygosity in the wild-type BRCA-1 allele, but interestingly mutations of BRCA-1 and BRCA-2 are uncommon in sporadic breast cancers (5,6).

Other genes involved in genetic predisposition to breast cancer include p53 (Li-Fraumeni syndrome) (7), AT (ataxia-telangiectasia, and PTEN (breast and thyroid cancer) (8). These high-risk genes only account for 2% of all breast cancers. The majority of family clusters are not attributable to any of these high-risk susceptibility genes and attention has recently turned to "low risk" genes such as FGFR2 and TNCR9, which may collectively be responsible for up to 25% of familial breast cancer overall.

Mutations within the mid portion of the BRCA-1 gene are associated with breast and ovarian cancer as opposed to breast cancer–specific disease. The overall risk of ovarian cancer for patients with a BRCA-1 mutation is between 20% and 40% (9). A single relative with both breast and ovarian cancer is sufficient to raise suspicion of a BRCA-1 gene mutation within a family in the absence of any other affected members. Similarly, BRCA-2 mutations are linked to male breast cancer and prostate cancer (10). Sometimes there are few female members within a family and this can conceal the clinical manifestation of any underlying genetic predisposition. It is also recognized that sporadic tumors can occur within families that harbor a known BRCA-1 or BRCA-2 gene mutation. This phenomenon of "phenocopy" can lead to overestimation of genetic risk, particularly if a mutation in these genes has yet to be identified.

The discovery and subsequent cloning of the breast cancer genes BRCA-1 and BRCA-2

has spawned demand for genetic testing. However, mutations within these two genes are relatively uncommon in sporadic forms of breast cancer and in consequence the prevalence within the population is only of the order 0.001% (11). The proportion of hereditary cancers is much higher in certain population groups such as the Ashkenazi Jews, where "founder" mutations are common (12). Genetic testing for BRCA-1 and BRCA-2 are therefore only relevant in a small percentage of individuals who belong to families with "hereditary" breast cancer. Within the United Kingdom, genetic testing is only undertaken after formal risk evaluation by clinical geneticists—it is not available "on demand." At least 300 different mutations have been found for each of these genes and genetic testing must screen for all the known mutations as well as searching for any potential "new" mutation for that family. Once a mutation has been characterized, it is easier to then screen other relatives for this specific change in nucleotide sequence. It is possible that no mutation will be found after exhaustive testing which can be frustrating for individuals who come from families where there is clearly a strong history of breast/ovarian cancer. Genetic testing is expensive ($2,500) and it is not feasible to carry out blanket screening of all interested women (13). Where "founder" mutations are present, genetic testing is easier and cheaper. The American Society of Clinical Oncology has issued guidelines for breast cancer predisposition testing, and the following criteria must be fulfilled:

- The individual has a strong family history of cancer and/or early age of onset.
- The test can be adequately interpreted.
- The results will guide management decisions for the patient or other family members (14).

A great advantage of genetic testing is provision of accurate risk quantitation. Once a mutation has been identified for a particular family, those members who test negative have no increased risk of developing breast cancer than an age-matched individual from the general population (no specific surveillance or treatment is indicated). By contrast, a family member with a documented mutation has a very high chance of developing the disease without some form of intervention. Herein lies a potential dilemma; when women consent to genetic testing, they must be counseled appropriately and be able to cope with the information gained from the test—whatever the result (15). Most women overestimate their risk, and genetic testing allows accurate risk assessment that more confidently informs any proposed management decisions (16).

Though MRI has much greater sensitivity than mammography for detecting cancer in younger women with denser breast tissue, there is no evidence for any reduction in mortality from enhanced radiological surveillance of high-risk women (17). MRI screening has a lower specificity and 10-fold higher cost compared with mammography (18). Moreover, chemoprevention with agents such as tamoxifen and raloxifene can reduce the incidence of breast cancer by up to 50%, but have no effect on survival from all causes of death (19–22). All chemopreventive agents have potential side effects and it should be remembered that these are administered to otherwise healthy women. The risk elevation for entry into chemoprevention trials is a projected risk of 1.66% at five years (23).

Bilateral prophylactic surgery reduces the expected risk of breast cancer by more than 90%. In a retrospective study of more than 600 women at moderate to high risk who had undergone bilateral prophylactic mastectomy, the incidence of breast cancer was reduced by 89.5% ($p < 0.001$) (24). An established Gail model for risk estimation was used to predict the number of breast cancer cases expected in these two groups without surgical intervention. This together with several smaller studies have validated bilateral prophylactic mastectomy as a management option for women at increased risk for development of breast cancer (25). Prophylactic surgery cannot remove all breast tissue and when the nipple-areolar complex is preserved (subcutaneous mastectomy) up

to 15% of breast tissue may remain. Interestingly, most women do not opt for prophylactic mastectomy even when good-quality immediate breast reconstruction is available. There can be profound psychological sequelae from this radical form of intervention and studies have shown that a small minority (3–6%) of women do regret their decision to choose a surgical option for risk reduction (26). This is more likely when women have been "talked into" the operation. Health professionals should inform rather than "sell" this option; there is a difference between offering and recommending bilateral prophylactic mastectomy and the final decision must be left to the patient (15). Women should be allowed plenty of time to reach a final decision and must fully understand the risks, benefits, and limitations of bilateral prophylactic surgery, which should probably not be undertaken under the age of about 25 years. Conversely, the older a women is when she has prophylactic surgery, the smaller are the absolute benefits due to a corresponding reduction in estimated lifetime risk (27). The mean age of patients in most studies of prophylactic mastectomy is 42 years, and there is minimal benefit from carrying out this procedure over the age of 60 years. The gains in life expectancy with bilateral prophylactic mastectomy are typically between three and five years and may be a matter of months for older patients (27). A patient with a BRCA-2 gene mutation who has a 70% to 80% lifetime risk of developing breast cancer would reduce her absolute risk of death from breast cancer by only 2.5%. Moreover, it should be remembered that survival rates from breast cancer have greatly improved, and these patients are likely to have a screen-detected lesion or at least a small palpable tumor.

Patients undergoing bilateral prophylactic mastectomy within the Cambridge Breast Unit do not have preservation of the nipple-areolar complex, though it is acknowledged that this practice is acceptable. However, patients must be warned of the finite risk of subsequent cancer development, particularly when a sliver of breast tissue is left deep to the nipple-areolar complex. It is preferable to employ a laterally placed incision for nipple-sparing mastectomy to minimize the chance of nipple ischemia. There is no role for routine sentinel lymph node biopsy in the absence of any evidence of cancer on preoperative investigations.

This patient elected to undergo prophylactic oophorectomy in addition to bilateral prophylactic mastectomy. BRCA-2 mutations are associated with a 10% to 20% risk for development of ovarian cancer (lower than for BRCA-1 mutations) (9). Oophorectomy not only reduces the risk of ovarian cancer by removal of ovarian tissue, but significantly impacts on the subsequent risk of breast cancer—irrespective of any genetic predisposition to the latter. Indeed, iatrogenic oophorectomy in women under the age of 40 years reduces breast cancer risk by approximately two-thirds. Studies have shown that among women who carry mutations of BRCA-1 and BRCA-2, oophorectomy reduces breast cancer risk between 50% and 75% (28,29). Therefore, prophylactic oophorectomy can potentially reduce the incidence of both breast and ovarian cancer and this should be discussed in those women with a hereditary predisposition. Studies suggest that bilateral salpingo-oophorectomy is more "acceptable" as a risk-reducing strategy than bilateral prophylactic mastectomy and is chosen by more than 85% of heterozygotes for the major susceptibility genes BRCA-1 and BRCA-2. There are uncertain issues relating to hormone replacement for control of menopausal symptoms in these relatively young women. A limited period of usage at the lowest dose compatible with control of acute climacteric symptoms seems sensible. Calcium and vitamin D supplements should be recommended in the longer term for maintenance of bone health.

Related Cases

Contralateral prophylactic mastectomy—*Case Study 39*

Implant-only based reconstruction—*Case Study 4*

Learning Points

1. Approximately 5% to 10% of all breast cancers have a recognized genetic predisposition, with the majority of these having mutations in the BRCA-1 or BRCA-2 genes.

2. For women with a genetic predisposition for breast cancer, there are three options available: surveillance (including breast MRI), prophylactic surgery (bilateral mastectomy may reduce breast cancer risk by 90% and bilateral salpingo-oophorectomy before age 40 may reduce breast cancer risk by 50% and ovarian cancer risk by 90%), and chemoprevention (with tamoxifen). However, there are no randomized prospective trials that have specifically addressed the impact of these interventions in mutation carriers.

3. If a patient decides to undergo bilateral mastectomy to reduce breast cancer risk, then skin-sparing mastectomy (removal of the breast and nipple-areolar complex with preservation of the overlying skin) is the procedure of choice. Alternatively, total mastectomy is an acceptable option. However, nipple-sparing mastectomy (subcutaneous mastectomy) should be discouraged because the patient would remain at risk for developing breast cancer within the ducts of the nipple-areolar complex.

References

1. Knudson AG Jr. Genetics of human cancer. Ann Rev Genet 1986; 20: 231–251.
2. Knudson AG Jr. Hereditary cancer, oncogenes, and antioncogenes. Cancer Res 1985; 45:1437–1443.
3. Hall JM, Lee MK, Newman B, et al. Linkage of early onset familial breast cancer to chromosome 17q21. Science 1990; 250:1684.
4. Wooster R, Neuhausen S, Mangion J, et al. Localisation of a breast cancer susceptibility gene, BRCA-2 to chromosome 13q12-13. Science 1994; 265:2088.
5. Ford D, Easton DF. The genetics of breast and ovarian cancer. Br J Cancer 1995; 72(4):805–812.
6. Ford D, Easton DF, Stratton M, et al. Genetic heterogeneity and penetrance analysis of the BRCA-1 and BRCA-2 genes in breast cancer families. Am J Hum Genet 1998; 62:676–689.

7. Borresen AL, Andersen TI, Garber J, et al. Screening for germline TP53 mutations in breast cancer patients. Cancer Res 1992; 52:3234–3236.

8. Tsou HC, Teng DH, Ping XL, et al. The role of MMAC1 mutations in early-onset breast cancer: causative in association with Cowden syndrome and excluded in BRCA-1 negative cases. Am J Hum Genet 1997; 61:1036–1043.

9. Ford D, Easton DF, Bishop DT, et al. Breast Cancer Linkage Consortium. Risks of cancer in BRCA-1 mutation carriers. Lancet 1994; 343:692–695.

10. Breast Cancer Linkage Consortium. Cancer risks in BRCA-2 mutation carriers. J Natl Cancer Inst 1999; 91:1310–1316.

11. Claus EB, Risch N, Thompson WD. Genetic analysis of breast cancer in the Cancer and Steroid Hormone study. Am J Hum Genet 1991; 48:232–242.

12. Struewing JP, Hartge P, Wacholder S, et al. The risk of cancer associated with specific mutations of BRCA-1 and BRCA-2 among Ashkenazi Jews. N Engl J Med 1997; 336:1401–1408.

13. Gauthier-Villars M, Gad S, Caux V, et al. Genetic testing for breast cancer predisposition. Surg Clin North Am 1999; 79:1171–1187.

14. Statement of the American Society of Clinical Oncology. Genetic testing for cancer susceptibility, adopted on February 20, 1996. J Clin Oncol 1996; 14:1730–1736.

15. Geller G, Bernhardt BA, Doksum T, et al. Decision-making about breast cancer susceptibility testing: how similar are the attitudes of physicians, nurse practitioners and at risk women? J Clin Oncol 1998; 16:2868–2876.

16. Black WC, Nease RF Jr., Toteson ANA. Perceptions of breast cancer risk and screening effectiveness in women younger women than 50 years of age. J Natl Cancer Inst 1995; 87:720–731.

17. MARIBS study group. Screening with magnetic resonance imaging and mammography of a UK population at high familial risk of breast cancer: a prospective multicentre cohort study (MARIBS). Lancet 2005; 365: 1769–1778.

18. Warner E, Causer PA. MRI surveillance for hereditary breast cancer. Lancet 2005; 365:1747–1749.

19. Fisher B, Constantino JP, Wickerman DL, et al. Tamoxifen for prevention of breast cancer: report of the National Surgical Adjuvant Breast and Bowel Project P-1 study. J Natl Cancer Inst 1998; 90: 1371–1388.

20. Veronesi U, Maisonneuve P, Costa A, et al. Prevention of breast cancer with tamoxifen: preliminary findings from the Italian randomized trial among hysterectomised women. Lancet 1998; 352:93–99.

21. Powles T, Eeles R, Ashley S, et al. Interim analysis of the incidence of breast cancer in the Royal Marsden Hospital tamoxifen randomized chemoprevention trial. Lancet 1998; 362:98–101.

22. Wickerham DL, Costantino JP, Vogel V, et al. The study of tamoxifen and raloxifene (STAR): initial findings from the NSABP P-2 breast cancer prevention study. 2006 ASCO Annual Meeting Proceedings Part 1. J Clin Oncol 2006; 24: No. 18S LBA5.

23. Cheblowski R, Col N, Weiner E, et al. American Society of Clinical Oncology technology assessment of pharmacological interventions for breast cancer risk reduction including tamoxifen, raloxifene and aromatase inhibition. J Clin Oncol 2002; 20: 3328–3343.

24. Hartmann LC, Schaid DJ, Woods JE, et al. Efficacy of bilateral prophylactic mastectomy in women with a family history of breast cancer. N Engl J Med 1999; 340:77–84.

25. Bilimoria MM, Morrow M. The woman at increased for breast cancer: evaluation and management strategies. CA Cancer J Clin 1995; 45: 263–278.

26. Montgomery LL, Tran KN, Heelan MC, et al. Issues of regret in women with contralateral prophylactic mastectomies. Ann Surg Oncol 1999; 6:546–552.

27. Schrag D, Kuntz KM, Garber JE, et al. Decision analysis—effects of prophylactic mastectomy and oophorectomy on life expectancy among women with BRCA-1 and BRCA-2 mutations. N Engl J Med 1997; 336:1465–1471.

28. Kauff ND, Satagopan JM, Robson ME, et al. Risk reducing salpingo-oophorectomy in women with a BRCA-1 or BRCCA-2 mutation. N Engl J Med 2002; 346:1609–1615.

29. Rebbeck TR, Lynch HT, Neuhausen SL, et al. Prophylactic oophorectomy in carriers of BRCA-1 or BRCA-2 mutations. N Engl J Med 2002; 346:1616–1622.

Part II: Contralateral Prophylactic Mastectomy

CASE STUDY 39

History

A 60-year-old woman was found to have an area of microcalcification in the right breast on routine screening mammography. She had undergone a left modified radical mastectomy for a grade III node-negative invasive ductal carcinoma of the right breast eight years earlier and received adjuvant chemotherapy that was poorly tolerated. She sustained a deep vein thrombosis during treatment. She remained well with no evidence of recurrent disease, but tended to become anxious at the time of breast imaging lest any further malignancy be detected in the contralateral breast. There was no family history of breast or ovarian cancer.

Clinical Findings

A well-healed mastectomy scar was present on the left side with no evidence of any locoregional recurrence. No discrete mass lesion or areas of focal nodularity were detectable in the right breast, which was noted to be rather heavy and pendulous (E1).

Clinical Assessment

Asymptomatic screen-detected microcalcification of the right breast in a patient with a previous invasive cancer of the left breast.

Investigations

Mammography (Right)

A cluster of relatively coarse microcalcification was seen in the upper outer quadrant of the right breast with no associated mass lesion.

Breast Ultrasound

Breast ultrasound was not performed.

Mammotome Biopsy

Percutaneous biopsy of the left breast was carried out with a mammotome (11-gauge needle) that yields a larger volume of tissue than standard core biopsy. A radiograph of the biopsy material confirmed that calcification was present in the specimen (Fig. 1). Histopathological evaluation revealed localized fibrous sclerosis containing coarse microcalcification consistent with a zone of fat necrosis (B2) (Fig. 2).

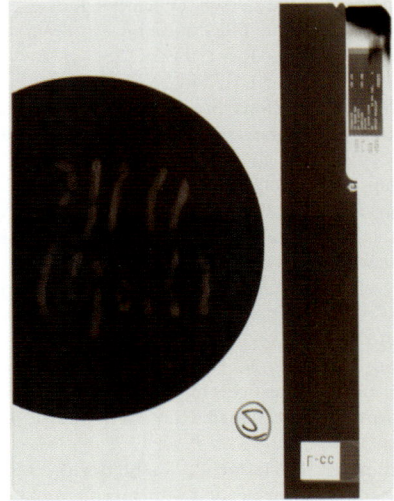

Figure 1

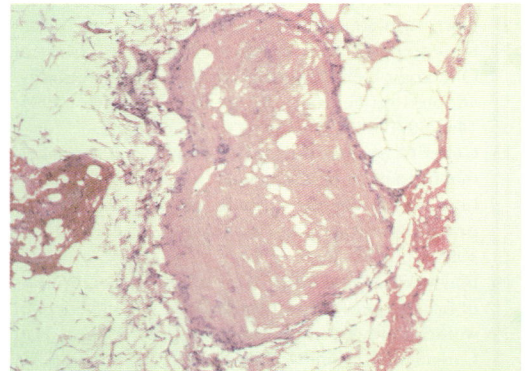

Figure 2

Diagnosis

Incidental area of fat necrosis of the right breast with no antecedent history of trauma.

Multidisciplinary Review 1

Following multidisciplinary review the patient was reassured and discharged back into the screening program. There was no indication for further tissue acquisition and open surgical biopsy was not necessary on the basis of the mammotome result.

Treatment and Progress

The patient accepted the results of the mammotome biopsy and was relieved that no malignancy had been detected. However, she felt unable to cope with fear of developing cancer in the contralateral breast and had been traumatized psychologically by the adjuvant treatments previously received for her left-breast cancer (namely chemotherapy). Moreover, she felt very lopsided with a single breast and had no desire for any reconstructive procedure to the left side. She therefore requested a contralateral prophylactic mastectomy and understood that though this would not prolong her life, it would minimize the chance of a second breast cancer and avoid the need for any further treatments such as chemotherapy. Interestingly, it was pointed out to the patient that a contralateral cancer is often of a more favorable grade and stage that makes the need for chemotherapy less likely. Despite these comments, the patient was adamant that she wished to proceed with a contralateral procedure and this was arranged within two months. A right simple mastectomy was carried out (without any form of axillary surgery) and the patient made an uneventful recovery. She was very pleased that she had undergone contralateral prophylactic surgery.

Definitive Histology

This revealed benign breast changes only with no evidence of atypia, in situ or invasive malignancy.

Discussion

The greatest risk factor for breast cancer is a personal history of the disease. The risk for development of contralateral breast cancer is approximately 0.7% per year and the risk of dying from a contralateral lesion about 0.2% per year (1). Between 4% and 15% of patients surviving breast cancer will develop cancer in the opposite breast (2). Patients who undergo breast conservation surgery have a risk of de novo cancer in both the contralateral and the remaining ipsilateral breast tissue. In the latter scenario, a true ipsilateral breast tumor recurrence must be distinguished from a new cancer. There is no evidence that scatter from external beam

radiotherapy (5–10% of total dosage) significantly increases the chance of malignant change in the remaining breast tissue. Systemic adjuvant chemohormonal therapies reduce ipsilateral breast tumor recurrence by approximately one-third (3–5) and hormonal therapies such as tamoxifen decrease the risk of contralateral disease by up to 40% (6). More women are now being successfully treated for breast cancer at an earlier stage of disease. For younger women who do not suffer from non–breast-cancer related deaths, survival is sufficiently prolonged to allow manifestation of a second, contralateral malignancy. For women with breast cancer diagnosed under the age of 50 years, the risk of contralateral breast cancer is 10- to 14-fold higher than for the general population. It has been estimated that fewer than 5% of women will have developed a contralateral breast cancer by 4 years and only 7% at 10 years (7). Patients with a known BRCA-1 mutation have at least a 60% risk of a contralateral breast cancer and usually bilateral mastectomy is recommended for this group of patients if breast cancer develops prior to any ipsilateral prophylactic procedure (8).

Some women will opt for a contralateral prophylactic mastectomy on the basis of a prior diagnosis of breast cancer in the absence of any strong family history or genetic predisposition. This is a personal choice and a woman has a right to choose her destiny. Nonetheless, it is important to emphasize to these patients that a contralateral procedure will not necessarily prolong their life, but will reduce the chance of further developing a breast cancer. A patient's fate is determined by the index tumor and second contralateral cancers are usually of a more favorable prognosis and probably contribute to only about 5% of breast cancer mortality (9). This is partly related to detection at an earlier stage from routine follow-up surveillance. However, with heightened public awareness and breast-screening programs, cancers are presenting at a smaller size and earlier stage. In consequence, any prognostic advantage of contralateral cancers will be eroded and therefore second cancers could become more important in the future. This would strengthen any argument for a contralateral prophylactic mastectomy in patients with an early-stage index lesion as it might confer an overall survival benefit for an individual patient and not just avoid further cancer treatment.

Many patients request a contralateral prophylactic mastectomy because they do not wish to endure further treatments for any new breast cancer. Such concerns often relate to chemotherapy rather than surgery per se despite prophylactic mastectomy being relatively radical surgery. Some patients feel very lopsided after a unilateral mastectomy for cancer and seek to be flat chested. Occasionally a single remaining heavy and pendulous breast can lead to back problems. Several of these factors pertained in the case described herein.

Contralateral prophylactic mastectomy may be requested because of a fear of further cancer per se and patients may seek to minimize the chance of any recurrence or second malignancies. It may be impossible to reassure patients that long-term survival is unlikely to be compromised in the event of a contralateral cancer. In younger women, increased density of breast tissue renders mammographic surveillance more difficult. Use of MRI as a screening tool may fail to reassure these younger patients that the opposite breast is tumor-free (there is no role for random contralateral biopsies) (10).

Though contralateral prophylactic mastectomy may be demanded by a patient from personal choice and in accordance with the principle of autonomy, there are situations where this may be surgically recommended:

1. Moderately strong family history of breast cancer.
2. The presence of florid lobular carcinoma in situ in association with a lobular phenotype in the ipsilateral breast cancer (higher chance of bilaterality).
3. Dense nodular breast parenchyma or a mammographically occult index lesion. This limits the sensitivity of clinical and radiological surveillance.
4. Patients who have received mantel irradiation for Hodgkin's disease are at high risk for bilateral breast cancers and a

contralateral prophylactic mastectomy should be considered when a unilateral tumor develops in this group of patients.

Related Cases

Bilateral prophylactic mastectomy—*Case Study 38*

Simple mastectomy without immediate breast reconstruction—*Case Study 44*

Learning Points

1. Women who have been diagnosed with breast cancer are at increased risk for developing contralateral breast cancer (0.7% per year). For women treated with endocrine therapy, this risk is halved. For some women, the fear of developing contralateral breast cancer is so great that contralateral prophylactic mastectomy is undertaken to reduce anxiety.

2. Recent retrospective studies have suggested that contralateral prophylactic mastectomy may improve breast cancer survival rates. However, there are no randomized prospective trials that have addressed this issue.

3. In the United States, the number of women electing to undergo contralateral prophylactic mastectomy following a breast cancer diagnosis has increased substantially in recent years. This may partly reflect the wider use of breast MRI, and the false-positives associated with it.

References

1. Robbins GF, Berg JW. Bilateral primary breast cancers: a prospective clinicopathological study. Cancer 1964; 17:1501–1527.
2. Wanebo HJ, Senofsky GM, Fechner RE, et al. Bilateral breast cancer: risk reduction of contralateral biopsy. Ann Surg 1985; 201:667–677.
3. Fisher B, Redmond C, Dimitrov NV, et al. A randomized clinical trial evaluating sequential methotrexate and fluorouracil in the treatment of patients with node negative breast cancer who have estrogen receptor negative tumours. N Engl J Med 1989; 320:473–478.
4. Early Breast Cancer Trialists Collaborative Group. Polychemotherapy for early breast cancer: an

overview of the randomized trial. Lancet 1998; 352:930–942.

5. Early Breast Cancer Trialists Collaborative Group. Tamoxifen for early breast cancer: an overview of the randomized trials. Lancet 1998; 351: 1451–1461.

6. Cuzik J, Baum M. Tamoxifen and contralateral breast cancer. Lancet 1985; 2:282.

7. Morrow M. Insurance policies for prophylactic surgery: to cover or not to cover?. Ann Surg Oncol 2000; 7:321–322.

8. Mann GB, Borgen PI. Breast cancer genes and the surgeon. J Surg Oncol 1998; 67:267–274.

9. Rosen PP, Groshen S, Kinne DW, et al. Contralateral breast carcinoma: an assessment of risk and prognosis in stage I and stage II patients with 20 year follow up. Surgery 1989; 106:904–910.

10. Cody HS. Routine contralateral breast biopsy: helpful or irrelevant? Experience in 871 patients, 1979–1993. Ann Surg 1997; 225:370–376.

Lymphedema

13

CASE STUDY 40

History

A 71-year-old woman presented with an eight-week history of a lump in the right breast. There was no associated nipple discharge but the patient had noticed recent inversion of the right nipple. The patient had no previous breast problems and had undergone a screening mammogram seven years earlier within the NHS Breast Screening Programme. There was no family history of breast or ovarian cancer. The patient had given birth to her first child at the age of 24 years and had never used either hormone replacement therapy or the oral contraceptive pill.

Clinical Findings

Examination revealed a hard irregular mass lying superior to the right nipple-areolar complex and measuring 3 cm in maximum diameter. There was associated tethering of the overlying skin and indrawing of the right nipple. A hard, fixed node was palpable in the right axilla (E5) (Fig. 1).

Clinical Assessment

Clinical carcinoma of the right breast (not conservable) with involved axillary lymph nodes.

Investigations

Mammography

A spiculated mass was seen in the right retroareolar region measuring 35 mm in

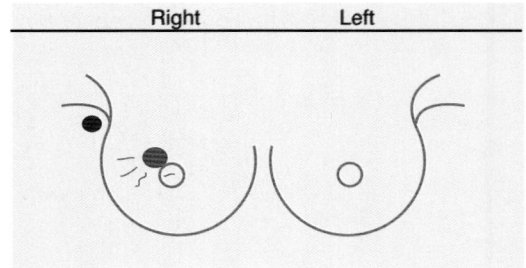

Figure 1

maximum diameter with the appearances of a carcinoma (R5) (Fig. 2A, B).

Breast Ultrasound

The sonographic correlate was a 34-mm ill-defined heterogeneous mass lesion, which was hypoechoic without posterior acoustic enhancement or attenuation (U5) (Fig. 3).

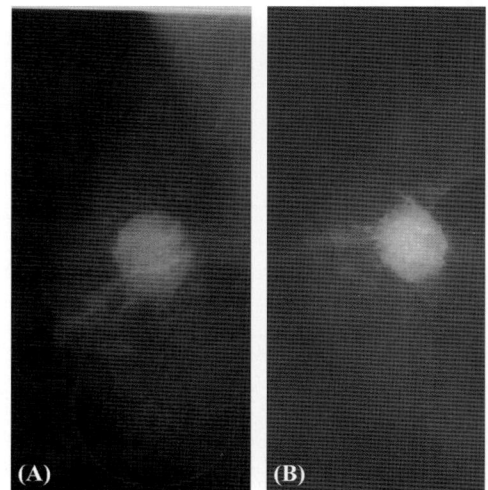

Figure 2

210

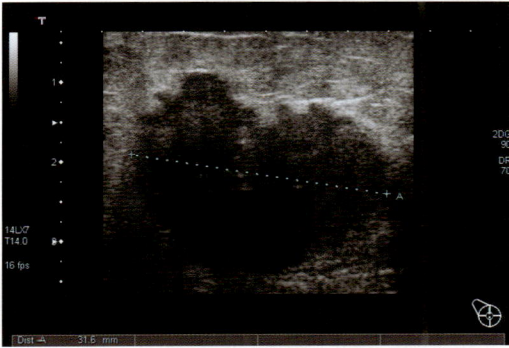

Figure 3

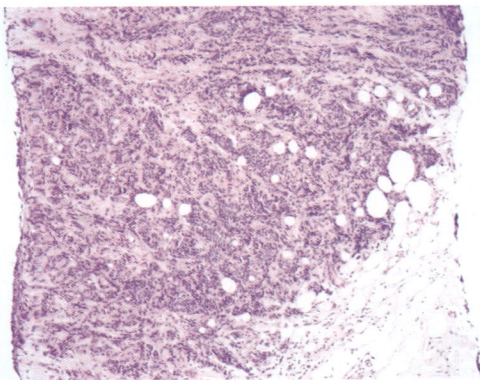

Figure 5

Core Biopsy

Ultrasound-guided core biopsy (16-gauge needle) of the breast mass confirmed an invasive carcinoma (provisionally grade II, but only a tiny fragment of tumor tissue present in core biopsy, ER positive[a]) (Fig. 4).

Diagnosis

Early-stage right-breast cancer (T2N2).

Multidisciplinary Review 1

It was recommended that the patient undergo a right modified radical mastectomy and a level II axillary lymph node dissection. The patient had a centrally located tumor exceeding 3 cm in size and associated with nipple indrawing, which precluded breast conservation. Moreover, the patient was not eligible for

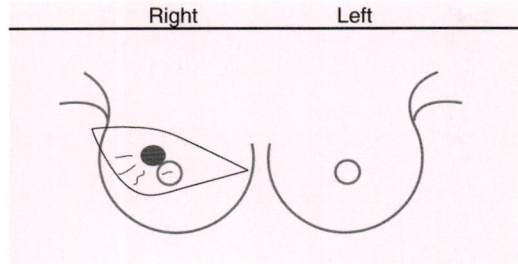

Figure 4

sentinel node biopsy due to the presence of a firm, fixed node in the right axilla. Radiotherapy to the chest wall would likely be required on account of the relatively large tumor size and clinically positive node.

Treatment and Progress

The patient proceeded to a right modified radical mastectomy within four weeks of initial presentation (2 weeks from tissue diagnosis). A wide skin excision was performed together with a level III axillary lymph node dissection (Fig. 5). The patient made an uneventful recovery and both drains were removed after 72 hours.

Definitive Histology

This revealed a multifocal invasive carcinoma, which was upgraded to III from the core biopsy [Fig. 6A (low power) and B (high power)]. There was associated high-grade cribriform and micropapillary DCIS and the largest lesion measured 32 mm in maximum extent (invasive and in situ component). Two other principle foci measuring 19 mm and 6.5 mm were identified lying just inferior to the main lesion and deep to the nipple, respectively. Lymphovascular invasion was present (Fig. 6C) and 7 of 26 lymph nodes contained metastatic tumor with evidence of extranodal spread (Fig. 6D).

Multidisciplinary Review 2

In view of the multifocality and extensive nodal involvement (>4 nodes positive),

[a] Allred score 8/8

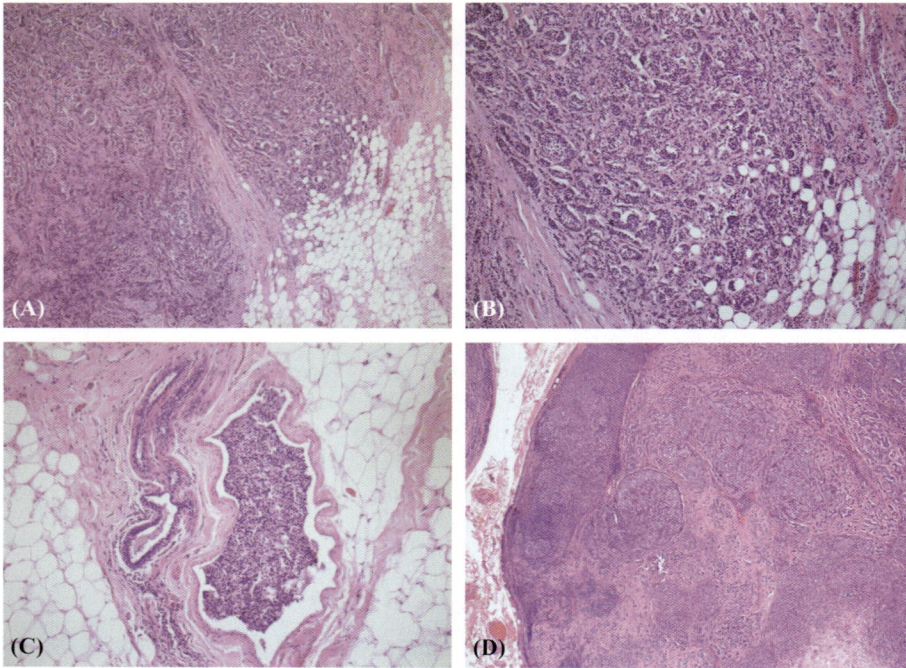

Figure 6

radiotherapy to the chest wall and supraclavicular fossa was recommended. Tamoxifen was commenced as adjuvant systemic hormonal therapy (tumor strongly ER positive) with a planned early switch to an aromatase inhibitor after two to three years (NPI ≥ 4.4).

Treatment and Progress

The patient underwent a course of radiotherapy to the chest wall and supraclavicular fossa commencing six weeks after surgery. She tolerated this well with no acute radiation sequelae. Four months following surgery, she presented with moderate lymphedema of the right arm and was referred to the lymphedema clinic (Fig. 7A–C). She was fitted with a standard sleeve and reviewed every six months (Fig. 8A, B). A routine contralateral mammogram performed at two years revealed no significant abnormality in the left breast.

Discussion

This patient developed moderately severe lymphedema four months following breast surgery, which incorporated a level III axillary lymph node dissection. Despite recent advances in treatments for breast cancer, lymphedema remains a common complication that can lead to major physical and psychological morbidity. Though it is often the nondominant upper limb that is affected (most breast cancers occur on the left side), lymphedema causes symptoms of heaviness and discomfort with associated functional impairment and an unsightly appearance (Fig. 6). The swelling of early lymphedematous change is soft with pitting on pressure and improvement with arm elevation. The accumulation of protein-rich fluid within the extracellular compartment renders the limb prone to recurrent superficial infection, which contributes to more chronic inflammatory changes with fibrosis. Disruption and blockage of the lymphatics raises hydrostatic pressure within other parts of the lymphatic system and promotes further tissue edema by hampering absorption of excess fluid back into the lymphatic vessels. The precise etiology of lymphedema remains unclear, but is related to the extent of axillary dissection. The latter disrupts lymphatic drainage pathways and thus compromised function is more likely when surgical dissection is more extensive. The overall incidence of lymphedema is cited as between 10% and 30% (1–4), though there are variations in the definition of lymphedema. Some reports are based on subjective assessment of arm swelling while others relate to measurements of limb volume excess. It is impractical to measure the latter by volume displacement techniques and the preferred method is serial circumferential measurements with calcula-

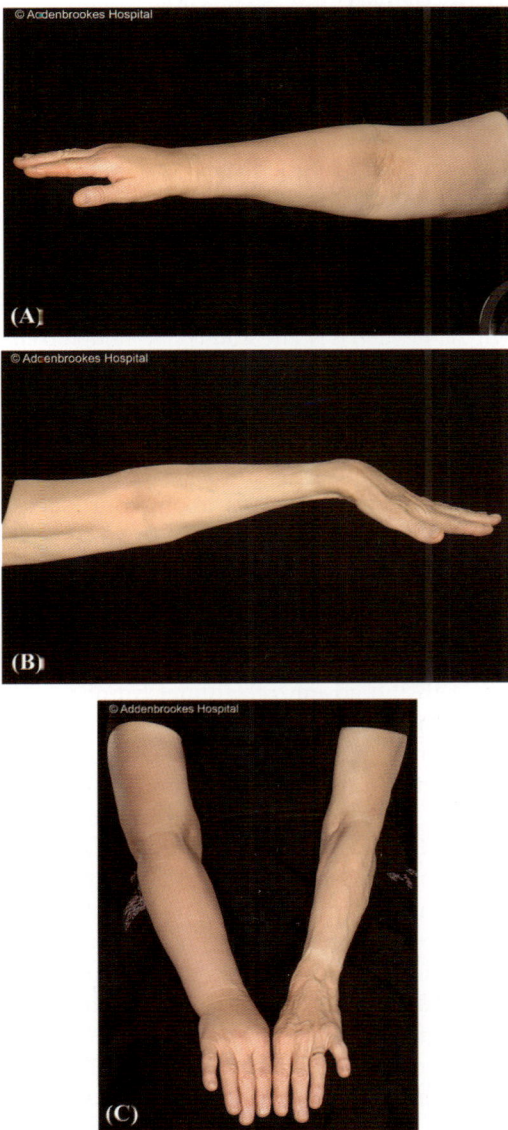

(A)
© Addenbrookes Hospital

(B)
© Addenbrookes Hospital

Figure 8

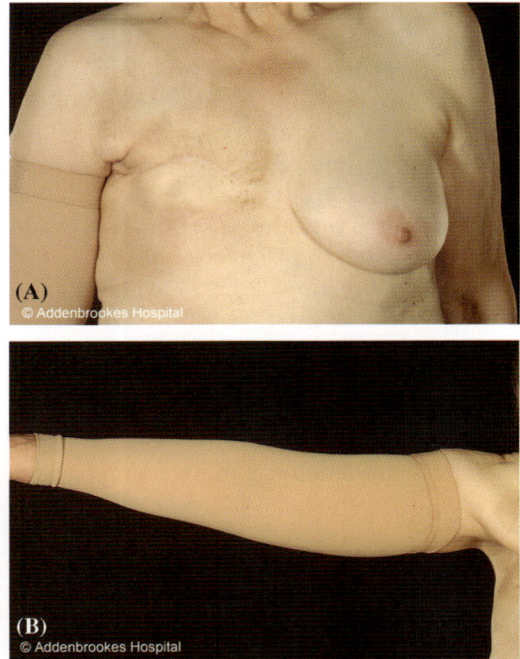

(A)
© Addenbrookes Hospital

(B)
© Addenbrookes Hospital

(C)
© Addenbrookes Hospital

Figure 7

tion of lymph volume using equations for a truncated cone (frustum) (5). A relatively simple method for assessing differential limb volume is to take measurements of limb circumference 10 cm above and below the olecranon; a difference of ≥ 2 cm is generally accepted as definition of lymphedema in a patient of average body habitus (6).

A level II axillary lymph node dissection involves clearance of all tissue below the axillary vein with no attempt to skeletonize the latter. Some fatty tissue remains inferior to the vein and this extent of dissection should be associated with lymphedema rates of less than 10% to 15%. When a level III dissection is undertaken, rates of lymphedema increase to approximately 25%, though some surgeons believe that removal of three to four nodes maximum at level III is unlikely to significantly impact on documented rates of lymphedema. Moreover, some surgeons loosely refer to level II/III dissection within the literature and this confounds interpretation of data on rates of lymphedema formation. The addition of axillary irradiation to a formal clearance can lead to rates in excess of 40%. There is rarely any justification for combined dissection and irradiation nowadays.

Lymphedema can develop many years after surgery (up to 20 years) and follow soon after an episode of heavy lifting or vigorous/prolonged usage of the arm. However, three-quarters of cases occur within the first 12 months and the onset may be insidious with a gradual progression to a severely swollen and impaired limb (7). Minor cuts and grazes and even venepuncture have been reported as precipitating factors. Lymphedema appears to be more common in patients who suffer postoperative infection and this may be related to obesity (8). Chronic lymphedema can be complicated by malignant change with development of secondary lymphangiosarcoma (Stewart–Treeves syndrome).

Lymphedema can be graded clinically as follows:

I—Swelling, which pits on pressure and may reduce with limb elevation;
II—Firmer, non-pitting edema; skin and nail changes with hair loss;
III—Elephantiasis of the limb with grossly thickened skin and large redundant folds.

Though a precipitating factor may be identified, there is usually no obvious reason why lymphedema has developed at a particular point in time after surgery. Duplex ultrasound should be carried out to exclude venous obstruction and a CT scan performed to determine whether an axillary mass (recurrent tumor) has a causative role. The majority of patients have mild to moderate lymphedema and conservative measures are the mainstay of treatment. Drug treatment and surgery are reserved for severe forms of chronic lymphedema with elephantiasis of the limb. The aims of treatment are to control edema, prevent infection, and maximize the function and appearance of the affected limb. Conservative treatment encompasses the following areas:

Hygiene—meticulous skin and nail care. Avoid breaks in skin and thorough antisepsis following minor cuts and abrasions. Commencement of antibiotics promptly or long-term prophylaxis.
Massage—manual lymphatic drainage (MLD) by a trained therapist initially. Gentle massage will facilitate lymph flow. MLD is a more formal type of massage that starts within non-lymphedematous zones of the trunk and moves more peripherally along the limb after these watershed areas have been "prepared" for receipt of extralymphatic fluid (9).
Elevation—this simple maneuver can effectively treat mild forms of chronic lymphedema. Ideally the limb should be elevated overnight but a nocturnal schedule is unlikely to be conducive to a good night's sleep.
Compression bandaging—this compensates for the loss of tissue elasticity in lymphedematous tissues. Most patients should wear compression garments, especially following a session of massage, to hinder reaccumulation of fluid. These compression sleeves can be custom made and class II or III provide an adequate level of support for upper limb lymphedema (30–40 mmHg and 40–50 mmHg), respectively. A compression sleeve should be worn day and night and a separate glove is available for the hand.
Exercise—flow of lymph within the lymphatic vessels is passive and contraction of the limb musculature stimulates onward movement of lymph in a proximal direction. Dynamic exercises are less likely to increase limb blood flow compared with static exercises and should be undertaken while wearing a compression garment.

Complex decongestive therapy is an integrated program that incorporates skin care, massage, compression devices, and regular exercise. The course lasts about four weeks and can lead to a 20% decrease in limb swelling (10). This patient was initially managed by a breast care nurse in a lymphedema clinic and was subsequently referred to a specialist lymphedema facility for more intensive therapy. With the advent of sentinel lymph node biopsy, the majority of clinically node-negative breast cancer patients no longer undergo routine axillary lymph node dissection at the outset. This is likely to reduce the number of cases of lymphedema in the future. There is no evidence at present that rates of lymphedema may ultimately be higher among patients who undergo a positive sentinel lymph node biopsy followed by a delayed axillary dissection (despite more technically challenging surgery). Those patients with involvement of a single sentinel lymph node (particularly when only micrometastases are present) should have axillary dissection confined to level II.

Related Cases

Learning Points

1. Lymphedema is associated with axillary surgery and radiation to the axilla. A review of several studies found that the risk of lymphedema was approximately 17% for breast cancer patients treated with axillary surgery alone and 41% for those treated with axillary radiation and surgery.
2. Reports concerning the incidence of lymphedema in breast cancer patients have varied considerably, largely due to the lack of uniform diagnostic criteria. Lymphedema is not detectable clinically until the interstitial volume is 30% above normal (11).

References

1. Kissin MW, Querci della Rovere G, Easton D, et al. Risk of lymphoedema following the treatment of breast cancer. Br J Surg 1986; 73:580–584.
2. Jacobsson S. Studies of the blood circulation in lymphoedematous limbs. Scan J Plast Reconstr Surg 1967; 3:1–81.
3. Schuneman J, Willich N. Lympheodema of the arm after primary treatment of breast cancer. Anticancer Res 1998; 18:2235–2236.
4. Mortimer PS, Bates DO, Brassington HD, et al. The prevalence of arm oedema following treatment for breast cancer. Q J Med 1996; 89:377–380.
5. Pain SJ, Purushotham AD. Lymphoedema following surgery for breast cancer. Br J Surg 2000; 87:1128–1141.
6. Gerber LH. A review of measures of lymphoedema. Cancer 1998; 83:2803–2804.
7. Olson JA, Petrek JA. Breast cancer–related lymphoedema. In: Singletary SE, Robb GL, eds. Advanced Therapy of Breast Disease. Ontario, California: BC Decker Inc., 2000:307–313.
8. Mozes M, Papa MZ, Karasik A, et al. The role of infection in post-mastectomy lymphoedema. Ann Surg 1982; 14:73–83.
9. Vodder E. Lymphdrainage ad modem Vodder. Aesthet Med 1965; 14:190–191.
10. Casely-Smith JR, Casely-Smith JR. Modern treatment of lymphoedema. Complex physical therapy: the dirst 200 Australian limbs. Australas J Dermatol 1992; 33:61–68.
11. Erickson VS, Pearson ML, Ganz PA, et al. Arm oedema in breast cancer patients. J Natl Cancer Inst 2001; 93:96–111.

Miscellaneous Conditions

14

Part I: Male Breast Cancer

CASE STUDY 41

History

A 77-year-old man presented to the breast unit with a one-week history of a lump in the left breast. He described the lump as being on the "edge of the nipple" and had noticed some indrawing thereof but no nipple discharge. His general health was otherwise good, and he reported no recent weight loss or unusual cough or back pain. He was taking no regular medication and had no family history of breast cancer.

Clinical Findings

Examination revealed a firm discrete lump lying close to the left nipple areolar complex and encroaching deep to this. There was dimpling of the periareolar skin and indrawing of the left nipple [Fig. 1A–C (post–core biopsy)]. The lump was partially fixed to the underlying pectoralis muscle and several hard, but mobile, nodes were palpable in the left axilla (E5) (Fig. 2).

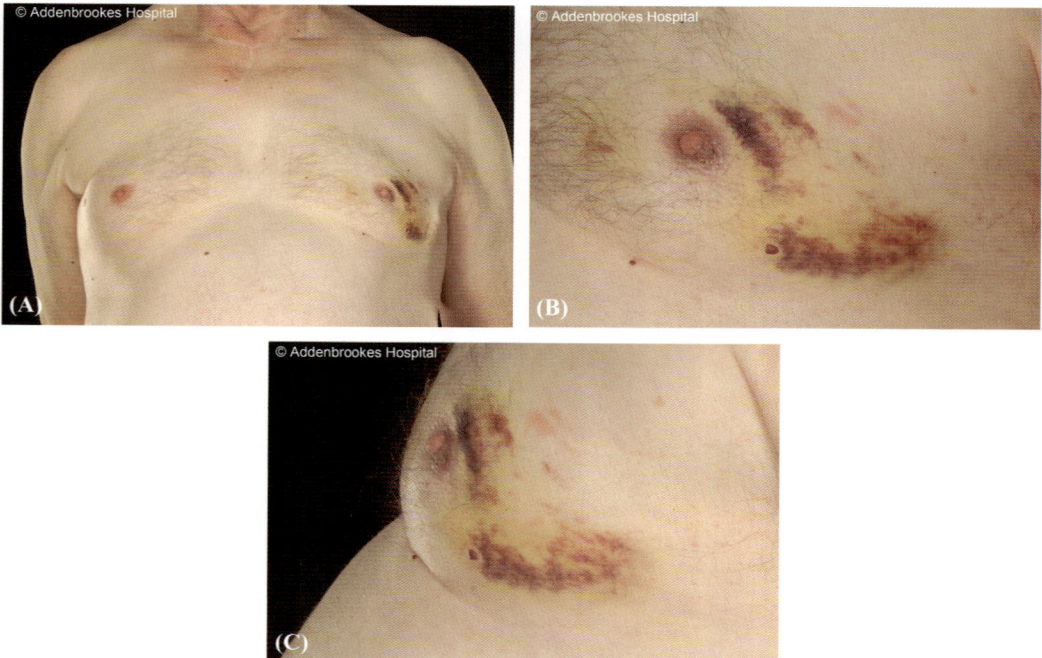

Figure 1

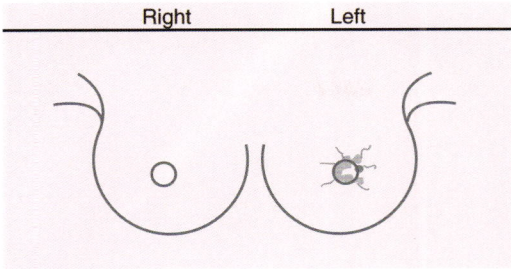

Figure 2

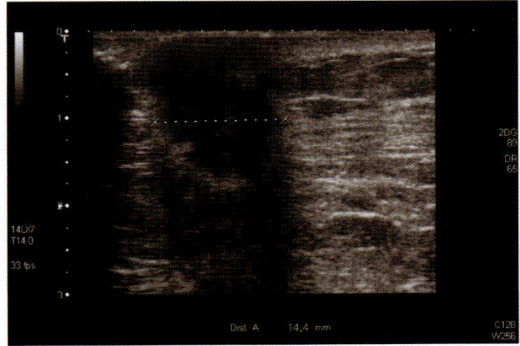

Figure 4

Clinical Assessment

Clinical carcinoma of the left breast in an elderly male with involved axillary lymph nodes.

Investigations

Mammography

A spiculate mass lesion was seen in the left retroareolar region measuring 15 mm in maximum diameter (R5) (Fig. 3A, B).

Ultrasound Breast/Axilla

The mammographic lesion corresponded to an ill-defined, heterogeneous mass measuring 15 mm on ultrasound. The echo pattern was hypoechoic with posterior acoustic attenuation (U5) (Fig. 4). The axilla was not interrogated sonographically.

Core Biopsy

Ultrasound-guided core biopsy (16-gauge needle) confirmed an invasive carcinoma (grade III, ER positive, HER2 negative) [Fig. 5A (low power), B (high power)].

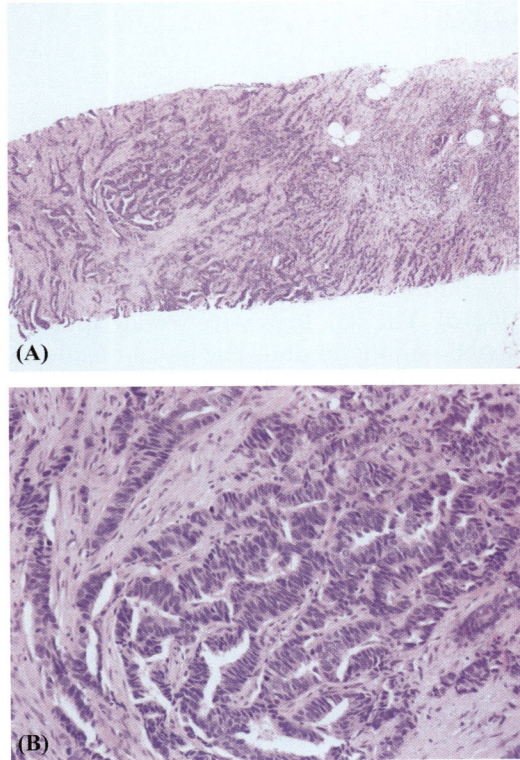

Figure 5

Diagnosis

Early-stage left-sided male breast cancer (T1N1).

Multidisciplinary Review 1

It was recommended the patient be offered a left modified radical mastectomy with a level

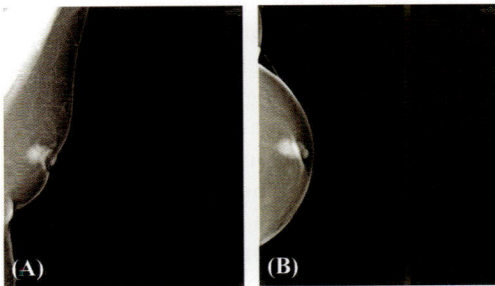

Figure 3

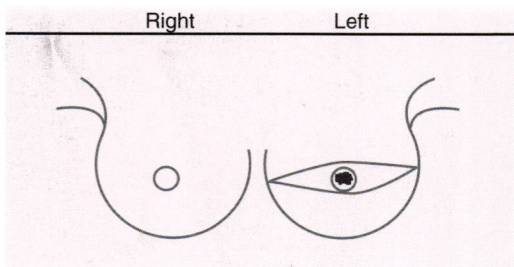

Figure 6

II/III axillary lymph node dissection (fit and healthy patient). Ultrasound assessment of the left axilla was not requested as the patient was ineligible for sentinel node biopsy in the presence of clinically palpable nodes.

Treatment and Progress

The patient underwent the proposed surgery and at operation there was macroscopic evidence of axillary lymph node involvement. A wide ellipse of skin was removed to incorporate the nipple areolar complex together with the skin overlying the tumor (Fig. 6). The skin flaps were readily approximated without tension. The patient made an uneventful recovery and was discharged home on the third postoperative day after removal of both drains. On subsequent review in the clinic 10 months after surgery, there was a well-healed mastectomy scar. However, the patient had recently developed lymphedema of the left upper limb, which necessitated the use of an elasticated sleeve (Fig. 7A, B).

Definitive Histology

This confirmed an invasive ductal carcinoma (grade III) measuring 18 mm in maximum diameter (Fig. 8A). The tumor was invading the overlying dermis, but not the underlying muscle (no muscle resected at the time of surgery) (Fig. 8B, C). There was associated high nuclear grade ductal carcinoma in situ (DCIS), but this did not extend beyond the invasive component. Lymphovascular invasion was present (Fig. 8D) and 10 of the 18 nodes removed were infiltrated with carcinoma (Fig. 8E).

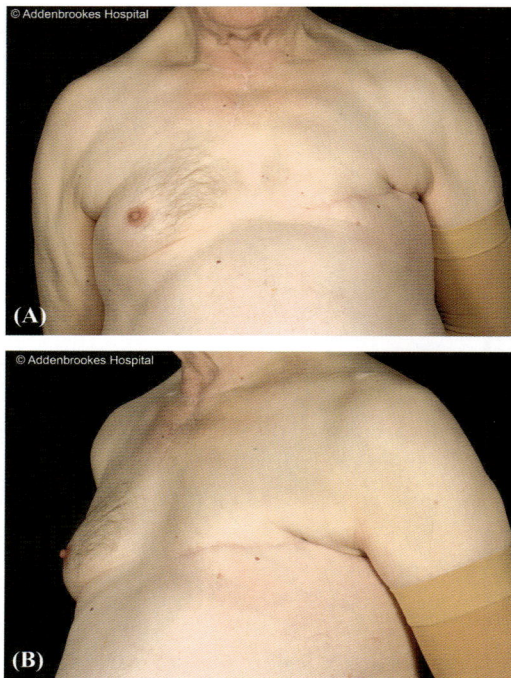

Figure 7

Multidisciplinary Review 2

It was recommended that the patient receive radiotherapy to the left chest wall and supraclavicular fossa on account of the extensive node involvement. The tumor was hormone sensitive, and tamoxifen for five years was advised as adjuvant systemic hormonal therapy.

Discussion

Male breast cancer is uncommon, representing 0.5% to 1% of all breast malignancies (1). The mean age at diagnosis is between 60 and 70 years, which is approximately 10 years more than that for female breast cancer. Nonetheless, men of all ages can be affected with this disease. Male breast cancer tends to present at a later stage with a higher incidence of axillary metastases at the time of diagnosis, though prognosis is similar to the disease in females when matched stage for stage (2–4). This may be attributable either to late clinical presentation or to earlier lymphatic infiltration consequent to the smaller volume of breast and fatty tissue.

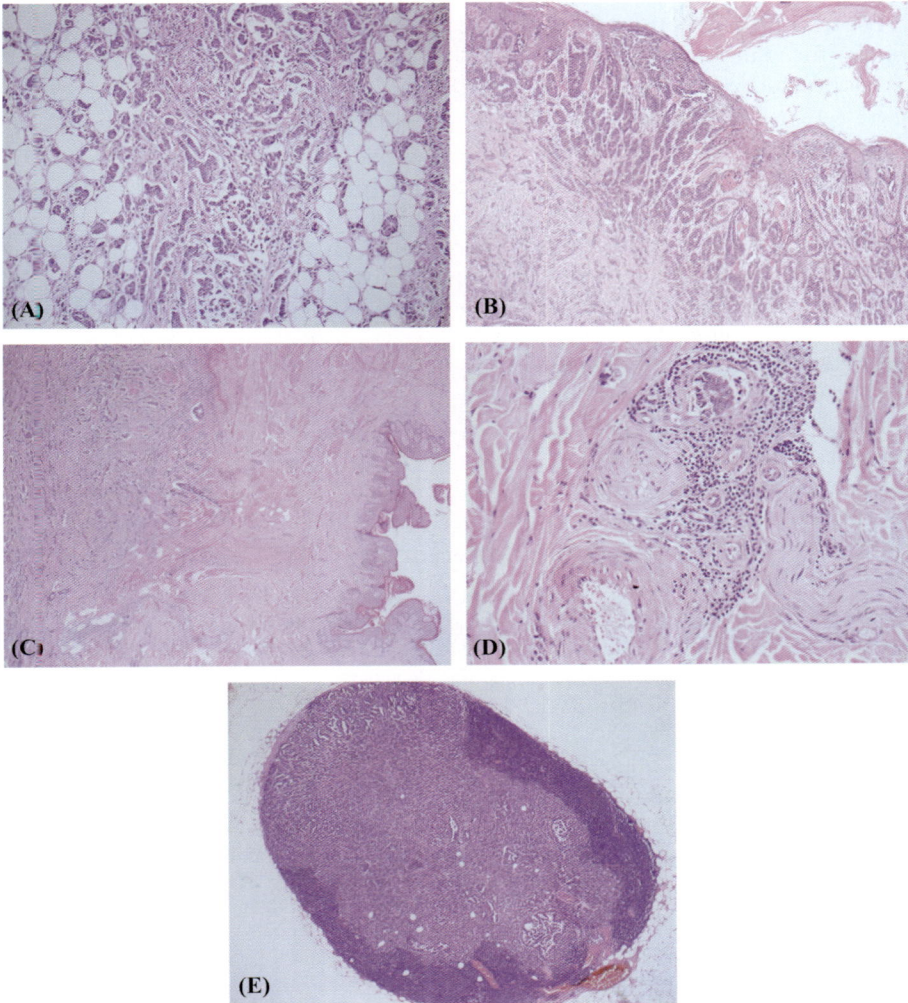

Figure 8

Predisposing risk factors include radiation exposure (4), estrogen administration, and diseases associated with hyperestrogenism such as cirrhosis of the liver and Kleinfelter's syndrome (5–8). Genetic predisposition occurs in some cases of male breast cancer, with an increased incidence in patients who have several female relatives affected with the disease. A higher risk of male breast cancer (6% risk) has been reported in families for whom a mutation in the BRCA-2 gene has been identified (9,10).

This man presented with overt signs of clinical carcinoma of the left breast. However, breast cancer in males can be difficult to distinguish clinically from gynecomastia, which is a much more common condition.

This is often bilateral and associated with a more generalized enlargement of the breast disc rather than a discrete lump. Gynecomastia may be tender whereas male breast cancer usually presents with a firm, slightly irregular, painless subareolar mass; the latter may be associated with skin changes and tethering to the overlying muscle.

The standard surgical treatment for male breast cancer is a modified radical mastectomy, which includes a level II axillary dissection (11). The paucity of breast tissue precludes any form of conservation due to the high tumor:breast size ratio and proximity of the cancer to the nipple. Where tumor is found to invade the pectoral muscle, a sliver of muscle can be removed at the time of mastectomy. There is little experience of sentinel node biopsy for male breast cancer, but this would be precluded for clinically positive axillae (12–14). The higher incidence of nodal involvement justifies formal axillary clearance at the outset for most patients. Male patients tend to present with more advanced stages of disease than females and often with a significant delay between onset of symptoms and diagnosis. Even though larger tumors may be more likely to be associated with nodal metastases, axillary ultrasound can be undertaken preoperatively in all clinically node-negative patients or confined to those with tumors >1.5 cm. Up to 60% of male breast cancer patients are reported to have nodal involvement at presentation (15), and axillary ultrasound can detect up to 40% of node-positive patients and permit axillary lymph node dissection (ALND) to be performed at the outset (16). With increasing awareness of the condition, men may seek medical attention at an earlier stage in the future.

Tamoxifen has been the standard adjuvant systemic treatment for ER-positive tumors. It is unclear whether aromatase inhibitors are effective for male breast cancer. The synthesis of estrogens by peripheral aromatization in fat tissue is probably quantitatively less important in males; it may therefore be more appropriate to use tamoxifen, which is a competitive antagonist for the ligand-binding site of the ER. For younger men with breast cancer, chemotherapy may be indicated. However, male breast cancer occurs in an older population in whom there may be significant comorbidities. Were this 77-year-old patient to have had an ER-negative tumor, no form of systemic therapy would have been given.

Related Cases

Male breast cancer—*Case Study 42*

Modified radical mastectomy in females—*Case Studies 1, 2, and 36*

Lymphedema—*Case Study 40*

Learning Points

1. Male breast cancer is extremely rare, accounting for about 1% of all breast cancer cases. The risk of male breast cancer increases with age, with a median age of approximately 67 years.
2. Infiltrating lobular carcinoma is rare in males, likely due to the rarity of terminal lobules in the male breast. Thus, the vast majority of male breast cancers are reported as either ductal or unclassified (93.7%).
3. Overall survival rates for men with breast cancer, when stratified by stage of disease, are lower than that for women. As in women, breast cancers in males tend to metastasize to the bone, lungs, and liver.

References

1. Greenlee RT, Murray T, Bolden S, et al. Cancer statistics, 2000. CA Cancer J Clin 2000; 50:7–33.
2. Heller S, Rosen PP, Schattenfeld DD, et al. Male breast cancer: a clinicopathological study of 97 cases. Ann Surg 1978; 188:60–65.
3. Borgen PI, Senie RT, McKinnon WMP, et al. Carcinoma of the male breast: analysis of prognosis compared to matched female patients. Ann Surg Oncol 1997; 4:385–388.
4. Goss PE, Reid C, Pintilie M, et al. Male breast carcinoma: review of 229 patients who presented to the Princess Margaret Hospital during 40 years: 1955–1996. Cancer 1999; 85:629–6639.
5. Visfeldt J, Shieke O. Male breast cancer. Histologic typing and grading of 187 Danish cases. Cancer 1973; 32:985–990.
6. Demers PA, Thomas BD, Rosenblatt KA, et al. Occupational exposure to electromagnetic fields and breast cancer in men. Am J Epidemiol 1991; 134:340–347.
7. Sasco AJ, Lowenfels AB, Pasker-deJong P. Epidemiology of male breast cancer. A meta-analysis of published case-control studies and discussion of selected aetiological factors. Int J Cancer 1993; 53:538–549.
8. Evans DB, Critchlow RW. Carcinoma of male breast and Kleinfelter's syndrome—is there an association? CA Cancer J Clin 1987; 37:246–250.
9. Couch FJ, Farid LM, DeShano ML, et al. BRCA-2 germline mutations in male breast cancer cases and breast cancer families. Nat Genet 1996; 13:123–125.
10. Thorlacius S, Tryggvadottir L, Olafsdottir GH, et al. Linkage to BRCA-2 region in hereditary male breast cancer. Lancet 1995; 346:544–545.
11. Donegan WL, Redlich PN, Lang PJ, et al. Carcinoma of the breast in males: a multi-institutional survey. Cancer 1998; 83:498–509.
12. Hill AD, Borgen PI, Cody HS III. Sentinel node biopsy in male breast cancer. Eur J Surg Oncol 1999; 25:442–443.

13. Gentilini O, Chagas E, Zurrida S, et al. Sentinel lymph node biopsy in male patients with early breast cancer. Oncologist 2007; 12:512–515.
14. Rusby JE, Smith BL, Dominguez FJ, et al. Sentinel lymph node biopsy in men with breast cancer: a report of 31 consecutive procedures and review of the literature. Clin Breast Cancer 2006; 7:406–410.
15. Joshi MG, Lee AK, Loda M, et al. Male breast carcinoma: an evaluation of prognostic factors contributing to a poorer outcome. Cancer 1996; 77:490–498.
16. MacMillan RD, Blamey RW. The case for axillary sampling. Adv Breast Cancer 2004; 1:9–10.

CASE STUDY 42

History

A 41-year-old man presented to the breast unit with a five-month history of intermittent bloodstained discharge from the right nipple. The discharge was spontaneous and associated with some tenderness of the right breast, but no lump therein. The patient had no previous history of any breast problems and no family history of breast, ovarian, or prostate cancer. The patient had a history of depression, and medication included citalopram (20 mg daily). He was otherwise fit and healthy with average alcohol consumption and reported no usage of tobacco products or recreational drugs.

Clinical Findings

On examination, there was an area of focal nodularity in the right retroareolar region but no discrete or dominant mass was palpable. A clear discharge could be elicited from the right nipple, which was positive for blood on chromogenic testing. There was no axillary lymphadenopathy.

Clinical Assessment

Though the findings on palpation were not suspicious, there was clinical concern about the history of bloodstained discharge, which was confirmed on formal assessment.

Investigations

Mammography

This revealed an area of asymmetrical density in the right breast with no focal mass lesion (Fig. 9A, B).

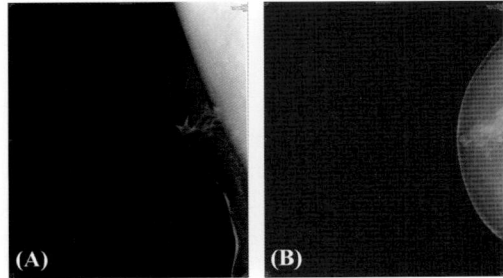

Figure 9

Ultrasound Breast/Axilla

The sonographic correlate of these indeterminate mammographic findings were two hypoechoic lesions measuring 6 and 9 mm in the right retroareolar region. These were partially cystic lesions and were suspicious for malignancy (U4) (Fig. 10).

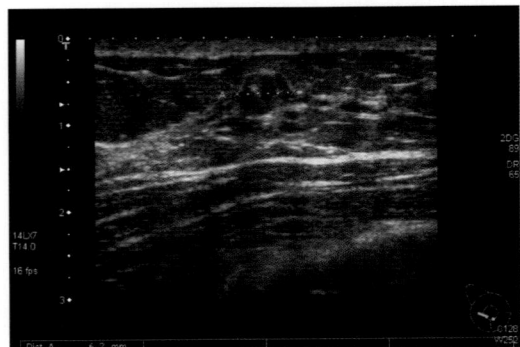

Figure 10

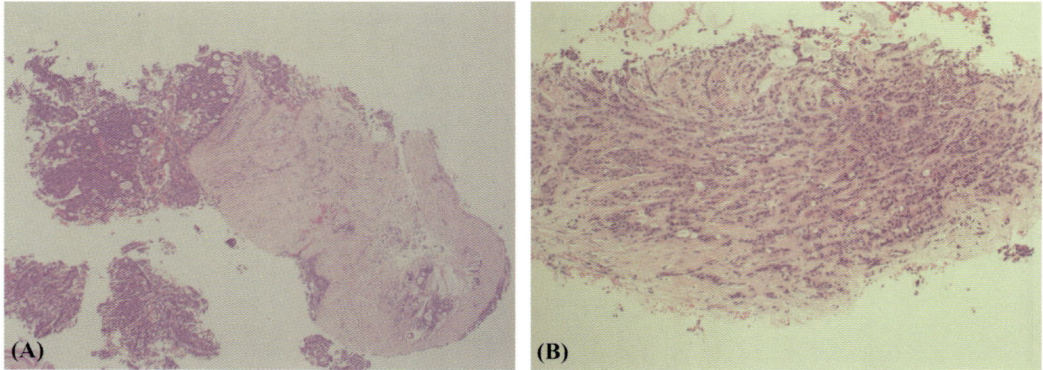

Figure 11

Core Biopsy

This showed features of an encapsulated papillary carcinoma with two foci of invasion just exceeding the 1 mm threshold [Fig. 11A (magnification 5×)]. The invasive component was too small (1.2 mm) to be graded but was strongly estrogen receptor positive (Allred score 8/8) [Fig. 11B (magnification 10×)].

Diagnosis

Early-stage right-sided male breast cancer (T1N0).

Multidisciplinary Review 1

Following multidisciplinary review, it was recommended the patient undergo a right simple mastectomy and sentinel lymph node (SLN) biopsy. A possible contralateral prophylactic mastectomy was discussed with the patient, but he chose to proceed with unilateral surgery in the first instance and consider a left mastectomy at a later date.

Treatment and Progress

The patient proceeded to a right mastectomy and SLN biopsy. Mastectomy was carried out with a narrow ellipse of skin that encompassed the nipple areolar complex and SLN biopsy was performed initially through the lateral one-third of the upper mastectomy incision. Dual localization methods were used with injection of technetium 99m–labeled nanocolloid (20 MBq) two hours (minimum) prior to surgery and 1 mL of patent blue dye at the time of surgery. Blue dye was injected in the 10 o'clock position (subareolar/intradermal)

with massage of the breast for five minutes. A single blue and very hot node was identified with an SLN:ex vivo count >10:1. No other blue nodes were seen, and there was no residual activity in the axilla following removal of the single SLN. A simple mastectomy was subsequently carried out using standard techniques and the wound was closed with two closed suction drains (Fig. 6). The skin flaps were readily approximated without tension. The patient made an uneventful recovery and was discharged home on the third postoperative day after removal of both drains.

Definitive Histology

This revealed an 18-mm grade I invasive ductal carcinoma with mucinous features (final histological size was comparable to the aggregate radiological estimate) [Fig. 12A (low power), B (high power)]. There was associated intermediate nuclear grade ductal carcinoma in situ with papillary and cribriform architecture. The latter extended along the main lactiferous ducts to the nipple. The single SLN was tumor-free.

Multidisciplinary Review 2

It was recommended the patient receive radiotherapy to the chest wall together with tamoxifen for five years as adjuvant systemic hormonal therapy. A contralateral prophylactic mastectomy remained an option at a later date.

Discussion

This patient had a small primary tumor that was unlikely to have spread to axillary lymph nodes (1). This together with his relatively

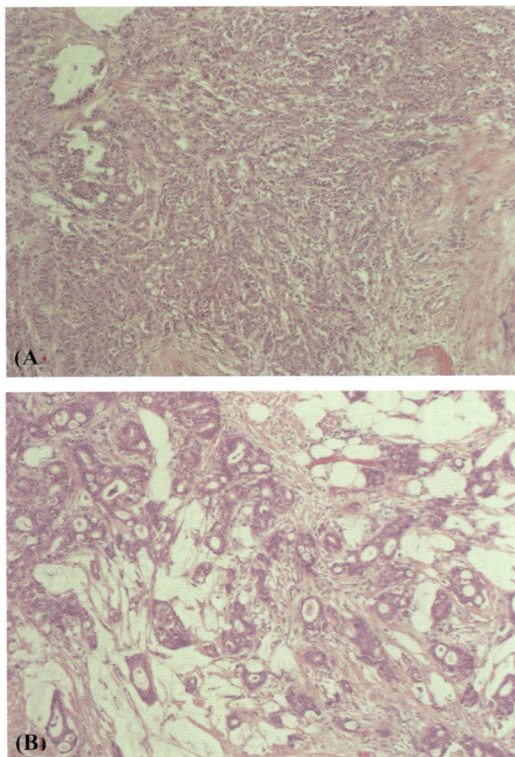

Figure 12

young age made him very suitable for SLN biopsy, which would potentially avoid ALND and concomitant morbidity. Lymphedema can develop in male patients just like their female counterparts and sentinel node biopsy should be considered for smaller, clinically node-negative tumors in men. There is clear evidence that SLN biopsy is associated with reduced arm morbidity, including lymphedema, shoulder stiffness, and paresthesia of the ipsilateral arm (2). This may be particularly relevant to the male population who constitute a high proportion of manual workers and up to 90% of those employed in heavy industries such as mining and construction (3). Male breast cancer patients are more likely to be sole breadwinners and there are economic consequences for upper limb morbidity at a personal level. In addition to a lower chance of long-term problems with impairment of upper limb function, SLN biopsy can shorten the duration of hospital stay and facilitate an earlier return to work.

A review by the American Society of Clinical Oncology Technology Assessment panel concluded that there was no a priori reason to suppose that SLN biopsy was intrinsically "less accurate in men than it is in women" (4). Cadaver studies have confirmed that the pattern of lymphatic distribution and drainage is similar in males and females (5); the cutaneous plexus of lymphatics is linked to lymphatics within the breast parenchyma via specialized subareolar and circumareolar plexuses, which drain directly to axillary nodes (6). On the basis of this common anatomy and physiology, SLN biopsy should be feasible in clinically node-negative male patients. A limited number of publications have emerged in the literature supporting this contention demonstrating high rates of detection and low rates of false negativity and axillary recurrence (7–12). However, the number of patients in these studies are necessarily very low, and calculations of relevant performance indicators must be interpreted with caution. Cimmino and colleagues reported on 18 male patients treated for breast cancer (mean tumor size 1.6 cm) of whom 6 underwent SLN biopsy (8). Most of these had a confirmatory ALND (4 of 6 patients) and half had a positive SLN biopsy. The authors concluded that SLN biopsy was suitable for male breast cancer patients with clinically node-negative tumors measuring ≤ 2 cm (T1). It was unclear whether the technique could be applied to larger tumors where the chance of nodal involvement and false negative rates were higher. Veronesi's group in Milan also reported an identification rate of 100% among a group of 32 male patients who underwent SLN biopsy for mainly T1 tumors (75%) (11). The mean number of SLNs removed at operation was 1.5 (range 1–3). Twenty-six of these 32 patients were SLN negative and were spared ALND. Among the six SLN biopsy–positive patients, only two had involvement of non-sentinel lymph nodes (NSLNs) and no axillary recurrences in SLN-negative patients had occurred at 30 months follow-up. Other studies have confirmed high rates of identification of the SLN in clinically node-negative male patients using dual localization techniques with or without lymphoscintigraphy; the latter may only identify SLNs in approximately two-thirds of patients (13). Boughey and colleagues emphasized that male patients present with larger tumors on average than females and are more likely to be SLN positive (37.0% vs. 22.3%, $p = 0.1$) and to harbor additional disease in NSLN (62.5% vs. 20.7%, $p = 0.01$) (10). These conclusions were echoed in a recent series of 78 male breast cancer patients from Memorial Sloan-Kettering Cancer Center. The SLN was successfully identified in 76 patients (97%) and the 37 of these had a positive SLN (node positivity rate 49%). Both patients with a failed SLN biopsy proceeded to ALND and were found to have nodal metastases. Further more, in three patients with a negative SLN (8%), a positive NSLN was found by digital palpation at operation (14). Goyal and colleagues investigated SLN biopsy in nine male patients with T1 (4) and T2 (5) cancers and documented an SLN positivity rate of 56%, with half of all SLN-positive patients having further involvement of NSLN on completion of ALND (14). The high proportion of SLN-positive patients in this study may be attributable to more than half having tumors exceeding 2 cm in size.

The overall benefits of SLN biopsy for men may be less than that for their female counterparts who may undergo regular breast screening and present with earlier stage disease or "minimal" breast cancer (15). Nonetheless, the procedure is feasible and appears safe and justified in a selected group of younger, clinically node-negative patients with tumors ≤ 2 cm.

Related Cases

Male breast cancer—*Case Study 41*

Sentinel lymph node biopsy in females—*Case Studies 5, 6, 7, 10, 11, 16, 24, and 26*

Learning Points

1. Although breast-conserving surgery (lumpectomy) is an option for most women with early breast cancer, it is rarely feasible in men because they have only a small amount of breast tissue and this is located immediately deep to the nipple. Therefore mastectomy is generally indicated for male breast cancer.

2. Sentinel node biopsy can be offered to most male breast cancer patients with clinically negative axillary nodes. However, breast cancer in males is often diagnosed at a more advanced stage, making sentinel node biopsy inappropriate.

3. Breast cancer in males is extremely rare, and management of this disease has not been assessed in large randomized trials. Thus, the optimal management of male breast cancer has not been fully delineated.

References

1. Querci della Rovere G, Bonomi R, Ashley S, et al. Axillary staging in women with small invasive breast tumours. Eur J Surg Oncol 2006; 32:733–737.
2. Purushotham AD, Upponi S, Klevesath M, et al. Morbidity following sentinel lymph node biopsy in primary breast cancer—a randomized controlled trial. J Clin Oncol 2005; 23:4312–4321.
3. Port ER, Fey JV, Cody HS III, et al. Sentinel lymph node biopsy in patients with male breast carcinoma. Cancer 2001; 91:319–323.
4. Lyman GH, Guiliano AE, Somerfield MR, et al. The Americal Society of Clinical Oncology guideline recommendations for sentinel lymph node biopsy in early stage breast cancer. J Clin Oncol 2005; 23:7703–7720.
5. Suami H, Pan WR, Mann GB, et al. The lymphatic anatomy of the breast and its implications for sentinel lymph node biopsy: a human cadaver study. Ann Surg Oncol 2008; 15:863–871.
6. Romrell LJ, Bland KI. Anatomy of the breast, axilla, chest wall and related metastatic sites. In: Bland KI, Copeland EM, eds. The Breast. Vol 1, 3rd ed. Philadelphia: Saunders, 2004.
7. Hill AD, Borgen PI, Cody HS III. Sentinel node biopsy in male breast cancer. Eur J Surg Oncol 1999; 25:442–443.
8. Cimmino VM, Degnim AC, Sabel MS, et al. Efficacy of sentinel lymph node biopsy in male breast cancer. J Surg Oncol 2004; 86:74–77.
9. Rusby JE, Smith BL, Dominguez FJ, et al. Sentinel lymph node biopsy in men with breast cancer: a report of 31 consecutive procedures and review of the literature. Clin Breast Cancer 2006; 7:406–410.
10. Boughey JC, Bedrosian I, Meric-Bernstam F, et al. Comparative analysis of sentinel lymph node operation in male and female breast cancer patients. J Am Coll Surg 2006; 203:475–480.
11. Gentilini O, Chagas E, Zurrida S, et al. Sentinel lymph node biopsy in male patients with early breast cancer. Oncologist 2007; 12:512–515.
12. Flynn LW, Park J, Patil SM, et al. Sentinel lymph node biopsy is successful and accurate in male breast carcinoma. J Am Coll Surg 2008; 206:616–621.
13. Albo D, Ames FC, Hunt KK, et al. Evaluation of lymph node status in male breast cancer patients: a

role for sentinel lymph node biopsy. Breast Cancer Res Treat 2003; 77:9–14.

14. Goyal A, Horgan K, Kissin M, et al. Sentinel node biopsy in male breast cancer patients. Eur J Surg Oncol 2004; 30:480–483.

15. Cady B, Stone MD, Schuler J, et al. The new era in breast cancer: invasion, size and nodal involvement dramatically decreasing as a result of mammographic screening. Arch Surg 1996; 131:301–308.

Part II: Paget's Disease

CASE STUDY 43

History

A 97-year-old woman presented with a six-month history of eczematous change and soreness of the left nipple. There was no palpable mass in the retro-areolar region of the breast. She had no previous breast problems and no family history of breast cancer. The patient was nulliparous and had never used any form of exogenous hormones.

Clinical Findings

There was an area of florid eczematous change involving the left nipple and areolar, which extended just beyond the margin of the latter. The area was weeping slightly but was not frankly ulcerated. There was no palpable mass in the retroareolar region and no axillary lymphadenopathy (E5). No eczematous changes were noted in the other nipple (nor elsewhere on the cutis) (Figs. 13 and 14A, B).

Clinical Assessment

Paget's disease of the left breast associated with an impalpable tumor.

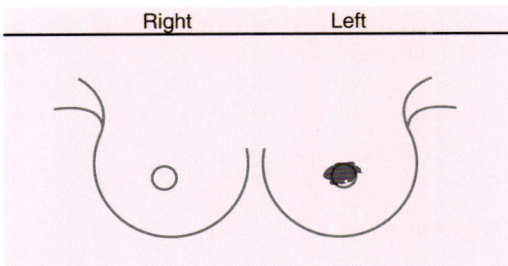

(A)
© Addenbrookes Hospital

(B)
© Addenbrookes Hospital

Figure 14

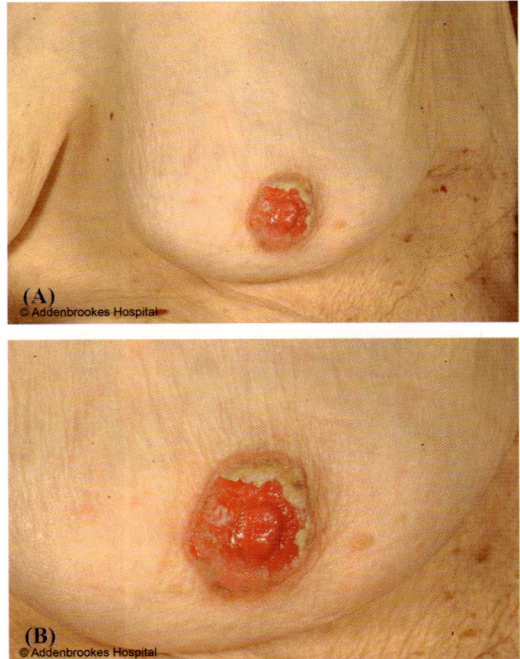

Figure 13

Investigations

Mammography

A normal parenchymal pattern was seen in both breasts with no focal lesion.

Breast Ultrasound

In view of the normal mammographic appearances, breast ultrasound was not performed.

Punch Biopsy

A punch biopsy of the left areola performed in the clinic showed infiltration of the

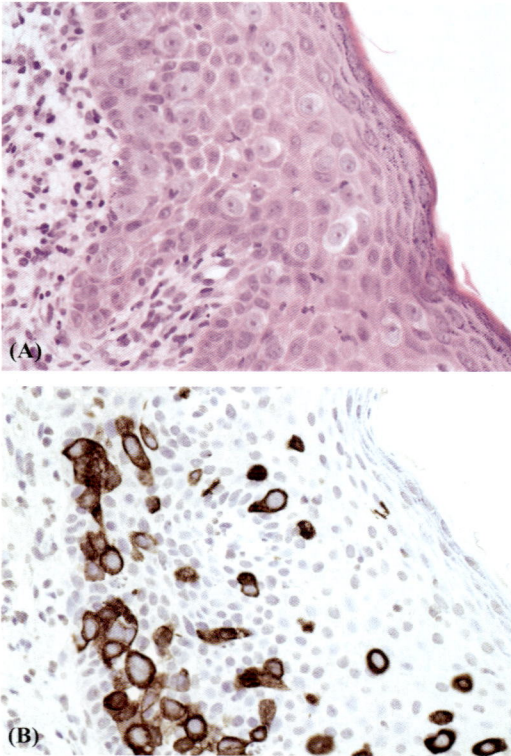

(A)

(B)

Figure 15

epidermis by nests of large epithelioid cells with abundant eosinophilic cytoplasm and marked nuclear pleomorphism (Fig. 15A (high power)). These cells were strongly positive for cytokeratin 5.2 (Fig. 15B) and negative for HMB45 and MelanA. The findings were consistent with Paget's disease of the nipple associated with DCIS.

Diagnosis

Paget's disease of the left breast with associated noninvasive breast cancer [Tis (Paget's)].

Multidisciplinary Review 1

It was recommended that this patient initially be managed expectantly. She was a frail lady of advanced age and surgical intervention was not deemed appropriate. There were concerns about commencing primary endocrine therapy with the aromatase inhibitor letrozole in the absence of documented hormone-sensitive (ER positive) invasive carcinoma. It was commented that there is no evidence for any benefit from either tamoxifen or aromatase inhibitors as primary endocrine treatment for in situ disease.

Treatment and Progress

The patient was therefore managed expectantly and the nipple was dressed regularly by the district nurse. Upon review after three months, the lesion appeared static and the patient was discharged back to the care of the general practitioner for further monitoring. Six months later, the general practitioner contacted the breast unit to specifically request further review.

On reassessment of the left nipple lesion, there was clear evidence of disease progression with frank ulceration of the lesion, but no underlying palpable mass. The patient reported some mild shortness of breath on exertion, but was otherwise generally well.

Multidisciplinary Review 2

Following further multidisciplinary review, it was recommended that the patient be commenced on letrozole (2.5 mg/day). A routine chest X ray was requested and revealed no evidence of metastatic pulmonary disease.

Treatment and Progress

The patient was reviewed in the clinic after three months, at which time she appeared well in her general self (she continued to live independently at home). Repeat clinical examination revealed a marked improvement in the appearance of the left nipple and areola with regression of the ulcerated areas and reduction in extent of the eczematous changes. The patient was instructed to continue taking letrozole and get the dressing changed by the district nurse every two to three days.

Discussion

The original description of this condition by Sir James Paget in 1874 referred to nipple changes as "a florid, intensely red, raw surface ... like the surface of a very acute eczema" (1). Paget's disease of the nipple is usually a unilateral lesion affecting one or other nipple, and this is an important feature serving to differentiate Paget's disease from simple eczema. Moreover, the condition primarily affects the nipple itself, with encroachment onto the adjacent areolar. The surface of the nipple is rough or "very finely granular" with erythema, ulceration, and scaling. Ulceration of the nipple occurs in 90% of cases and is more likely when the condition involves both the nipple and areolar (as in the case described here) (2). Patients usually complain of itching and burning of the nipple, together with bleeding and oozing from the surface. Nipple retraction may develop in more advanced cases. Delays in diagnosis are common; the condition may improve or heal temporarily and subsequently relapse (3). The differential diagnosis includes not only eczema, but also Bowen's disease (intraepithelial neoplasia) and the cutaneous manifestations of duct ectasia and periductal mastitis. Malignant melanoma and psoriasis should be considered clinically and can be excluded with immunohistochemical markers. Clinicians must maintain a high index of suspicion for Paget's disease among patients with an eczematous lesion of the nipple.

Paget's disease constitutes approximately 1.5% to 2.0% of all breast cancers and occurs in an age range from 26 to 88 years, but most commonly between 50 and 70 years of age (median age 56 years) (4). The condition is associated with an underlying breast cancer in >90% of cases, which can be either invasive or in situ carcinoma (invasive ductal more common than invasive lobular) and is usually centrally located and close to the nipple surface (5). The nipple changes characteristic of Paget's disease result from proliferation of cancer cells within the epidermis of the nipple. Pathognomonic cells infiltrating the dermis are readily distinguished from keratinocytes, especially when large numbers are present. These Pagetoid cells are relatively large with abundant cytoplasm and prominent, hyperchromatic, pleomorphic nuclei. They resemble melanocytes, and special markers may be needed to differentiate them from this cell type. Pagetoid cells contain mucin, which can be highlighted with periodic acid-Schiff (PAS) or mucicarmin stains (3,5). Staining for S-100 and HMB45 is positive in melanomas, while cytokeratins are positive for both Paget's and Bowen's disease. Pagetoid cells also stain positive for milk fat globulin, CAM 5.2, CEA, and CK7. Both ER and PgR are expressed in Paget's disease and interestingly HER2/neu tends to be overexpressed (6).

It is unclear whether Pagetoid cells result from migration of malignant ductal epithelial cells from an underlying breast cancer or from transformation of cells within the nipple itself. The immunohistochemical profile of Pagetoid cells supports the former theory with concordance observed in more than 90% of cases. However, pre-Paget cells have been identified with features of both keratinocytes and Paget's cells, which supports a transformation theory. Approximately half of all Paget's cases will have a radiological abnormality, and mammography should be performed in all patients with a suspicious eczematous lesion of the nipple (2,7). MRI can be helpful in confirming multifocality and distance of any unifocal lesion from the nipple.

Historically, all cases of Paget's disease have been managed with mastectomy (8); disease within the breast is often multifocal and the true extent of disease may be difficult to assess preoperatively. Central segmental mastectomy may be suitable for patients with a unifocal lesion in the vicinity of the nipple-areolar complex and who have large pendulous breasts (9–11). Resection margins must be clear histologically (2–3 mm microscopic margin width). Radiotherapy should be administered postoperatively and studies have shown a high rate of local recurrence (40% at 5 years) when wide local excision alone is performed for Paget's disease (12). An axillary staging procedure is essential in all patients with documented invasive disease on percutaneous biopsy. Sentinel lymph node biopsy should be undertaken in all patients with Paget's disease; approximately 50% of all patients with a palpable mass will have axillary nodal involvement compared with 11% for an impalpable lesion. Nonsurgical treatment of Paget's is appropriate in elderly and/or unfit patients. However, results of primary radiotherapy alone are variable with many patients having to undergo subsequent salvage mastectomy (13).

There is little data on the response of Paget's disease to primary endocrine treatment. Both ER and PgR are expressed in Paget's disease and can be useful markers to guide therapy. This patient did respond clinically to a course of letrozole with a marked improvement in appearance of the nipple after three months of treatment. It is likely that for most patients optimal local control will be achieved when primary radiotherapy or endocrine treatment is followed by local excision. Current trials are evaluating wide local excision followed by radiotherapy as an alternative to mastectomy in otherwise fit patients.

Related Cases

Primary endocrine treatment—*Case Studies 30, 31, and 32*

Breast cancer in the elderly—*Case Studies 33 and 34*

Learning Points

1. If Paget's disease of the nipple is suspected, then a punch biopsy of the nipple skin should be obtained. The diagnosis of Paget's disease is confirmed if Paget's cells are found on biopsy.
2. Approximately 95% of patients with Paget's disease of the nipple have an underlying breast cancer (either DCIS or invasive cancer). A careful physical examination and mammography are generally used to identify the underlying cancer.
3. In most patients, Paget's disease is treated with either a modified radical mastectomy (for invasive cancer) or mastectomy alone (for DCIS). Alternatively, if the disease is confined to the nipple and an area immediately around it, then breast-conserving surgery is feasible (the nipple, areola, and involved part of the breast is removed). For invasive breast cancer, a sentinel node biopsy/axillary clearance is also indicated. For patients treated with breast conservation, radiotherapy is generally administered afterward. Systemic therapy is administered using the same guidelines as that used for any patient who presents with invasive breast cancer or DCIS.

References

1. Paget J. Disease of the mammary areola preceding cancer of the mammary gland. St Bart Hosp Rep 1874; 10:89.
2. Kollmorgen DR, Varanasi JS, Edge SB, et al. Paget's disease of the breast: a 33 year experience. J Am Coll Surg 1998; 187:171–177.
3. Dixon AR, Galea NH, Ellis IO, et al. Paget's disease of the nipple. Br J Surg 1991; 78:722–723.
4. Wertheim U, Ozello L. Neoplastic involvement of nipple and skin flap in carcinoma of the breast. Am J Surg Pathol 1980; 4:543–549.
5. Chaudary MA, Millis RR, Lane EB, et al. Paget's disease of the nipple: a 10 year review including clinical, pathological and immunohistochemical findings. Breast Cancer Res Treat 1986; 8:139–146.
6. Ramachandra S, Machin L, Ashely S, et al. Immunohistochemical distribution of c-erbB-2 in situ breast carcinoma: a detailed morphological analysis. J Pathol 1990; 161:7–14.
7. Ikeda DM, Helvie MA, Frank TS, et al. Paget's disease of the nipple: radiologic-pathological correlation. Radiology 1993; 189:89–94.
8. Freund H, Maydovnik M, Laufer N, et al. Paget's disease of the breast. J Surg Oncol 1997; 9:93–98.
9. Lagios MD, Westdahl PR, Rose MR, et al. Paget's disease of the nipple: alternative management in cases without or with minimal extent of underlying carcinoma. Cancer 1984; 54:545–551.
10. Bijker N, Rutgers EJ, Duchateau L, et al. Breast conserving surgery for Paget's disease of the nipple: a prospective European Organisation for Research and Treatment of Cancer study of 61 patients. Cancer 2001; 91:472–477.
11. El-Sharkawi A, Waters JS. The place for conservative treatment in the management of Paget's disease of the nipple. Eur J Surg Oncol 1992; 18:301–303.
12. Jamali FR, Ricci A Jr, Deckers PJ. Paget's disease of the nipple areola complex. Surg Clin North Am 1996; 76:365–381.
13. Stockdale AD, Brierley JD, White WF, et al. Radiotherapy for Paget's disease of the nipple: a conservative alternative. Lancet 1989; 2:664–666.

Part III: Phyllodes Tumor

CASE STUDY 44

History

A 56-year-old woman was referred to the breast unit after she was admitted to hospital five days previously with a deep vein thrombosis of the right leg. She had been noted to have a huge mass in the right breast, which was not a presenting symptom. On direct questioning it transpired that the mass had been present for at least six months, but had recently become ulcerated and prone to bleeding on light contact. The patient reported weight loss of approximately 1 stone over this period, but no unusual cough or back pain. A recent chest X ray was normal with no evidence of any pulmonary lesions. The patient was taking low molecular weight heparin and had not been warfarinized. She otherwise had no history of any breast problems, and of note, had never undergone screening mammography. There was a weak family history of breast cancer with the patient's maternal grandmother developing the disease at 50 years of age. She had two children and was 19 years of age at the time of birth of her first child. She had never used any form of exogenous hormones.

Clinical Findings

On clinical examination there was a huge ulcerated tumor of the central right breast, which was partially fixed to the chest wall and measured at least 10 cm (Fig. 16). There was frank fungation over the inferior aspect of the breast, which bled on direct contact (Fig. 17A, B). There was no axillary lymphadenopathy. The mass was relatively mobile on the chest wall, and the skin of the breast around the mass was normal with no evidence of tumor infiltration (E5) (Fig. 18A, B).

Clinical Assessment

The clinical impression was of a large locally advanced cancer of the right breast. The

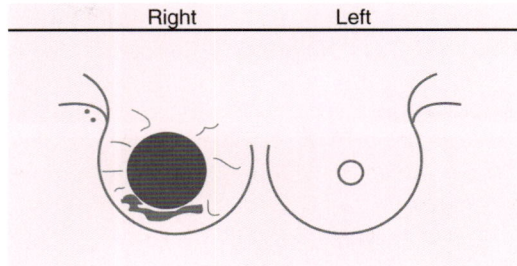

Figure 16

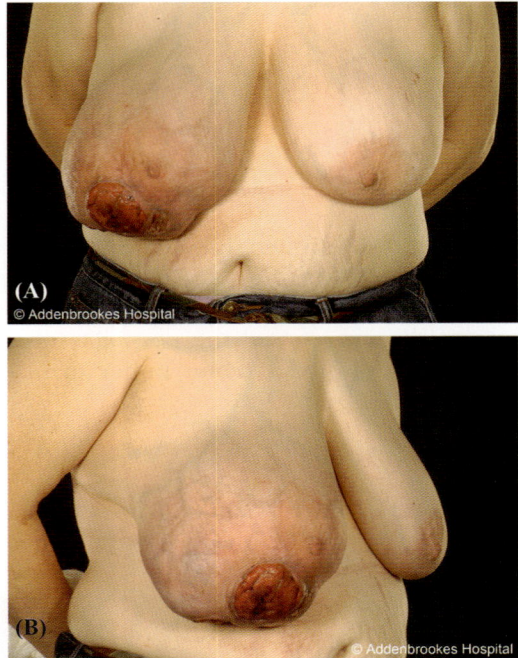

Figure 17

mass was perhaps unusually mobile on the chest wall and well circumscribed.

Investigations

Mammography

It was not possible to compress the right breast between the plates of a mammogram machine. Mammography of the contralateral breast was normal (Fig. 19A, B).

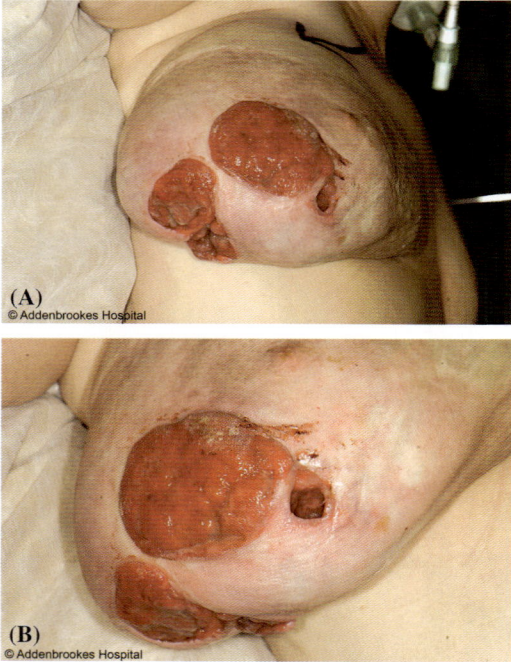

Figure 18

Breast Ultrasound

Ultrasound confirmed the presence of a huge tumor of the right breast, which was impossible to measure. Interestingly, the texture of the mass raised the possibility of a sarcoma or phyllodes tumor rather than a carcinoma (U4).

Core Biopsy

Biopsy of the mass was undertaken with two passes of a 16-gauge needle (patient not warfarinized and therefore no contraindication to biopsy). Histology supported the sonographic images and revealed a fibroepithelial lesion with no evidence of in situ or invasive malignancy. There were no mitotic figures in the biopsy material which was classified as a benign phyllodes tumor (B3) [Fig. 20A (low power), B (high power)].

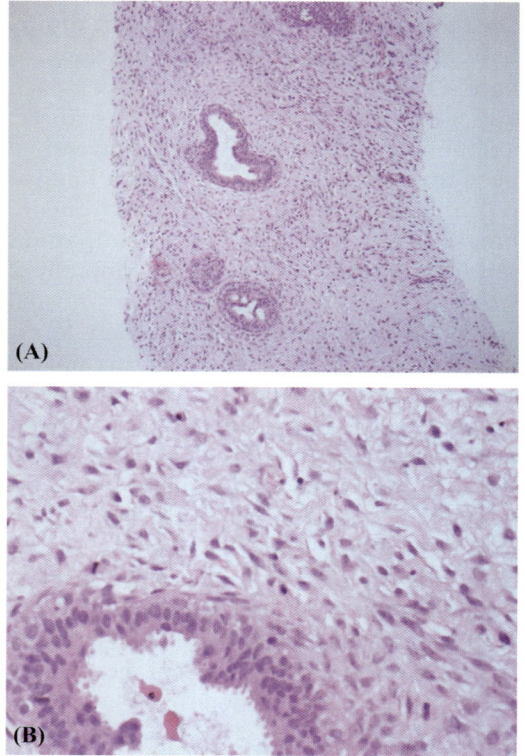

Figure 20

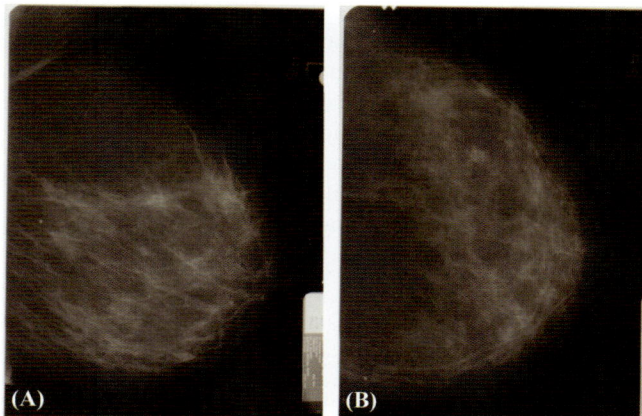

Figure 19

Diagnosis

Benign phyllodes tumor of the right breast.

Multidisciplinary Review 1

In view of the relatively large size of the mass, excision and complete pathological evaluation was mandatory. In practical terms, this necessitated a right simple mastectomy with primary skin closure (plenty of healthy, mobile skin around the lesion). Despite results of core biopsy, there were concerns about the patient's recent DVT and weight loss. A staging CT scan was therefore requested to exclude any distant (metastatic) disease.

Investigations

1. Hepatic ultrasound (Fig. 20C)—normal
2. CT chest, abdomen, and pelvis—normal

Treatment and Progress

The patient proceeded with a right simple mastectomy. At the time of operation, the mass was found to be well circumscribed with a clear plane of dissection between the mass and surrounding tissues (including pectoral/serratus anterior muscles). Large feeding vessels were individually ligated. Mastectomy flaps were easily apposed without tension and skin closed with interrupted sutures (to facilitate evacuation of any postoperative hematoma). The patient made an excellent recovery and was warfarinized on the fourth postoperative day.

Definitive Histology

This confirmed a massive phyllodes tumor of the right breast with ulceration through the skin (Fig. 21A). A fibroepithelial lesion was seen with moderate stromal cellularity (Fig. 21B) and a prominent leaf-like architecture [Fig. 21C (low power)]. The stromal component consisted of spindle cells with focal mild cytological atypia and a low mitotic index [Fig. 21D (high power)]. Though the lesion had an infiltrative pattern

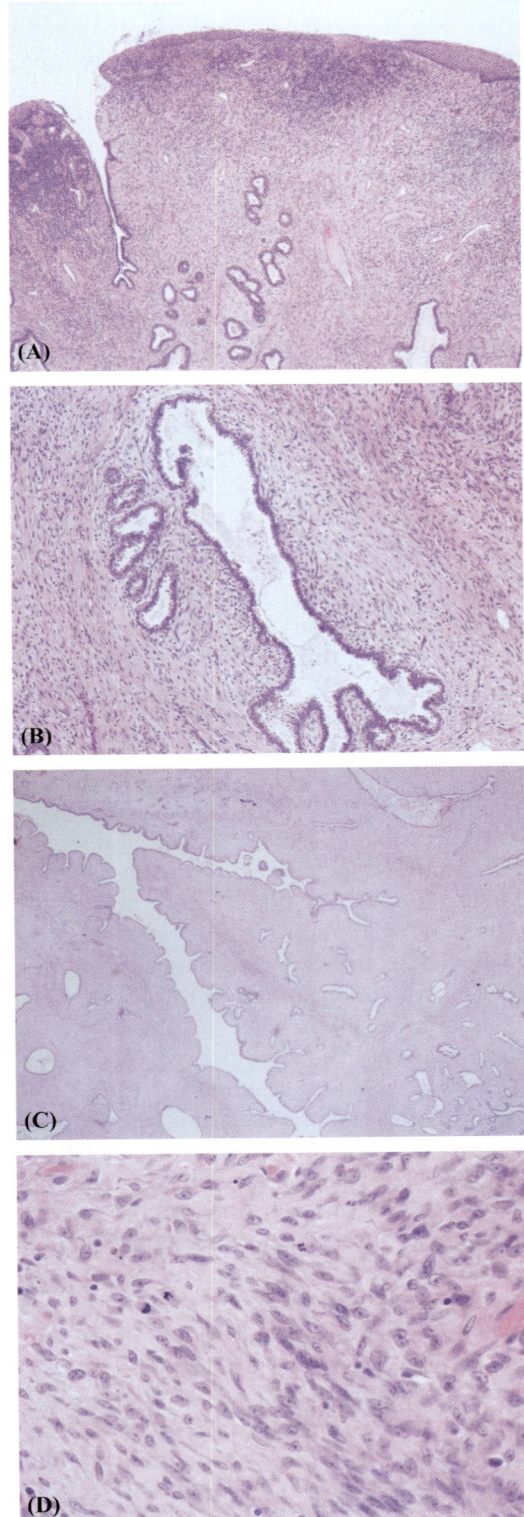

Figure 21

of growth and involved the surrounding fat, there was no evidence of overtly malignant features. The lesion was considered border-line between benign and malignant.

Multidisciplinary Review 2

As this patient had undergone a right simple mastectomy, no further resection of breast tissue was indicated. In the absence of any frank malignancy, no adjuvant therapies were indicated and the patient was discharged from formal clinical follow-up. She would undergo contralateral follow-up mammography within the NHS Breast Screening Programme.

Discussion

Cystosarcoma phyllodes is a tumor with the basic structure of a fibroadenoma, but is characterized by marked proliferation of con-nective tissue stroma and have potential for local recurrence and metastasis. The name cystosarcoma phyllodes was coined by Muller in 1938, describing a large fleshy tumor with a papillary "leaf-like" appearance on its cut sur-face (1). The biological behavior of these tumors is unpredictable; even the histological appearance is not a good prediction of subse-quent behavior, but these lesions are usually classified as benign (80%) or malignant (20%). The principle histological features are (*i*) the number of mitoses, (*ii*) a pushing or infiltrative margin, and (*iii*) nuclear pleio-morphism (2). The tumors occur in middle-aged women, with the maximum incidence in the fifth decade. However, the tumors have been reported in adolescent as well as elderly women. Phyllodes tumors characteristically grow slowly initially and then rapidly attain a large size. Although they are usually larger than a typical fibroadenoma, size alone is not a reliable diagnostic criterion, and there is no way of differentiating a fibroadenoma from a benign phyllodes tumor on gross appearance. They present clinically as a large circum-scribed tumor within the breast, which can measure up to 10 to 20 cm in maximum

diameter. Cutaneous ulceration may occur, but is a late manifestation (3).

This patient presented with a huge fun-gating tumor of the right breast. She came from the Fenland community and had not been particularly troubled by the mass. It was unclear why she had never attended for routine screening mammography or why she had not sought a medical opinion ear-lier. Though it was unusually mobile on the chest wall, the lesion otherwise had the mac-roscopic appearance of an invasive carci-noma (E5). Interestingly, the sonographic texture was more suggestive of a phyllodes tumor or sarcoma rather than a carcinoma. Core biopsy revealed a fibroepithelial lesion with no mitotic activity. This accorded with the final histopathological evaluation of the resected tumor. Staging investigations were requested preoperatively despite a benign core biopsy result in view of the patient's history of recent DVT, anemia, and weight loss. No formal follow-up or adjuvant therapy was indicated and the patient made an excel-lent recovery with a well-healed and neat mastectomy scar.

Related Cases

Simple mastectomy—*Case Study 39*

Learning Points

1. Approximately 80% of phyllodes tumors are benign and 20% are malignant. Although the benign tumors do not metastasize, they do have a tendency to grow aggressively and recur locally. The malignant tumors metastasize hemato-genously, similar to other sarcomas.

2. In most cases, phyllodes tumors should be treated with wide local excision, and a rim of normal tissue obtained around it. Phyllodes tumors should not be "shelled out" (as is often done for a fibroadenoma). For large phyllodes tumors, a simple mastectomy is war-ranted. An axillary node dissection

should only be performed if clinically suspicious nodes are evident.

References

1. Muller J. Uber den feinern Bau und die Formen der Krankhaften Geschwulste. Berlin: G Reimer, 1838:54–60.

2. Norris HJ, Taylor HB. Relationship of histological features to behaviour of cystosarcoma phyllodes: analysis of 94 cases. Cancer 1967; 20:2090–2099.

3. Moffat C, Pinder S, Dixon AR, et al. Phyllodes tumour of the breast: a clinicopathological review of thirty two cases. Histopathology 1995; 27:205–218.

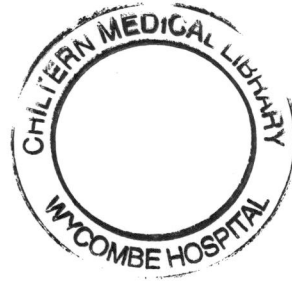

CHILTERN MEDICAL LIBRARY
WYCOMBE HOSPITAL

Appendices

The Nottingham prognostic index (NPI) divides patients into five prognostic groups based on scores calculated as follows:

$$\text{NPI} = 0.2 \times \text{tumour size} + \text{grade}$$
$$(1 \text{ to } 3) + \text{lymph node status } (1 \text{ to } 3)$$

where grade I = 1; grade II = 2; grade III = 3 and node negative = 1; 1 to 3 nodes positive = 2; ≥ 4 nodes = 3)

The five prognostic groups have 10-year survival figures as follows:

Excellent	≤ 2.4	94%
Good	≤ 3.4	83%
Moderate 1	≤ 4.4	70%
Moderate 2	≤ 5.4	51%
Poor	> 5.4	19%

APPENDIX II

- Adjuvantonline.com is a decision support tool that is now widely used in many countries. It allows for a more objective (rather than intuitive) estimates of benefits from hormonal and chemotherapy.
- Information on individual patients (including age, tumour size, tumour grade, and nodal status) is fed into a validated computerized program and absolute mortality benefits are calculated for chemotherapy, hormonal therapy, and combined chemohormonal therapy.
- Chemotherapy would be recommended for patients with an absolute benefit of $\geq 5\%$ and discussed for those with benefits of $\geq 3\%$ and $< 5\%$.
- It is the policy of the Cambridge Breast Unit not to mention chemotherapy to patients whose benefit falls below the 3% discussion threshold.

APPENDIX III

Adjuvant Chemotherapy Regimens

Drug	Dose	Route	Days	Frequency
CMF				
Cyclophosphamide	600 mg/m^2	i.v.	Day1 and day 8 every 28 days	For 6 cycles
Methotrexate	40 mg/m^2	i.v.	Day1 and day 8 every 28 days	For 6 cycles
5-Fluorouracil	600 mg/m^2	i.v.	Day1 and day 8 every 28 days	For 6 cycles, 3 weekly, cycles 1–4

Drug	Dose	Route	Days	Frequency
E-CMF				
Epirubicin	100 mg/m^2	i.v.	Day 1	
Cyclophosphamide	600 mg/m^2	i.v.	Day 1 and day 8	4 weekly, from day 1, cycles 5–8
Methotrexate	40 mg/m^2	i.v.	Day 1 and day 8	4 weekly, from day 1, cycles 5–8
5-Fluorouracil	600 mg/m^2	i.v.	Day 1 and day 8	4 weekly, from day 1, cycles 5–8
AC				
Doxorubicin*	60 mg/m^2	i.v.	Day 1	Every 3 weeks (4 or 6 cycles)
Cyclophosphamide	600 mg/m^2	i.v.	Day 1	Every 3 weeks (4 or 6 cycles)

Maximum cumulative lifetime dose of Doxorubicin (Adriamycin*) = 450 mg/m^2.

Neoadjuvant Chemotherapy Regimens

Drug	Dose	Route	Days	Frequency
EC				
Epirubicin	90 mg/m^2	i.v. bolus	Day 1	21 days × 6
Cyclophosphamide	600 mg/m^2	i.v. bolus	Day 1	21 days × 6
EC/Docetaxel				
Epirubicin	90 mg/m^2	i.v. bolus	Day 1	21 days × 4
Cyclophosphamide	600 mg/m^2	i.v. bolus	Day 1	21 days × 4
Docetaxel	100 mg/m^2	i.v. infusion[a]	Day 1	21 days × 4

[a]0.9% sodium chloride 250 mL over one hour.

Neoadjuvant/Adjuvant Chemotherapy Regimens

Drug	Dose	Route	Days	Frequency
FEC/Docetaxel				
5-Fluorouracil	500 mg/m^2	i.v.	Day 1	Cycles 1, 2, and 3 every 3 weeks
Epirubicin	100 mg/m^2	i.v.	Day 1	Cycles 1, 2, and 3 every 3 weeks
Cyclophosphamide	500 mg/m^2	i.v.	Day 1	Cycles 1, 2, and 3 every 3 weeks
Docetaxel	100 mg/m^2	i.v.	Day 1	Cycles 4, 5, and 6 every 3 weeks

Adjuvant Trastuzumab (Herceptin)

Drug	Dose	Route	Days	Frequency
Trastuzumab (initial cycle)	100 mg/m^2	i.v.	Day 1	Cycle 1 only
Trastuzumab (subsequent cycles)	100 mg/m^2	i.v.	Day 1	Cycles 2–18 every 3 weeks

Assessment of cardiac function [left ventricular ejection fraction (LVEF)] at baseline and three monthly

Index